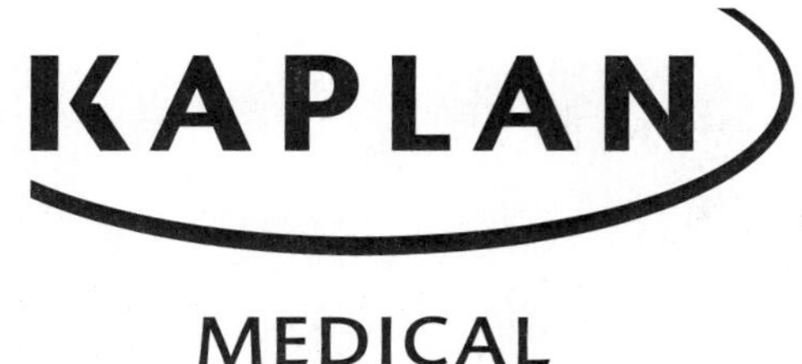

USMLE® STEP 1 Lecture Notes 2017

Physiology

Published by Kaplan Medical, a division of Kaplan, Inc.
750 Third Avenue
New York, NY 10017

8 7 6 5 4 3 2 1

e ISBN: 978-1-5062-0876-3

Retail IS : 978-1-5062-0840-4

Editor

L. Britt Wilson, Ph.D.
Professor
Department of Pharmacology, Physiology, and Neuroscience
University of South Carolina School of Medicine
Columbia, SC

Contributors

Raj Dasgupta M.D., F.A.C.P., F.C.C.P., F.A.A.S.M.
Assistant Professor of Clinical Medicine
Department of Medicine, Division of Pulmonary, Critical Care and Sleep Medicine
Keck School of Medicine of USC, University of Southern California
Los Angeles, CA

Frank P. Noto, M.D.
Assistant Professor of Internal Medicine
Site Director, Internal Medicine Clerkship and Sub-Internship
Icahn School of Medicine at Mount Sinai
New York, NY

Hospitalist
Elmhurst Hospital Center
Queens, NY

The editors would like to thank **Wazir Kudrath, M.D.,** for his invaluable commentary, review, and contributions.

We want to hear what you think. What do you like or not like about the Notes?
Please email us at **medfeedback@kaplan.com**.

Contents

Section VIII: Renal Physiology

Section IX: Acid–Base Disturbances

Section X: Endocrinology

Section XI: Gastrointestinal Physiology

SECTION I

Fluid Distribution and Edema

Fluid Distribution and Edema 1

Learning Objectives

- ❑ Interpret scenarios on distribution of fluids within the body
- ❑ Answer questions about review and integration
- ❑ Use knowledge of microcirculation
- ❑ Interpret scenarios on edema (pathology integration)
- ❑ Interpret scenarios on volume measurement of compartments

DISTRIBUTION OF FLUIDS WITHIN THE BODY

Total Body Water

- Intracellular fluid (ICF): approximately 2/3 of total of body water
- Extracellular fluid (ECF): approximately 1/3 of total body water
- Interstitial fluid (ISF): approximately 3/4 of the extracellular fluid
- Plasma volume (PV): approximately 1/4 of the extracellular fluid
- Vascular compartment: contains the blood volume which is plasma and the cellular elements of blood, primarily red blood cells

It is important to remember that membranes can serve as barriers. The 2 important membranes are illustrated in Figure I-1-1. The **cell membrane** is a relative barrier for Na^+, while the **capillary membrane** is a barrier for plasma proteins.

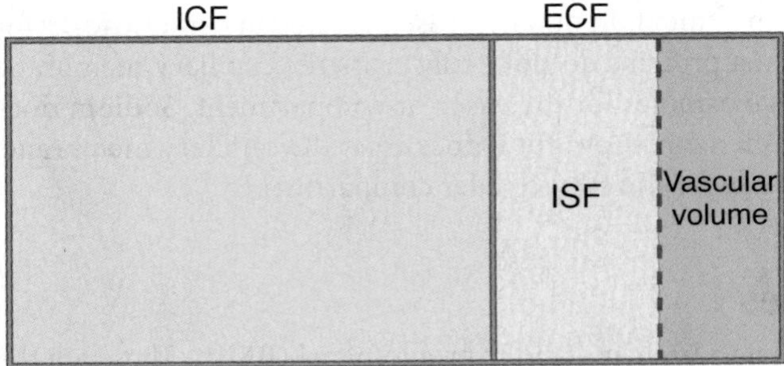

Solid-line division represents cell membrane

Dashed line division represents capillary membranes

Figure I-1-1.

Osmosis

The distribution of fluid is determined by the osmotic movement of water. Osmosis is the diffusion of water across a semipermeable or selectively permeable membrane. Water diffuses from a region of higher water concentration to a region of lower water concentration. The concentration of water in a solution is determined by the concentration of solute. The greater the solute concentration is, the lower the water concentration will be.

The osmotic properties are defined by:

- **Osmolarity:**

  mOsm (milliosmoles)/L = concentration of particles per liter of solution

- **Osmolality:**

  mOsm/kg = concentration of particles per kg of solvent (water being the germane one for physiology/medicine)

It is the **number of particles** that is crucial. The basic principles are demonstrated in Figure I-1-2.

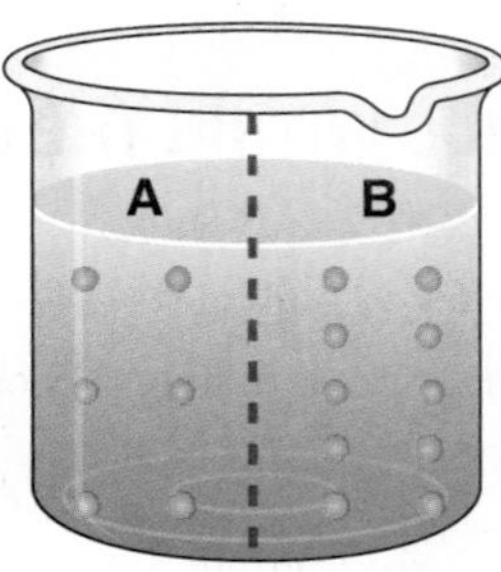

Figure I-1-2.

This figure shows 2 compartments separated by a membrane that is permeable to water but not to solute. Side B has the greater concentration of solute (circles) and thus a lower water concentration than side A. As a result, water diffuses from A to B, and the height of column B rises, and that of A falls.

Effective osmole: If a solute doesn't easily cross a membrane, then it is an "effective" osmole for that compartment. In other words, it creates an osmotic force for water. For example, plasma proteins do not easily cross the capillary membrane and thus serve as effective osmoles for the vascular compartment. Sodium does not easily penetrate the cell membrane, but it does cross the capillary membrane, thus it is an effective osmole for the extracellular compartment.

Extracellular Solutes

The figure below represents a basic metabolic profile/panel (BMP). These are the common labs provided from a basic blood draw. The same figure to the right represents the normal values corresponding to the solutes. Standardized exams provide normal values and thus knowing these numbers is not required. However, knowing them can be useful with respect to efficiency of time.

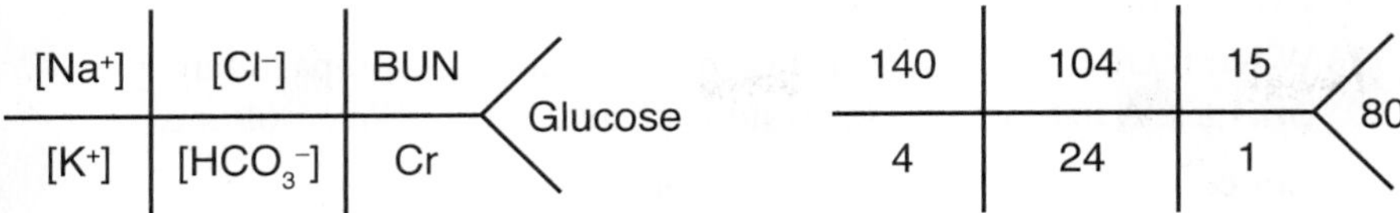

Figure I-1-3.

Osmolar Gap

The osmolar gap is defined as the difference between the **measured** osmolality and the **estimated** osmolality using the equation below. Using the data from the BMP, we can estimate the extracellular osmolality using the following formula:

$$\textbf{ECF estimated osmolality} = 2(\text{Na}^+)\ \text{mEq/L} + \frac{\text{glucose mg \%}}{18} + \frac{\text{urea mg \%}}{2.8}$$

The basis of this calculation is:

- Na^+ is the most abundant osmole of the extracellular space.
- Na^+ is doubled because it is a positive charge and thus for every positive charge there is a negative charge, chloride being the most abundant, but not the only one.
- The 18 and 2.8 are converting glucose and BUN into their respective osmolarities (note: their units of measurement are mg/dL).
- Determining the osmolar gap (normal ≤15) aids in narrowing the differential diagnosis. While many things can elevate the osmolar gap, some of the more common are: ethanol, methanol, ethylene glycol, acetone, and mannitol. Thus, an inebriated patient has an elevated osmolar gap.

Graphical Representation of Body Compartments

It is important to understand how body osmolality and the intracellular and extracellular volumes change in clinically relevant situations. Figure I-1-4 is one way to present this information. The y axis is solute concentration or osmolality. The x axis is the volume of intracellular (2/3) and extracellular (1/3) fluid.

If the solid line represents the control state, the dashed lines show a decrease in osmolality and extracellular volume but an increase in intracellular volume.

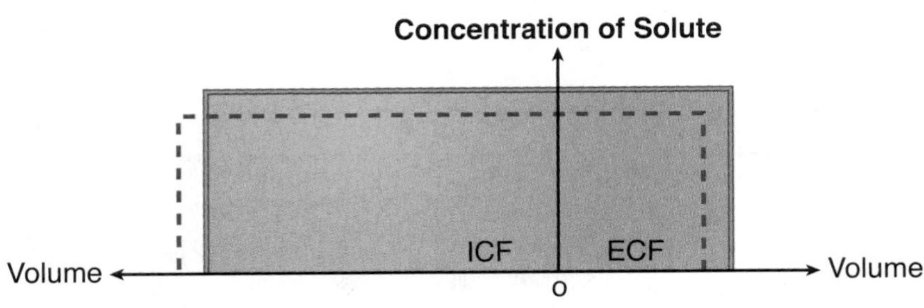

Figure I-1-4. Darrow-Yannet Diagram

Note

The value provided for chloride is the one most commonly used, but it can vary depending upon the lab.

Ranges:

Na^+: 136–145 mEq/L

K^+: 3.5–5.0 mEq/L

Cl^-: 100–106 mEq/L

HCO_3^-: 22–26 mEq/L

BUN: 8–25 mg/dl

Cr (creatinine): 0.8–1.2 mg/dl

Glucose: 60–100 mg/dl

- **Extracellular volume**

  When there is a net gain of fluid by the body, this compartment always enlarges. A net loss of body fluid decreases extracellular volume.
- **Concentration of solutes**

  This is equivalent to body osmolality. At steady-state, the intracellular concentration of water equals the extracellular concentration of water (cell membrane is not a barrier for water). Thus, the intracellular and extracellular osmolalities are the same.
- **Intracellular volume**

  This varies with the effective osmolality of the extracellular compartment. Solutes and fluids enter and leave the extracellular compartment first (sweating, diarrhea, fluid resuscitation, etc.). Intracellular volume is only altered if extracellular osmolality changes.
- If ECF osmolality increases, cells lose water and shrink. If ECF osmolality decreases, cells gain water and swell.

Below are 6 Darrow-Yannet diagrams illustrating changes in volume and/or osmolality. You are encouraged to examine the alterations and try to determine what occurred and how it could have occurred. Use the following to approach these alterations (answers provided on subsequent pages):

Does the change represent net water and/or solute gain or loss?

Indicate various ways in which this is likely to occur from a clinical perspective, i.e., the patient is hemorrhaging, drinking water, consuming excess salt, etc.

Changes in volume and concentration (dashed lines)

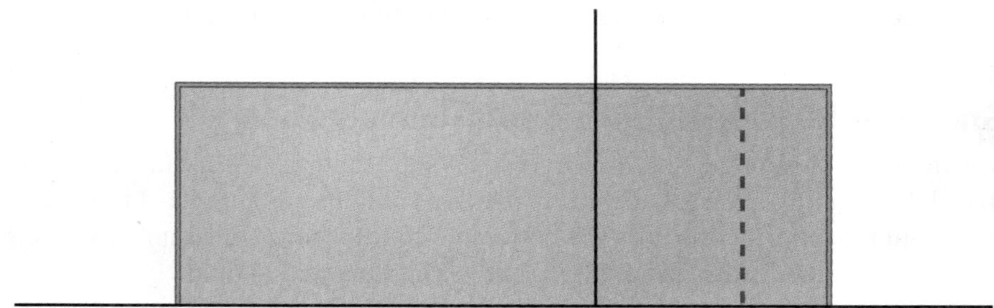

Figure I-1-5.

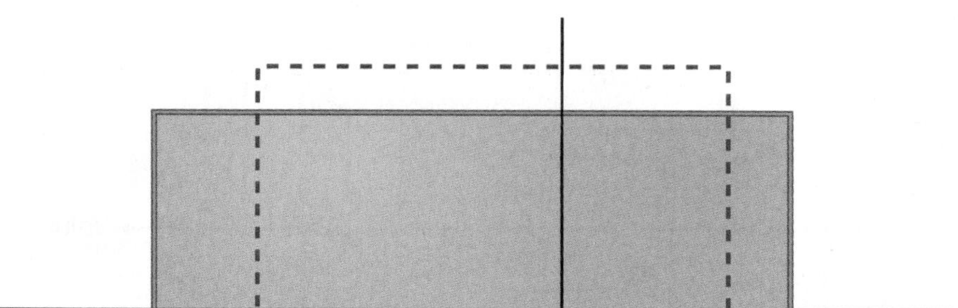

Figure I-1-6.

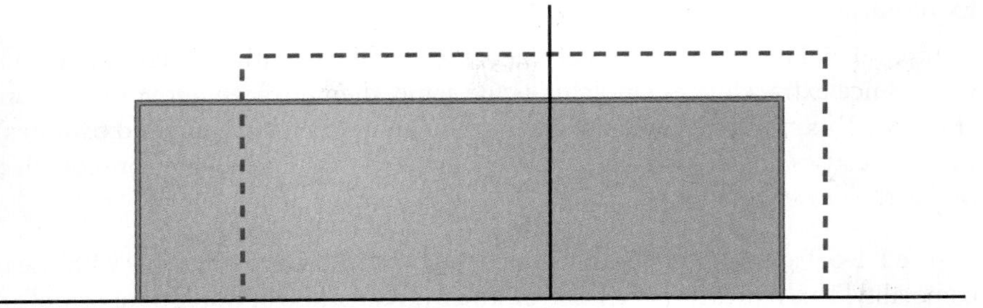

Figure I-1-7.

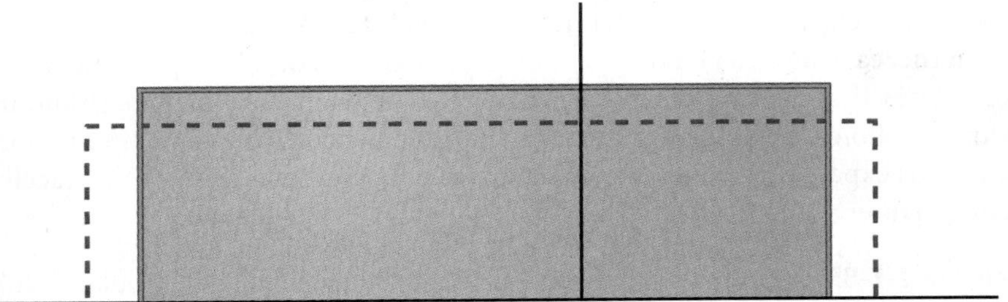

Figure I-1-8.

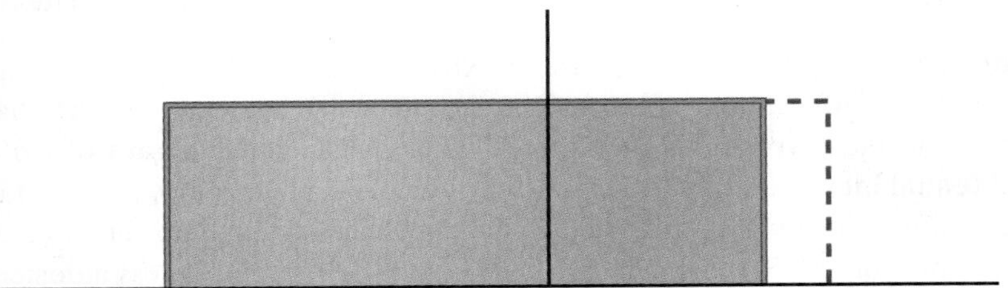

Figure I-1-9.

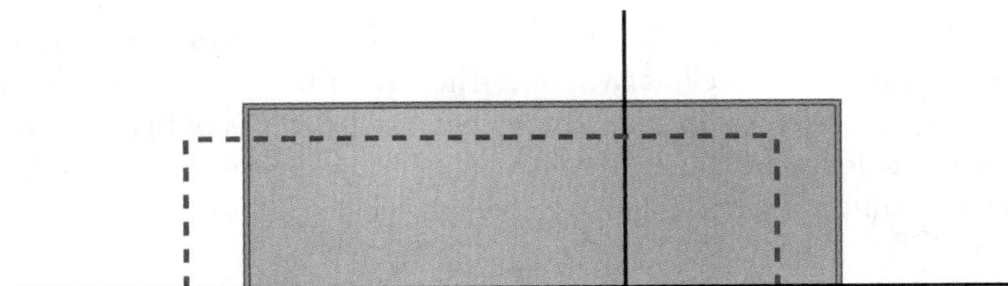

Figure I-1-10.

Explanations

Figure I-1-5: Patient shows loss of extracellular volume with no change in osmolality. Since extracellular osmolality is the same, then intracellular volume is unchanged. This represents an **isotonic fluid loss (equal loss of fluid and osmoles)**. Possible causes are hemorrhage, isotonic urine, or the immediate consequences of diarrhea or vomiting.

Figure I-1-6: Patient shows loss of extracellular and intracellular volume with rise in osmolality. This represents a **net loss of water (greater loss of water than osmoles)**. Possible causes are inadequate water intake or sweating. Pathologically, this could be hypotonic water loss from the urine resulting from diabetes insipidus.

Figure I-1-7: Patient shows gain of extracellular volume, increase in osmolality, and a decrease in intracellular volume. The rise in osmolality shifted water out of the cell. This represents a **net gain of solute (increase in osmoles greater than increase in water)**. Possible causes are ingestion of salt, hypertonic infusion of solutes that distribute extracellularly (saline, mannitol), or hypertonic infusion of colloids. Colloids, e.g. dextran, don't readily cross the capillary membrane and thus expand the vascular compartment only (vascular is part of extracellular compartment).

Figure I-1-8: Patient shows increase in extracellular and intracellular volumes with a decrease in osmolality. The fall in osmolality shifted water into the cell. Thus, this represents **net gain of water (more water than osmoles)**. Possible causes are drinking significant quantities of water (could be pathologic primary polydipsia), drinking significant quantities of a hypotonic fluid, or a hypotonic fluid infusion (saline, dextrose in water). Pathologically this could be abnormal water retention such as that which occurs with syndrome of inappropriate ADH.

Figure I-1-9: Patient shows increase in extracellular volume with no change in osmolality or intracellular volume. Since extracellular osmolality didn't change, then intracellular volume is unaffected. This represents a **net gain of isotonic fluid (equal increase fluid and osmoles)**. Possible causes are isotonic fluid infusion (saline), drinking significant quantities of an isotonic fluid, or infusion of an isotonic colloid. Pathologically this could be the result of excess aldosterone. Aldosterone is a steroid hormone that causes Na^+ retention by the kidney. At first glance one would predict excess Na^+ retention by aldosterone would increase the concentration of Na^+ in the extracellular compartment. However, this is rarely the case because water follows Na^+, and even though the total body mass of Na^+ increases, its concentration doesn't.

Figure I-1-10: Patient shows decrease in extracellular volume and osmolality with an increase in intracellular volume. The rise in intracellular volume is the result of the decreased osmolality. This represents a **net loss of hypertonic fluid (more osmoles lost than fluid)**. The only cause to consider is the pathologic state of adrenal insufficiency. Lack of mineralcorticoids, e.g., aldosterone causes excess Na^+ loss.

Table I-1-1. Summary of Volume Changes and Body Osmolarity Following Changes in Body Hydration

	ECF Volume	Body Osmolarity	ICF Volume	D-Y Diagram
Loss of isotonic fluid Hemorrhage Diarrhea Vomiting	↓	no change	no change	
Loss of hypotonic fluid Dehydration Diabetes insipidus Alcoholism	↓	↑	↓	
Gain of isotonic fluid Isotonic saline	↑	no change	no change	
Gain of hypotonic fluid Hypotonic saline Water intoxication	↑	↓	↑	
Gain of hypertonic fluid Hypertonic saline Hypertonic mannitol	↑	↑	↓	

ECF = extracellular fluid; ICF = intracellular fluid; D-Y = Darrow-Yannet

REVIEW AND INTEGRATION

Although the following is covered in more detail later in this book (Renal and Endocrine sections), let's review 2 important hormones involved in volume regulation: aldosterone and anti-diuretic hormone (ADH), also known as arginine vasopressin (AVP).

Aldosterone

One of the fundamental functions of aldosterone is to increase sodium reabsorption in principal cells of the kidney. This reabsorption of sodium plays a key role in regulating extracellular volume. Aldosterone also plays an important role in regulating plasma potassium and increases the secretion of this ion in principal cells. The 2 primary factors that stimulate aldosterone release are:

- Plasma angiotensin II (Ang II)
- Plasma K^+

Note

ADH secretion is primarily regulated by plasma osmolality and blood pressure/volume. However, it can also be stimulated by Ang II and corticotropin-releasing hormone (CRH). This influence of CRH is particularly relevant to clinical medicine, because a variety of stresses (e.g., surgery) can increase ADH secretion.

ADH (AVP)

ADH stimulates water reabsorption in principal cells of the kidney via the V_2 receptor. By regulating water, ADH plays a pivotal role in regulating extracellular osmolality. In addition, ADH vasoconstricts arterioles (V_1 receptor) and thus can serve as a hormonal regulator of vascular tone. The 2 primary regulators of ADH are:

- Plasma osmolality (directly related): an increase stimulates, while a decrease inhibits
- Blood pressure/volume (inversely related): an increase inhibits, while a decrease stimulates

Renin

Although renin is an enzyme, not a hormone, it is important in this discussion because it catalyzes the conversion of angiotensinogen to angiotensin I, which in turn is converted to Ang II by angiotensin converting enzyme (ACE). This is the renin-angiotensin-aldosterone system (RAAS). The 3 primary regulators of renin are:

- Perfusion pressure to the kidney (inversely related): an increase inhibits, while a decrease stimulates
- Sympathetic stimulation to the kidney (direct effect via β-1 receptors)
- Na^+ delivery to the macula densa (inversely related): an increase inhibits, while a decrease stimulates

Negative Feedback Regulation

Examining the function and regulation of these hormones one should see the feedback regulation. For example, aldosterone increases sodium reabsorption, which in turn increases extracellular volume. Renin is stimulated by reduced blood pressure (perfusion pressure to the kidney; reflex sympathetic stimulation). Thus, aldosterone is released as a means to compensate for the fall in arterial blood pressure. As indicated, these hormones are covered in more detail later in this book.

Application

Given the above, you are encouraged to review the previous Darrow-Yannet diagrams and predict what would happen to levels of each hormone in the various conditions. Answers are provided below.

Figure I-1-5: Loss of extracellular volume stimulates RAAS and ADH.

Figure I-1-6: Decreased extracellular volume stimulates RAAS. This drop in extracellular volume stimulates ADH, as does the rise osmolarity. This setting would be a strong stimulus for ADH.

Figure I-1-7: The rise in extracellular volume inhibits RAAS. It is difficult to predict what will happen to ADH in this setting. The rise in extracellular volume inhibits, but the rise in osmolality stimulates, thus it will depend upon the magnitude of the changes. In general, osmolality is a more important factor, but significant changes in vascular volume/pressure can exert profound effects.

Figure I-1-8: The rise in extracellular volume inhibits RAAS and ADH. In addition, the fall in osmolality inhibits ADH.

Figure I-1-9: The rise in extracellular volume inhibits both.

Figure I-1-10: Although the only cause to consider is adrenal insufficiency, if this scenario were to occur, then the drop in extracellular volume stimulates RAAS. It is difficult to predict what happens to ADH in this setting. The drop in extracellular volume stimulates, but the fall in osmolality inhibits, thus it depends upon the magnitude of the changes.

MICROCIRCULATION

Filtration and Absorption

Fluid flux across the capillary is governed by the 2 fundamental forces that cause water flow:

- Hydrostatic, which is simply the pressure of the fluid
- Osmotic (oncotic) forces, which represents the osmotic force created by solutes that don't cross the membrane (discussed earlier in this section)

Each of these forces exists on both sides of the membrane. Filtration is defined as the movement of fluid from the plasma into the interstitium, while absorption is movement of fluid from the interstitium into the plasma. The interplay between these forces is illustrated in Figure I-1-11.

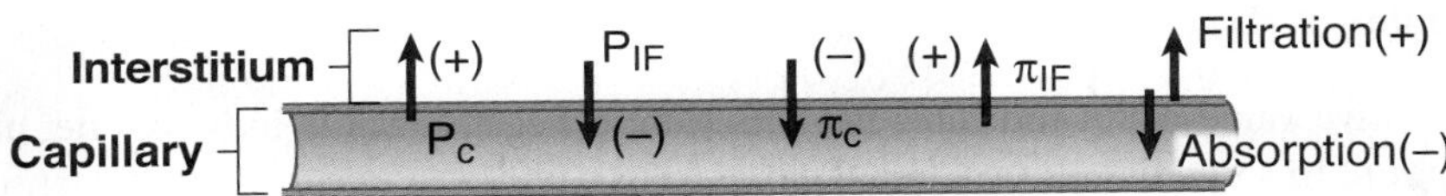

Figure I-1-11. Starling Forces

P = Hydrostatic pressure
π = Osmotic (oncotic) pressure (mainly proteins)

Forces for filtration

P_C = hydrostatic pressure (blood pressure) in the capillary

This is directly related to:

- Blood flow (regulated at the arteriole)
- Venous pressure
- Blood volume

π_{IF} = oncotic (osmotic) force in the interstitium

- This is determined by the concentration of protein in the interstitial fluid.
- Normally the small amount of protein that leaks to the interstitium is minor and is removed by the lymphatics.
- Thus, under most conditions this is not an important factor influencing the exchange of fluid.

Forces for absorption

π_C = oncotic (osmotic) pressure of plasma

- This is the oncotic pressure of plasma solutes that cannot diffuse across the capillary membrane, i.e., the plasma proteins.
- Albumin, synthesized in the liver, is the most abundant plasma protein and thus the biggest contributor to this force.

P_{IF} = hydrostatic pressure in the interstitium

- This pressure is difficult to determine.
- In most cases it is close to zero or negative (subatmospheric) and is not a significant factor affecting filtration versus reabsorption.
- However, it can become significant if edema is present or it can affect glomerular filtration in the kidney (pressure in Bowman's space is analogous to interstitial pressure).

Starling Equation

These 4 forces are often referred to as Starling forces. Grouping the forces into those that favor filtration and those that oppose it, and taking into account the properties of the barrier to filtration, the formula for fluid exchange is the following:

> Qf: fluid movement
>
> k: filtration coefficient

$$Qf = k\,[(P_c + \pi_{IF}) - (P_{IF} + \pi_C)]$$

The filtration coefficient depends upon a number of factors but for our purposes permeability is most important. As indicated below, a variety of factors can increase permeability of the capillary resulting in a large flux of fluid from the capillary into the interstitial space.

A positive value of Qf indicates net filtration; a negative value indicates net absorption. In some tissues (e.g., renal glomerulus), filtration occurs along the entire length of the capillary; in others (intestinal mucosa), absorption normally occurs along the whole length. In other tissues, filtration may occur at the proximal end until the forces equilibrate.

Lymphatics

The lymphatics play a pivotal role in maintaining a low interstitial fluid volume and protein content. Lymphatic flow is directly proportional to interstitial fluid pressure, thus a rise in this pressure promotes fluid movement out of the interstitium via the lymphatics.

The lymphatics also remove proteins from the interstitium. Recall that the lymphatics return their fluid and protein content to the general circulation by coalescing into the lymphatic ducts, which in turn empty into to the subclavian veins.

Questions

1. Given the following values, calculate a net pressure:

   $P_C = 25$ mm Hg

   $P_{IF} = 2$ mm Hg

   $\pi_C = 20$ mm Hg

   $\pi_{IF} = 1$ mm Hg

2. Calculate a net pressure if the interstitial hydrostatic pressure is –2 mm Hg.

Answers

1. +4 mm Hg
2. +8 mm Hg

EDEMA (PATHOLOGY INTEGRATION)

Edema is the accumulation of fluid in the interstitial space. It expresses itself in peripheral tissues in 2 different forms:

- **Pitting edema**: In this type of edema, pressing the affected area with a finger or thumb results in a visual indentation of the skin that persists for some time after the digit is removed. This is the "classic," most common type observed clinically. It generally responds well to diuretic therapy.
- **Non-pitting edema**: As the name implies, a persistent visual indentation is absent when pressing the affected area. This occurs when interstitial oncotic forces are elevated (proteins for example). This type of edema does not respond well to diuretic therapy.

Primary Causes of Peripheral Edema

Significant alterations in the Starling forces which then tip the balance toward filtration, increase capillary permeability (k), and/or interrupted lymphatic function can result in edema. Thus:

- **Increased capillary hydrostatic pressure (P_C):** causes can include the following:
  - Marked increase in blood flow, e.g., vasodilation in a given vascular bed
  - Increasing venous pressure, e.g., venous obstruction or heart failure
  - Elevated blood volume (typically the result of Na^+ retention), e.g., heart failure
- **Increased interstitial oncotic pressure (π_{IF}):** primary cause is thyroid dysfunction (elevated mucopolysaccharides in the interstitium)
  - These act as osmotic agents resulting in fluid accumulation and a non-pitting edema. Lymphedema (see below) can also increase π_{IF}.
- **Decreased vascular oncotic pressure (π_C):** causes can include the following:
  - Liver failure
  - Nephrotic syndrome

- **Increased capillary permeability (k):** Circulating agents, e.g., tumor necrosis factor alpha (TNF-alpha), bradykinin, histamine, cytokines related to burn trauma, etc., increase fluid (and possibly protein) filtration resulting in edema.
- **Lymphatic obstruction/removal (lymphedema):** causes can include the following:
  - Filarial (*W. bancrofti*—elephantitis)
  - Bacterial lymphangitis (streptococci)
  - Trauma
  - Surgery
  - Tumor

  Given that one function of the lymphatics is to clear interstitial proteins, lymphedema can produce a non-pitting edema because of the rise in π_{IF}.

Pulmonary Edema

Edema in the interstitium of the lung can result in grave consequences. It can interfere with gas exchange, thus causing hypoxemia and hypercapnia (see Respiration section). A low hydrostatic pressure in pulmonary capillaries and lymphatic drainage helps "protect" the lungs against edema. However, similar to peripheral edema, alterations in Starling forces, capillary permeability, and/or lymphatic blockage can result in pulmonary edema. The most common causes relate to elevated capillary hydrostatic pressure and increased capillary permeability.

- **Cardiogenic (elevated P_C)**
  - Most common form of pulmonary edema
  - Increased left atrial pressure, increases venous pressure, which in turn increases capillary pressure
  - Initially increased lymph flow reduces interstitial proteins and is protective
  - First patient sign is often orthopnea (dyspnea when supine), which can be relieved when sitting upright
  - Elevated pulmonary wedge pressure provides confirmation
  - Treatment: reduce left atrial pressure, e.g., diuretic therapy
- **Non-cardiogenic (increased permeability): adult respiratory distress syndrome (ARDS)**
  - Due to direct injury of the alveolar epithelium or after a primary injury to the capillary endothelium
  - Clinical signs are severe dyspnea of rapid onset, hypoxemia, and diffuse pulmonary infiltrates leading to respiratory failure
  - Most common causes are sepsis, bacterial pneumonia, trauma, and gastric aspirations
  - Fluid accumulation as a result of the loss of epithelial integrity
  - Presence of protein-containing fluid in the alveoli inactivates surfactant causing reduced lung compliance
  - Pulmonary wedge pressure is normal or low

VOLUME MEASUREMENT OF COMPARTMENTS

To measure the volume of a body compartment, a tracer substance must be easily measured, well distributed within that compartment, and not rapidly metabolized or removed from that compartment. In this situation, the volume of the compartment can be calculated by using the following relationship:

$$V = \frac{A}{C}$$

V = volume of the compartment to be measured

C = concentration of tracer in the compartment to be measured

A = amount of tracer

For example, 300 mg of a dye is injected intravenously; at equilibrium, the concentration in the blood is 0.05 mg/mL. The volume of the compartment that contained the dye is volume $= \frac{300 \text{ mg}}{0.05 \text{ mg/mL}} = 6{,}000$ mL.

This is called the volume of distribution (VOD).

Properties of the Tracer and Compartment Measured

Tracers are generally introduced into the vascular compartment, and they distribute throughout body water until they reach a barrier they cannot penetrate. The 2 major barriers encountered are **capillary membranes** and **cell membranes.** Thus, tracer characteristics for the measurement of the various compartments are as follows:

- Plasma: tracer not permeable to capillary membranes, e.g., albumin
- ECF: tracer permeable to capillary membranes but not cell membranes, e.g., inulin, mannitol, sodium, sucrose
- Total body water: tracer permeable to capillary and cell membranes, e.g., tritiated water, urea

Blood Volume versus Plasma Volume

Blood volume represents the plasma volume plus the volume of RBCs, which is usually expressed as hematocrit (fractional concentration of RBCs).

The following formula can be utilized to convert plasma volume to blood volume:

$$\textbf{Blood volume} = \frac{\textbf{plasma volume}}{\textbf{1 - hematocrit}}$$

For example, if the hematocrit is 50% (0.50) and plasma volume = 3 L, then:

$$\text{Blood volume} = \frac{3 \text{ L}}{1 - 0.5} = 6 \text{ L}$$

If the hematocrit is 0.5 (or 50%), the blood is half RBCs and half plasma. Therefore, blood volume is double the plasma volume.

Blood volume can be estimated by taking 7% of the body weight in kgs. For example, a 70 kg individual has an approximate blood volume of 5.0 L.

The distribution of intravenously administered fluids is as follows:

- Vascular compartment: whole blood, plasma, dextran in saline
- ECF: saline, mannitol
- Total body water: D5W–5% dextrose in water
  - Once the glucose is metabolized, the water distributes 2/3 ICF, 1/3 ECF

Chapter Summary

- ECF/ICF fluid distribution is determined by osmotic forces.
- ECF sodium creates most of the ECF osmotic force because it is the most prevalent dissolved substance in the ECF that does not penetrate the cell membrane easily.
- The BMP represents the plasma levels of 7 important solutes and is a commonly obtained plasma sample.
- If ECF sodium concentration increases, ICF volume decreases. If ECF sodium concentration decreases, ICF volume increases. Normal extracellular osmolality is about 290 mOsm/kg (osmolarity of 290 mOsm/L).
- Vascular/interstitial fluid distribution is determined by osmotic and hydrostatic forces (Starling forces).
- The main factor promoting filtration is capillary hydrostatic pressure.
- The main factor promoting absorption is the plasma protein osmotic force.
- Pitting edema is the result of altered Starling forces.
- Non-pitting edema results from lymphatic obstruction and/or the accumulation of osmotically active solutes in the interstitial space (thyroid).
- Pulmonary edema can be cardiogenic (pressure induced) or non-cardiogenic (permeability induced).

SECTION II

Excitable Tissue

Ionic Equilibrium and Resting Membrane Potential

1

Learning Objectives

- ❑ Explain information related to overview of excitable tissue
- ❑ Interpret scenarios on ion channels
- ❑ Explain information related to equilibrium potential

OVERVIEW OF EXCITABLE TISSUE

Figure II-1-1 provides a basic picture of excitable cells and the relative concentration of key electrolytes inside versus outside the cell. The intracellular proteins have a negative charge.

In order to understand and apply what governs the conductance of ions as it relates to the function of excitable tissue (nerves and muscle), it is important to remember this relative difference in concentrations for these ions. In addition, it is imperative to understand the following 5 key principles.

1. **Membrane potential (E_m)**
   - There is a separation of charge across the membrane of excitability tissue at rest. This separation of charge means there is the potential to do work and is measured in volts. Thus, E_m represents the measured value.
2. **Electrochemical gradient**
   - Ions diffuse based upon chemical (concentration) gradients (high to low) and electrical gradients (like charges repel, opposites attract). Electrochemical gradient indicates the combination of these 2 forces.
3. **Equilibrium potential**
   - This is the membrane potential that puts an ion in electrochemical equilibrium, i.e., the membrane potential that results in no NET diffusion of an ion. If reached, the tendency for an ion to diffuse in one direction based upon the chemical gradient is countered by the electrical force in the opposite direction. The equilibrium potential for any ion can be calculated by the Nernst equation (see below).
4. **Conductance (g)**
   - Conductance refers to the flow of an ion across the cell membrane. Ions move across the membrane via channels (see below). Open/closed states of channels determine the relative permeability of the membrane to a given ion and thus the conductance. Open states create high permeability and conductance, while closed states result in low permeability and conductance.

5. **Net force (driving force)**
   - This indicates the relative "force" driving the diffusion of an ion. It is estimated by subtracting the ions equilibrium potential from the cell's membrane potential. In short, it quantitates how far a given ion is from equilibrium at any membrane potential.

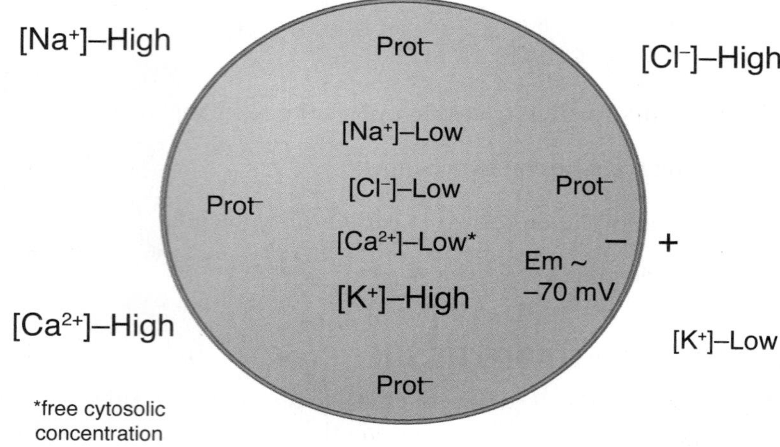

Figure II-1-1. Basic Schematic of an Excitable Cell

ION CHANNELS

Ions diffuse across the membrane via ion channels. There are 3 basic types of ion channels (Figure II-1-2).

Ungated (Leak)

- Always open
- Direction the ion moves depends upon electrochemical forces
- Important for determining resting membrane potential of a cell

Voltage-Gated

- Open/closed state is determined primarily by membrane potential (voltage)
- Change in membrane potential may open or close the channel

Ligand-Gated

- Channel contains a receptor
- State of the channel (open or closed) is influenced by the binding of a ligand to the receptor
- Under most circumstances, the binding of the ligand opens the channel

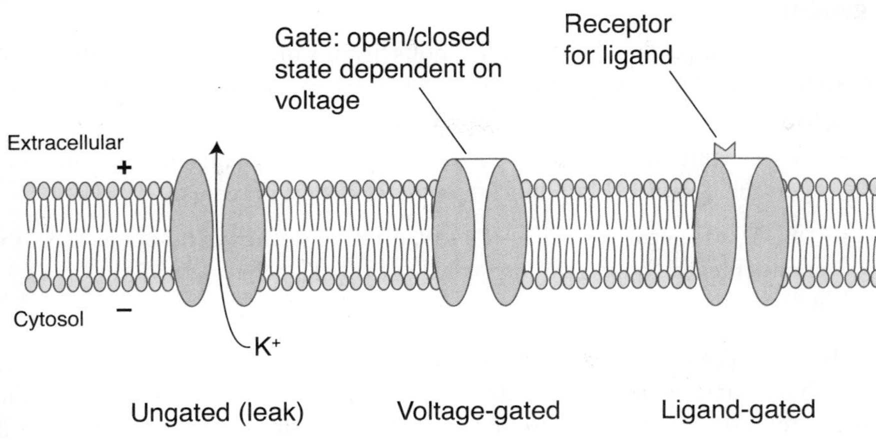

Figure II-1-2. Classes of Ion Channels

NMDA Receptor (Exception to the Rule)

Above, we defined the 3 basic classes into which ion channels fall. The NMDA (N-methyl-D-aspartic acid) is an exception because it is both voltage- and ligand-gated.

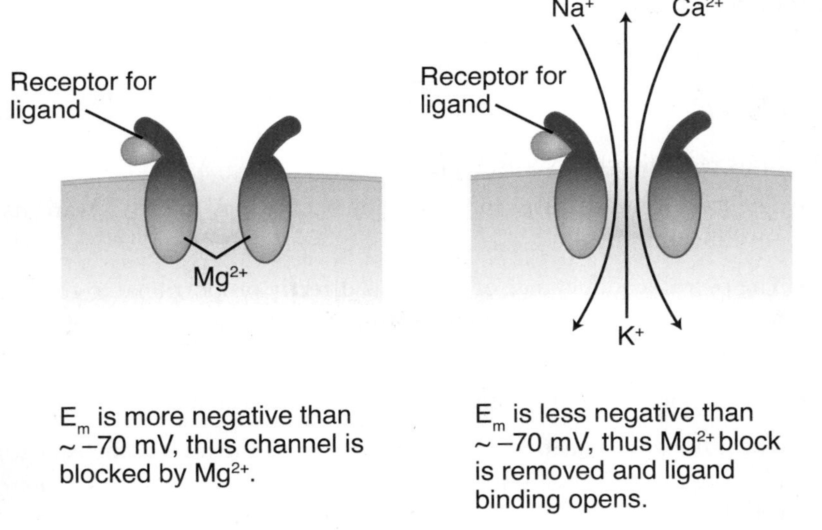

Figure II-1-3. NMDA Receptor

Voltage-gated

- The pore of the NMDA receptor is blocked by Mg^{2+} if E_m is more negative than ~ –70 mV.
- This Mg^{2+} block is removed if E_m becomes less negative than ~ –70 mV.
- Thus, the NMDA receptor exhibits characteristics of a voltage-gated channel.

Ligand-gated

Glutamate and aspartate are the endogenous ligands for this receptor. Binding of one of the ligands is **required** to open the channel, thus it exhibits characteristics of a ligand-gated channel.

- If E_m is more negative than ~ –70 mV, binding of the ligand does **not** open the channel (Mg^{2+} block related to voltage prevents).
- If E_m is less negative than ~ –70 mV, binding of the ligand opens the channel (even though no Mg^{2+} block at this E_m, channel will not open without ligand binding).

The NMDA receptor is a non-selective cation channel (Na^+, K^+, and Ca^{2+} flux through it). Thus, opening of this channel results in depolarization. Although the NMDA receptor is likely involved in a variety of functions, the 2 most important are (1) memory and (2) pain transmission. With respect to memory, NMDA has been shown to be involved in long-term potentiation of cells, thought to be an important component of memory formation. With respect to pain transmission, NMDA is expressed throughout the CNS and has been proven in numerous studies to play a pivotal role in the transmission and ultimate perception of pain.

EQUILIBRIUM POTENTIAL

E_{X^+} = equilibrium potential

$[X^+]_o$ = concentration outside (extracellular)

$[X^+]_i$ = concentration inside (intracellular)

Z = value of the charge

Equilibrium potential is the membrane potential that puts an ion in electrochemical equilibrium, and it can be calculated using the **Nernst equation**. This equation computes the equilibrium potential for any ion based upon the concentration gradient.

$$E_{X^+} = \frac{60}{Z} \log_{10} \frac{[X^+]_o}{[X^+]_i}$$

Key points regarding the Nernst equation:

- The ion always diffuses in a direction that brings the E_m toward its equilibrium.
- The overall conductance of the ion is directly proportional to the net force and the permeability (determined by ion channel state) of the membrane for the ion.
- The E_m moves toward the E_X of the most permeable ion.
- The number of ions that actually move across the membrane is negligible. Thus, opening of ion channels does not alter intracellular or extracellular concentrations of ions under normal circumstances.

Approximate Equilibrium Potentials for the Important Ions

It is difficult to measure the intracellular concentration of the important electrolytes, thus equilibrium potentials for these ions will vary some across the various references. The following represent reasonable equilibrium potentials for the key electrolytes:

E_{K+} ~ -95 mV $\quad$ E_{Na+} ~ +70 mV

E_{Cl-} ~ -76 mV $\quad$ E_{Ca2+} ~ +125 mV

Definitions

In **depolarization**, E_m becomes less negative (moves toward zero). In **hyperpolarization,** E_m becomes more negative (further from zero).

Resting Membrane Potential

Potassium (K^+)

There is marked variability in the resting membrane potential (rE_m) for excitable tissues, but the following generalizations are applicable.

- rE_m for nerves is ~ -70 mV while rE_m for striated muscle is ~ –90 mV.
- Excitable tissue has a considerable number of leak channels for K^+, but not for Cl^-, Na^+, or Ca^{2+}. Thus, K^+ conductance (g) is high in resting cells.
- Because of this high conductance, rE_m is altered in the following ways by changes in the extracellular concentration of K^+:
  - **Hyperkalemia depolarizes the cell.** If acute, excitability of nerves is increased (nerve is closer to threshold for an action potential) and heart arrhythmias may occur.
  - **Hypokalemia hyperpolarizes the cell.** This decreases the excitability of nerves (further from threshold) and heart arrhythmias may occur.

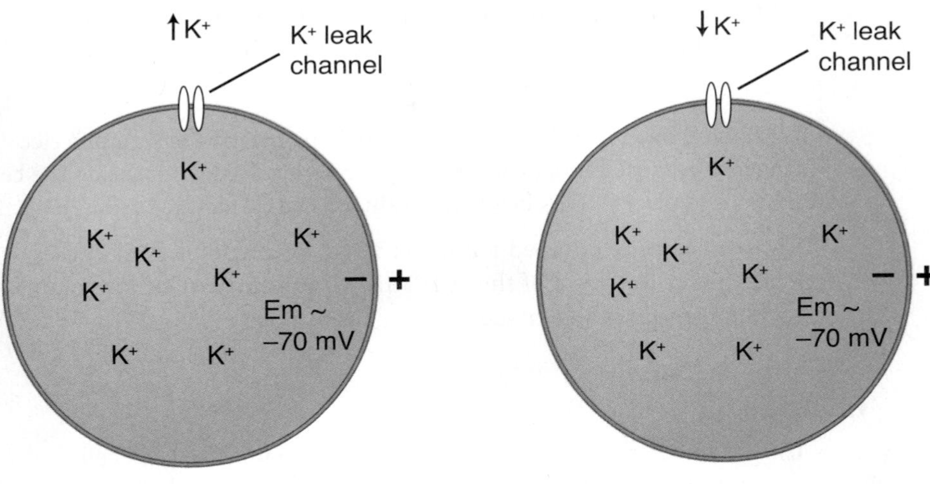

Figure II-1-4. Effect of Changes in Extracellular K^+ on Resting Membrane Potential

Altering the g for K^+ has the following effects:

- Increasing g causes K^+ to leave the cell, resulting in hyperpolarization of the cell. Recall that increasing g for an ion causes the E_m to move toward the equilibrium potential for that ion. Thus, the cell will move from -70 mV toward -95 mV.
- Decreasing g depolarizes the cell (cell moves away from K^+ equilibrium). This applies to K^+ because of its high resting g.

The Na^+/K^+ ATPase

Although the cell membrane is relatively impermeable to Na^+, it is not completely impervious to it. Thus, some Na^+ does leak into excitable cells. This Na^+ leak into the cells is counterbalanced by pumping it back out via the Na^+/K^+ ATPase. Important attributes of this pump are:

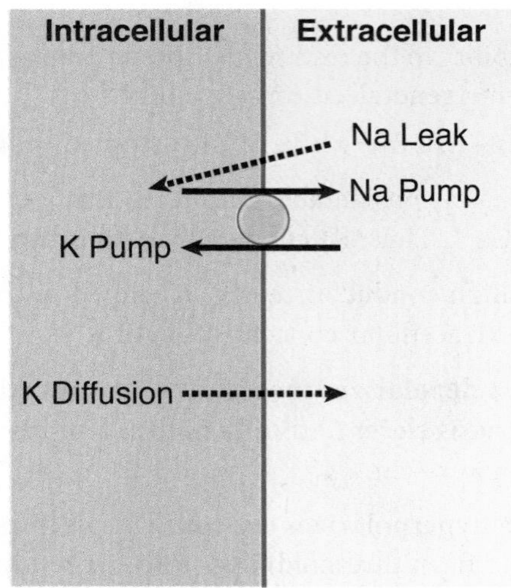

Figure II-1-5. Steady-State Resting Relationship between Ion Diffusion and Na/K-ATPase Pump

- The stoichiometry is 3 Na^+ out, 2 K^+ in. This means the pump is electrogenic because more positive charges are removed from inside the cell than are replaced. This helps maintain a negative charge inside the cell.
- Three solutes are pumped out in exchange for 2 solutes. This causes a net flux of water out of the cell. This pump is important for volume regulation of excitable tissue.

Chloride (Cl^-)

- Cl^- g is low at rest. Thus, decreasing g or changing the extracellular concentration has minimal effect on rE_m.
- Assuming rE_m is -70 mV, increasing Cl^- g hyperpolarizes the cell (E_m moves toward equilibrium for Cl^-, which is –76 mV, see also Figure II-1-6).
- If rE_m is -80 mV or more negative, increasing Cl^- g depolarizes the cell.

Sodium (Na^+)

- Na^+ g is very low at rest. Thus decreasing g or changing the extracellular concentration has no effect on rE_m.
- Increasing Na^+ g depolarizes the cell (E_m moves to equilibrium for Na^+, which is +70 mV, see also Figure II-1-6).

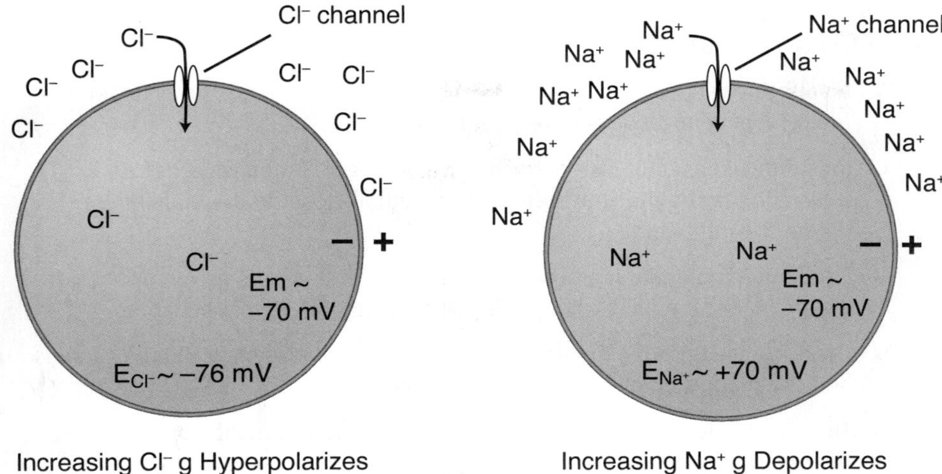

Figure II-1-6. Effect of Increase Cl^- g (left) or Na^+ g (right)

Calcium (Ca^{2+})

- Similar to Na^+, Ca^{2+} g is very low at rest. Thus decreasing g or changing the extracellular concentration has no effect on rE_m.
- Increasing Ca^{2+} g depolarizes the cell (E_m moves toward equilibrium for Ca^{2+}, which is +125 mV).

Chapter Summary

- A voltage exists across the membrane of excitable tissue, with the inside of the cell being negative with respect to the outside.
- Ions diffuse based upon electrochemical gradients and always diffuse in a direction that brings the membrane potential closer to the equilibrium potential for that ion.
- Equilibrium potential is the membrane potential that puts an ion in electrochemical equilibrium and is computed by the Nernst equation.
- Conductance (g) of an ion is determined by the relative state of ion channels and the proportion of ion channels in a given state.
- The further the membrane potential is from the ion's equilibrium potential, the greater the net force for that ion.
- Ion channels are either ungated (leak), voltage-gated, or ligand-gated. The NMDA receptor is the exception, because it is both ligand and voltage-gated.
- Resting cells have a relatively high K^+ conductance. Thus, changing the conductance of K^+ and/or altering the extracellular concentration of K^+ changes membrane potential.
- Alterations in extracellular Cl^- and Na^+ do not significantly change resting membrane potential.
- The Na^+—K^+ ATPase plays a crucial role in maintaining a low intracellular concentration of Na^+, keeping the inside of the cell negative, and regulating intracellular volume.

The Neuron Action Potential and Synaptic Transmission 2

Learning Objectives

- ❑ Explain information related to overview of the action potential
- ❑ Solve problems concerning voltage-gated ion channels
- ❑ Demonstrate understanding of the action potential
- ❑ Use knowledge of properties of action potentials
- ❑ Answer questions about synaptic transmission
- ❑ Interpret scenarios on review and integration

OVERVIEW OF THE ACTION POTENTIAL

The action potential is a rapid depolarization followed by a repolarization (return of membrane potential to rest). The function is:

- **Nerves**: conduct neuronal signals
- **Muscle**: initiate a contraction

Figure II-2-1 shows the action potential from 3 types of excitable cells. Even though there are many similarities, there are differences between these cell types, most notably the duration of the action potential. In this chapter, we discuss the specific events pertaining to the nerve action potential, but the action potential in skeletal muscle is virtually the same. Thus, what is stated here can be directly applied to skeletal muscle. Because the cardiac action potential has several differences, it will be discussed in the subsequent chapter.

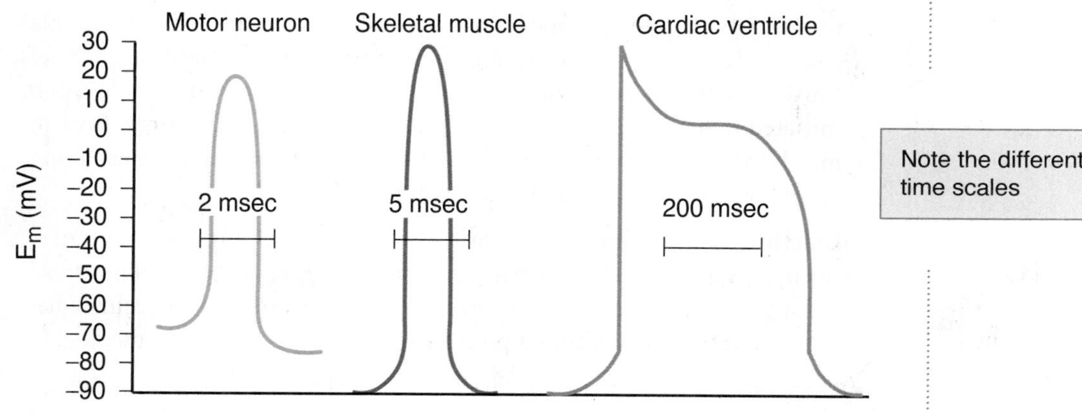

Note the different time scales

Figure II-2-1. Action Potentials from 3 Vertebrate Cell Types

(Redrawn from Flickinger, C.J., et al.: Medical Cell Biology, Philadelphia, 1979, W.B. Saunders Co.)

VOLTAGE-GATED ION CHANNELS

In order to understand how the action potential is generated, we must first discuss the ion channels involved.

Voltage-Gated (Fast) Na^+ Channels

The opening of these channels is responsible for the rapid depolarization phase (upstroke) of the action potential. Figure II-2-2 shows the details of the fast Na^+ channel. It has 2 gates and 3 conformational states:

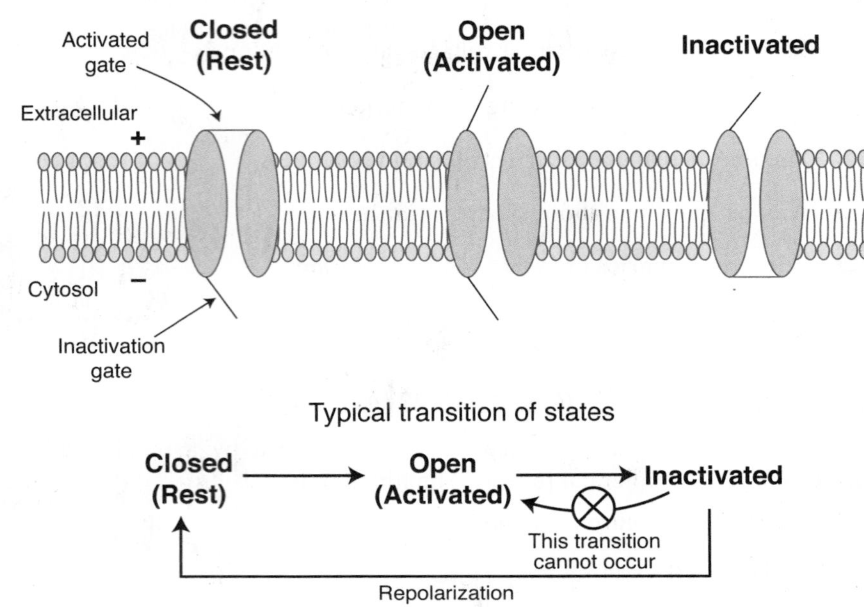

Figure II-2-2. Voltage-Gated (Fast) Na^+ Channel

- **Closed:** In the closed state, the activation gate (m-gate) is closed and the inactivation gate (h-gate) is open. Because the activation gate is closed, Na^+ conductance (g) is low.
- **Open:** Depolarization causes the channel to transition to the open state, in which both gates are open and thus Na^+ g increases. The elevated Na^+ g causes further depolarization, which in turn opens more Na^+ channels, causing further depolarization. In short, a positive-feedback cycle can be initiated if enough Na^+ channels open at or near the same time. Bear in mind, there are numerous fast Na^+ channels in every cell, and each one has its own threshold voltage for opening.
- **Inactivated:** After opening, the fast Na^+ channel typically transitions to the inactivated state. In this state, the activation gate is open and inactivation gate (h-gate) is closed. Under normal circumstances, this occurs when membrane potential becomes positive as a result of the action potential.
- Once the cell repolarizes, the fast Na^+ channel transitions back to the closed state, and is thus ready to reopen to cause another action potential.

Clinical Correlate

As indicated in the previous chapter, hyperkalemia depolarizes neurons. Acutely, this increases excitability because the cell is closer to threshold. However, this depolarization opens some fast Na^+ channels. Over time, these channels transition into the inactivated state. Because E_m never returns to its original resting E_m (hyperkalemia keeps cell depolarized), the fast Na^+ channel is unable to transition back to the closed state and is thus "locked" in the inactivated state. This reduces the number of fast Na^+ channels available to open, resulting in the reduced neuronal excitability seen with chronic hyperkalemia.

Key point: Once a Na^+ channel inactivates, it cannot go back to the open state until it transitions to the closed state (see Figure II-2-2). The transition to the closed state typically occurs when the cell repolarizes. However, there are conditions in which this transition to the closed state doesn't occur.

Important fact: Extracellular Ca^{2+} blocks fast Na^+ channels.

Voltage-Gated K^+ Channels

- Closed at resting membrane potential
- Depolarization opens, but kinetics are much slower than fast Na^+ channels
- Primary mechanism for repolarization

THE ACTION POTENTIAL

Subthreshold Stimulus

The blue and purple lines in Figure II-2-3 show changes in membrane potential (E_m) to increasing levels of stimuli, but neither result in an action potential. Thus, these are subthreshold stimuli. Important points regarding these stimuli are:

- The degree of depolarization is related to the magnitude of the stimulus.
- The membrane repolarizes (returns to rest).
- It can summate, which means if another stimulus is applied before repolarization is complete, the depolarization of the second stimulus adds onto the depolarization of the first (the 2 depolarizations sum together).

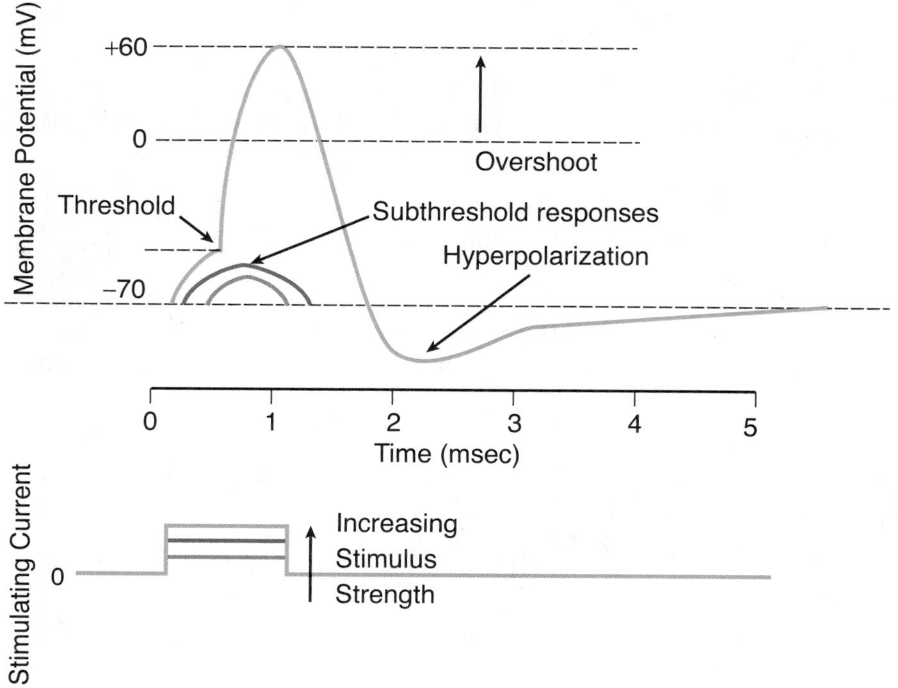

Figure II-2-3. The Neuron Action Potential

Bridge to Pharmacology

Tetrodotoxin (TTX), saxitoxin (STX), and local anesthetics ("caine drugs") block fast Na^+ channels, thereby preventing an action potential.

Bridge to Pharmacology

Ciguatoxin (CTX: fish) and batrachotoxin (BTX: frogs) are toxins that block inactivation of fast Na^+ channels.

Threshold Stimulus

The green line in Figure II-2-3 depicts the action potential. Provided the initial stimulus is great enough to depolarize the neuron to threshold, then an action potential results. The following represents the events that occur during an action potential, which is an application of the aforementioned discussion on ion channels.

- At threshold, a critical mass of fast Na^+ channels open, resulting in further depolarization and the opening of more fast Na^+ channels.
- Because Na^+ g is high (see also Figure II-2-4), the E_m potential rapidly approaches the equilibrium potential for Na^+ (~ +70 mV)
- As membrane potential becomes positive, fast Na^+ channels begin to inactivate (see above), resulting in a rapid reduction in Na^+ conductance (see also Figure II-2-4).
- Voltage-gated K^+ channels open in response to the depolarization, but since their kinetics are much slower, the inward Na^+ current (upstroke of the action potential) dominates initially.
- K^+ g begins to rise as more channels open. As the rise in E_m approaches its peak, fast Na^+ channels are inactivating, and now the neuron has a high K^+ g and a low Na^+ g (see also Figure II-2-4).
- The high K^+ g drives E_m toward K^+ equilibrium (~ -95 mV) resulting in a rapid repolarization.
- As E_m becomes negative, K^+ channels begin to close, and K^+ g slowly returns to its original level. However, because of the slow kinetics, a period of hyperpolarization occurs.

Key Points

- The upstroke of the action potential is mediated by a Na^+ current (fast Na^+ channels).
- Although the inactivation of fast Na^+ channels participates in repolarization, the dominant factor is the high K^+ g due to the opening of voltage-gated K^+ channels.
- The action potential is all or none: Occurs if threshold is reached, doesn't occur if threshold is not reached.
- The action potential cannot summate.
- Under normal conditions, the action potential regenerates itself as it moves down the axon, thus it is propagated (magnitude is unchanged).

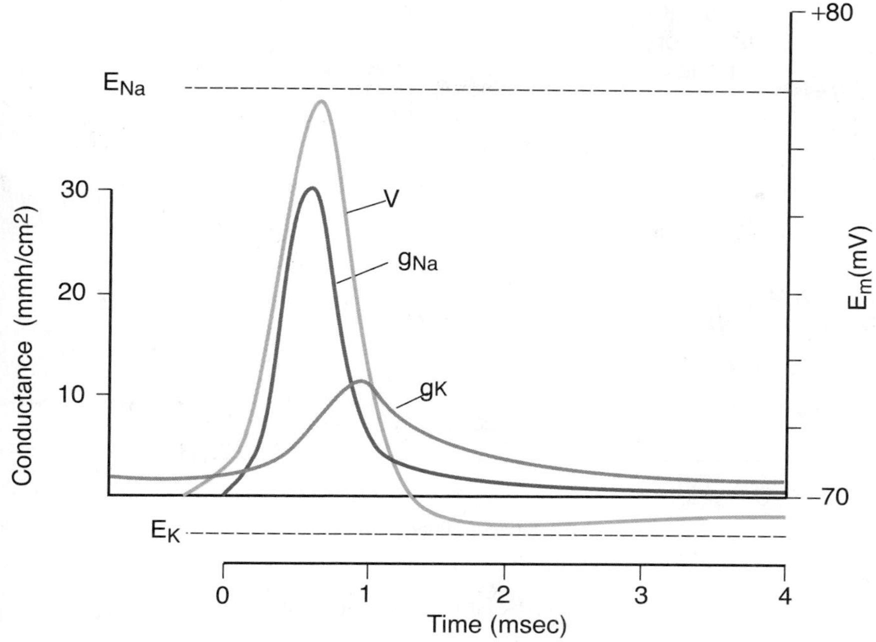

V = Membrane potential (action potential)
g_{Na} = Sodium ion conductance
g_K = Potassium ion conductance

Figure II-2-4. Axon Action Potential and Changes in Conductance

PROPERTIES OF ACTION POTENTIALS

Refractory Periods

Absolute refractory period

The absolute refractory period is the period during which no matter how strong the stimulus, it cannot induce a second action potential. The mechanism underlying this is the fact that during this time, most fast Na^+ channels are either open or in the inactivated state. The approximate duration of the absolute refractory period is illustrated in Figure II-2-5. The length of this period determines the maximum frequency of action potentials.

Relative refractory period

The relative refractory period is that period during which a greater than threshold stimulus is required to induce a second action potential (see approximate length in Figure II-2-5). The mechanism for this is the elevated K^+ g.

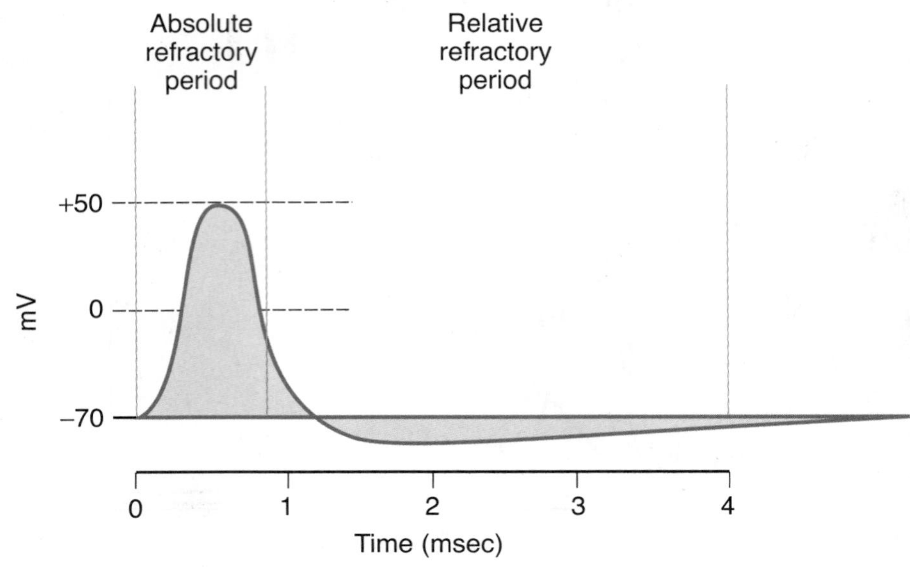

Figure II-2-5. Refractory Periods

Bridge to Pathology

Multiple sclerosis (MS) and Guillain-Barre syndrome (GBS) are demyelinating diseases. Loss of myelin results in current leakage across the membrane. Because of this, the magnitude of current reaching the cluster of fast Na^+ channels is unable to cause threshold depolarization, resulting in a conduction block. MS preferentially demyelinates neurons in the CNS, while GBS acts on peripheral neurons.

Conduction Velocity of the Action Potential

The 2 primary factors influencing conduction velocity in nerves are:

- **Cell diameter**: The greater the cell diameter, the greater the conduction velocity. A greater cross-sectional surface area reduces the internal electrical resistance.
- **Myelination**: Myelin provides a greater electrical resistance across the cell membrane, thereby reducing current "leak" through the membrane. The myelination is interrupted at the nodes of Ranvier where fast Na^+ channels cluster. Thus, the action potential appears to "bounce" from node to node with minimal decrement and greater speed (saltatory conduction).

SYNAPTIC TRANSMISSION

Neuromuscular Junction (NMJ)

The synapse between the axons of an alpha-motor neuron and a skeletal muscle fiber is called the neuromuscular junction (NMJ). The terminals of alpha-motor neurons contain acetylcholine (Ach), thus the synaptic transmission at the neuromuscular junction is one example of cholinergic transmission. The basics of neurotransmitter release described in this section are applicable to synaptic transmission for all synapses.

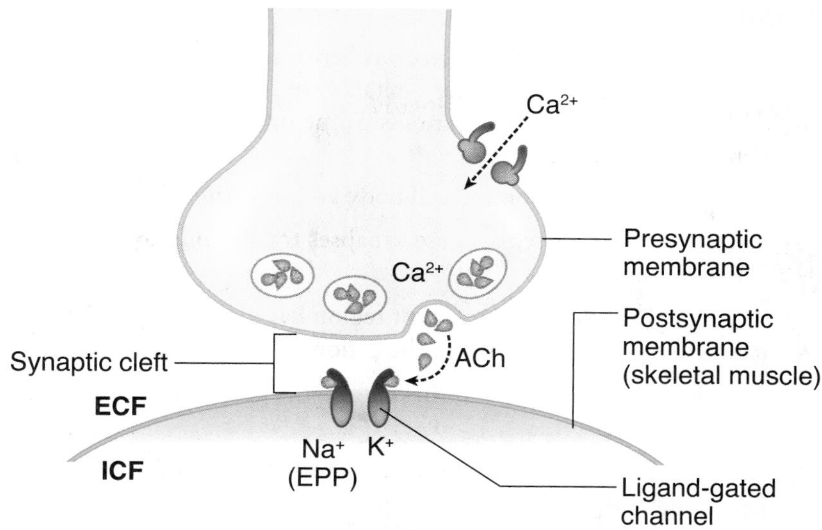

Figure II-2-6. Neuromuscular Transmission and Nicotinic Synapses

Sequence of events

1. The action potential travelling down the motor neuron depolarizes the presynaptic membrane.
2. This depolarization opens voltage-gated Ca^{2+} channels in the presynaptic membrane, resulting in Ca^{2+} influx into the presynaptic terminal.
3. The rise in Ca^{2+} causes synaptic vesicles to release their contents, in this case, Ach. The amount of neurotransmitter release is **directly related** to the rise in cytosolic Ca^{2+}, i.e., the more Ca^{2+} that enters, the more neurotransmitter released.
4. Ach binds to a nicotinic receptor located on the muscle membrane (N_M receptor). The N_M receptor is a non-selective monovalent cation channel (both Na^+ and K^+ can traverse). Given that Na^+ has a much greater net force (see Chapter 1 of this section), depolarization occurs. This depolarization is called an end-plate potential (EPP). The magnitude of the EPP is directly related to the amount of Ach released.
5. The resulting depolarization opens fast Na^+ channels on the muscle membrane (sarcolemma) causing an action potential in the sarcolemma. Under normal circumstances, an action potential in the motor neuron releases enough Ach to cause an EPP that is at least threshold for the action potential in the skeletal muscle cell. In other words, there is a one-to-one relationship between an action potential in the motor neuron and an action potential in the skeletal muscle cell.
6. The actions of Ach are terminated by acetylcholinesterase (AchE), an enzyme located on the postsynaptic membrane that breaks down Ach into choline and acetate. Choline is taken back into the presynaptic terminal (reuptake), hence providing substrate for re-synthesis of Ach.

Synapses Between Neurons

Figure II-2-7 illustrates synaptic junctions between neurons. In general, the synaptic potentials produced are either excitatory or inhibitory (see below) and are produced by **ligand-gated ion channels**. Some other important aspects associated with these synapses are:

- Synapses are located on the cell body and dendrites.
- The currents produced at these synapses travel along the dendritic and cell body membranes.
- The axon hillock–initial segment region has a high density of fast Na^+ channels and is the origin for the action potential of the axon.
- The closer the synapse is to this region, the greater its influence in determining whether an action potential is generated.
- If the sum of all the inputs reaches threshold, an action potential is generated and conducted along the axon to the nerve terminals.

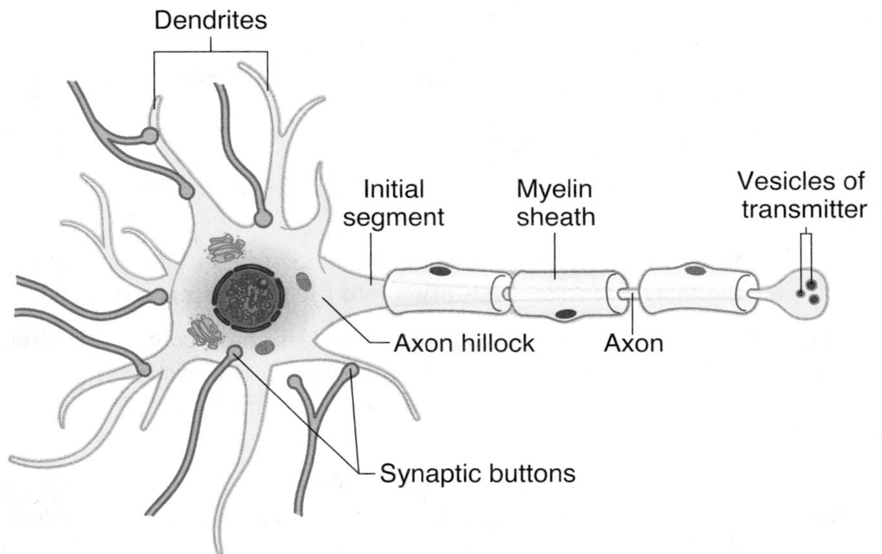

Figure II-2-7. Synapse Transmission between Neurons

Excitatory postsynaptic potential (EPSP)

EPSP is excitatory if it increases the excitability of the postsynaptic neuron, i.e., it is more likely to fire an action potential.

- It is primarily the result of increased Na^+ g.
- It is similar to the EPP found at the neuromuscular junction.
- Important receptors that produce:
  - Nicotinic: Endogenous ligand is Ach and include N_M and N_N.
  - Non-NMDA (N-methyl-D-aspartic acid): Endogenous ligands are glutamate and aspartate (excitatory amino acid transmitters), and Na^+ g is increased when they bind.
  - NMDA: Endogenous ligands are the excitatory amino acids and it is a non-selective cation channel (discussed in the preceding chapter).

Inhibitory postsynaptic potential (IPSP)

IPSP is inhibitory if it decreases the excitability of the postsynaptic neuron, i.e., it is less likely to fire an action potential.

- It is primarily the result of increased Cl^- g.
- Important receptors that produce:
  - $GABA_{A\&C}$: Endogenous ligand is GABA (gamma-aminobutryic acid).
  - Glycine: Endogenous ligand is glycine.

Electrical Synapses

- In contrast to chemical synaptic transmission, there is a direct flow of current from cell to cell.
- This cell-to-cell communication occurs via gap junctions; because the cells are electrically coupled, there is no synaptic delay.
- Cardiac and single-unit smooth muscle cells have these electrical synapses.

Overview of the Peripheral Nervous System

Motor

- Alpha-motor neurons release Ach, which binds to the NM (nicotinic muscle) receptor.
- These are large, well-myelinated neurons—i.e., they exhibit fast conduction.

Parasympathetic nervous system

- Preganglionic neurons release Ach, which binds to NN (nicotinic neuronal) receptor.
- Postganglionic fibers release Ach, which binds to muscarinic receptor (G-protein coupled).

Sympathetic nervous system

- Preganglionic neurons release Ach, which binds to NN receptor.
- Postganglionic neurons (most) release norepinephrine (NE): Binds to alpha and beta (β-1 & β-3) receptors (G-protein coupled).

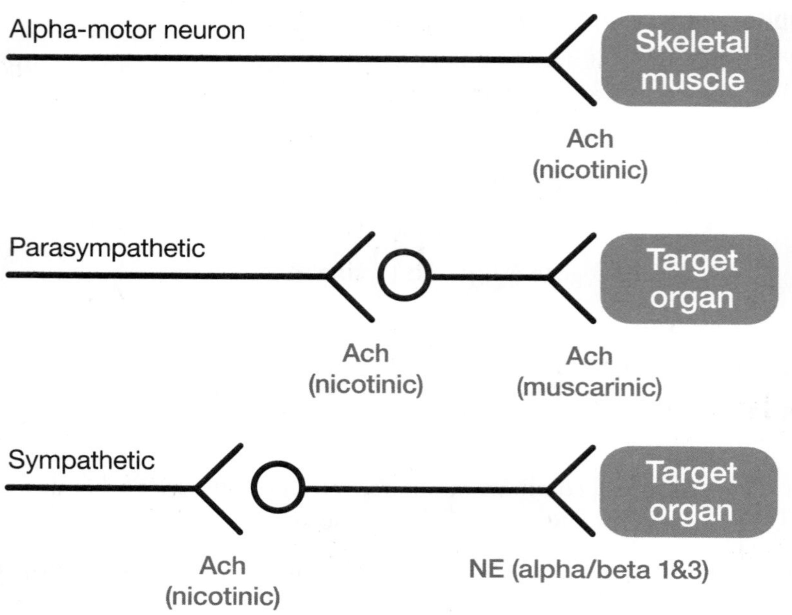

Figure II-2-8. Peripheral Nervous System

Bridge to Pharmacology

Botulinum toxin is a protease that destroys proteins needed for the fusion and release of synaptic vesicles. This toxin targets cholinergic neurons, resulting in flaccid paralysis.

Bridge to Pharmacology

Latrotoxin, the venom from the black-widow spider, opens presynaptic Ca^{2+} channels, resulting in excess Ach release.

Bridge to Pharmacology

Many pesticides, as well as some therapeutic agents, block AchE, resulting in the prolonged action of Ach in cholinergic synapses.

REVIEW AND INTEGRATION

In this section, we review much of the preceding information and add in applicable new information as it pertains to clinical signs indicative of alterations in the normal physiological function just discussed. These are clinical signs intended to help further reinforce the important physiology and thus aid the student in recognizing possible causes of these clinical signs. This is not intended to fully represent all the specific signs/symptoms related to each and every condition indicated.

Decreased Neuronal Excitability/Conduction

Clinical signs could include: weakness; ataxia; hyporeflexia; paralysis; sensory deficit. Possible causes include the following.

Table II-2-1

Ion Disturbances	Loss of Neurons/ Demyelination	Toxins/Drugs	NMJ
Hypokalemia	Guillian-Barre	Local anesthetics ("caine" drugs)	Depolarizing N_M blockers
Chronic hyperkalemia	ALS (amyotrophic lateral sclerosis)	TTX	Non-depolarizing N_M blockers
Hypercalcemia	Aging	STX	Lambert-Eaton
			Myasthenia gravis
			Botulinum

Increased Neuronal Excitability/Conduction

Clinical signs could include hyperreflexia, spasms, muscle fasciculations, tetany, tremors, paresthesias, and convulsions. Possible causes include the following.

Table II-2-2

Ion Disturbances	Loss of Neurons/ Demyelination	Toxins/Drugs	NMJ
Acute hyperkalemia	Multiple sclerosis	CTX	AchE inhibitors
Hypocalcemia		BTX	Latrotoxin

Bridge to Pharmacology

A variety of compounds can block N_M receptors (non-depolarizing neuromuscular blockers), while succinylcholine binds to this receptor causing the channel to remain open (depolarizing neuromuscular blocker).

Bridge to Pathology

Two important pathologies related to neuromuscular junctions are **myasthenia gravis** and **Lambert-Eaton** syndrome. The most common form of myasthenia gravis is an autoimmune condition in which antibodies are created that block the N_M receptor. Lambert-Easton is also an autoimmune condition, but the antibodies block the presynaptic voltage-gated Ca^{2+} channels.

Chapter Summary

- The action potential is an explosive change in membrane potential. It carries electrical impulses from one nerve to the next or from the nerve to a target tissue. In muscle, it initiates contraction.
- The depolarization phase is sodium influx through voltage-gated, fast Na^+ channels. These channels are required for neuronal and skeletal muscle action potentials.
- The positive membrane potential produced the upstroke of the action potential causes fast Na^+ channels to transition into the inactivated state.
- Repolarization is primarily mediated by voltage-gated K^+ channels. Blocking these channels greatly slows the repolarization process.
- The absolute refractory period is the result of fast Na^+ channels being in either the open or inactivated state.
- Conduction velocity of the neuronal action potential is determined by diameter of the neuron, and the level of myelination.
- Synaptic transmission involves the entry of extracellular calcium into the nerve terminal. This calcium triggers the release of the transmitter.
- The postsynaptic membrane is dominated by ligand-gated ion channels. In most cases, this allows either an influx of sodium (EPP or EPSP) or an influx of chloride (IPSP).
- Termination of acetylcholine's action is mainly by enzymatic destruction, whereas with other neurotransmitters, it is reuptake by the presynaptic membrane and/or diffusion away from the site of action.
- Electrical synapses are bidirectional and faster than chemical synapses, which are unidirectional.
- Motor neurons release Ach, which depolarizes skeletal muscle via nicotinic muscle (N_M) receptors.
- Preganglionic neurons release Ach, causing depolarization of postganglionic neurons via the nicotinic neuronal (N_N) receptor.
- Postganglionic parasympathetic neurons release Ach acting on muscarinic receptors (G-protein coupled), while postganglionic sympathetic fibers primarily release NE, which acts on adrenergic receptors (G-protein coupled), specifically α and β-1/β-3 receptors.

Electrical Activity of the Heart 3

Learning Objectives

- ❑ Use knowledge of properties of cardiac tissue
- ❑ Answer questions about cardiac action potentials
- ❑ Use knowledge of control of nodal excitability
- ❑ Answer questions about electrocardiology
- ❑ Explain information related to arrhythmias/ECG alterations

PROPERTIES OF CARDIAC TISSUE

Different cells within the heart are specialized for different functional roles. In general, these specializations are for automaticity, conduction, and/or contraction.

Automaticity

Cardiac cells initiate action potentials spontaneously. Further, the cells are electrically coupled via gap junctions. Thus, when a cell fires an action potential, it typically sweeps throughout the heart. Although all cardiac tissue shows spontaneous depolarization, only the following 3 are germane.

- **Sinoatrial (SA) node cells** are specialized for automaticity. They spontaneously depolarize to threshold and have the highest intrinsic rhythm (rate), making them the pacemaker in the normal heart. Their intrinsic rate is ~ 100/min.
- **Atrioventricular (AV) node cells** have the second highest intrinsic rhythm (40-60/min). Often, these cells become the pacemaker if SA node cells are damaged.
- Although not "specialized" for automaticity per se, **Purkinje cells** do exhibit spontaneous depolarizations with a rate of ~ 35/min.

Conduction

All cardiac tissue conducts electrical impulses, but the following are particularly specialized for this function.

- AV node: These cells are specialized for slow conduction. They have small diameter fibers, a low density of gap junctions, and the rate of depolarization (phase 0, see below) is slow in comparison to tissue that conducts fast.

- Purkinje cells: These cells are specialized for rapid conduction. Their diameter is large, they express many gap junctions, and the rate of depolarization (phase 0, see below) is rapid. These cells constitute the HIS-Purkinje system of the ventricles.

Contraction

Although myocytes have a spontaneous depolarization and they conduct electrical impulses, they contain the protein machinery to contract.

Conduction Pathway

Because cells are electrically coupled via gap junctions, excitation to threshold of one cell typically results in the spread of this action potential throughout the heart. In the normal heart, the SA node is the pacemaker because it has the highest intrinsic rhythm. Below is the normal conduction pathway for the heart.

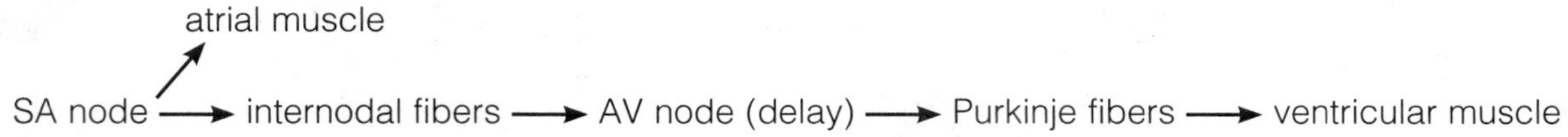

CARDIAC ACTION POTENTIALS

Resting Membrane Potential (Non-Nodal Cells)

Potassium conductance is high in resting ventricular or atrial myocytes. This is also true for Purkinje cells. Because of this, resting membrane potential is close to K^+ equilibrium potential. This high-resting K^+ conductance is the result to 2 major types of channels.

Ungated potassium channels

Always open and unless the membrane potential reaches the potassium equilibrium potential (~ –95 mV), a potassium flux (efflux) is maintained through these channels.

Inward K^+ rectifying channels (IK_1)

- Voltage-gated channels that are open at rest.
- Depolarization closes.
- They open again as the membrane begins to repolarize.

Action Potential (Non-Nodal Cells)

Understanding the ionic basis of cardiac action potentials is important for understanding both cardiac physiology and the electrocardiogram (ECG), which is a recording of the currents produced by these ionic changes. In addition, antiarrhythmic drugs exert their effects by binding to the channels that produce these ionic currents.

In this section, we go through the various phases of the action potentials that occur in myocytes and Purkinje cells. Action potentials generated by nodal cells (SA and AV) are discussed later. Although there are slight differences in the action potentials generated by atrial and ventricular myocytes, as well as Purkinje cells, these differences are not included here. Furthermore, it is important to remember that cardiac cells are electrically coupled by gap junctions. Thus, when a cell fires an action potential, it spreads and is conducted by neighboring cells.

Figure II-3-1 shows the labeled phases of the action potential from a ventricular myocyte and the predominant ionic currents related to the various phases.

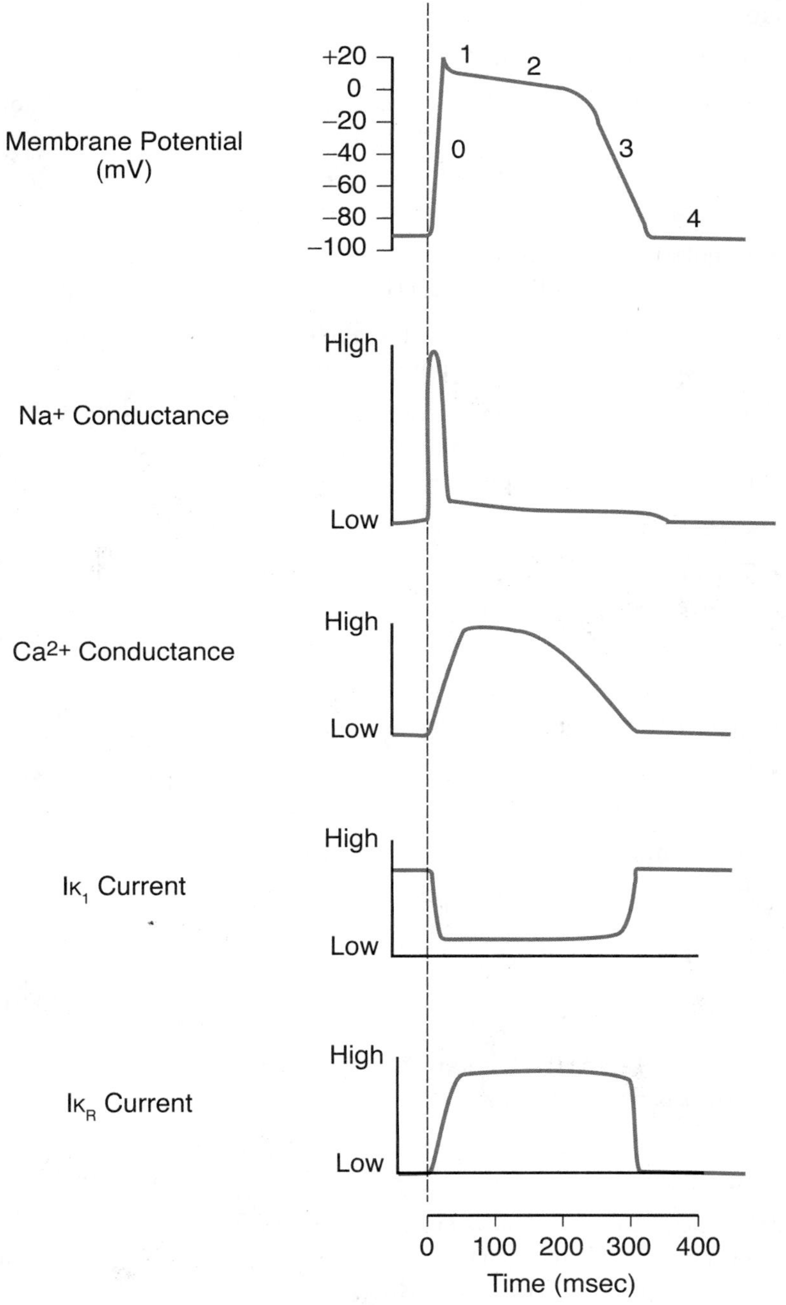

Figure II-3-1. Action Potential in a Ventricular Myocyte

Bridge to Pathology

In Figure II-3-1, note that Na^+ conductance during phase 2 is still slightly elevated. Some of these channels are very slow to inactivate and data suggest that genetic alterations can result in a significant Na^+ current during phase 2. This Na^+ current delays repolarization, resulting in a prolonged QT. This genetic alteration appears to play a role in congenital long QT syndrome.

A prolonged QT interval can cause a form of ventricular tachycardia known as **torsade de pointes**. Other factors can increase the QT interval, thus possibly producing torsade de pointes.

Phase 0

- Upstroke of the action potential
- Similar to nerve and skeletal muscle, mediated by the opening of voltage-gated, fast Na^+ channels (note high Na^+ conductance)
- Conduction velocity is directly related to rate of change in potential (slope). Stimulation of β-1 receptors, e.g., epinephrine and norepinephrine, increases the slope and thus increases conduction velocity.
- Creates the QRS complex of the ECG

Bridge to Pharmacology

Class I antiarrhythmic agents block fast Na^+ channels, resulting in a change in phase 0. Blocking these channels reduces conduction velocity, an action that can be beneficial, e.g., use of lidocaine to reduce conduction and stabilize the heart when the tissue becomes ischemic.

Phase 1

- Slight repolarization mediated by a transient potassium current
- Sodium channels transition to the inactivated state (note reduction in Na^+ conductance).

Phase 2 (plateau)

- Depolarization opens voltage-gated Ca^{2+} channels (primarily L-type) and voltage-gated K^+ channels (IK_R current being one example).
- The inward Ca^{2+} current offset by the outward K^+ current results in little change in membrane potential (plateau).
- The influx of Ca^{2+} triggers the release of Ca^{2+} from the SR (Ca^{2+} induced Ca^{2+} release), resulting in cross-bridge cycling and muscle contraction (see next chapter).
- Creates the ST segment of the ECG
- The long duration of the action potential prevents tetany in cardiac muscle (see next chapter).

Bridge to Pharmacology

Class III antiarrhythmic drugs block K^+ channels. This delays repolarization, resulting in a long QT interval.

Phase 3

- Repolarization phase
- L-type channels begin closing, but rectifying K^+ currents (IK_R current being one example) still exist resulting in repolarization.
- IK_1 channels reopen and aid in repolarization.
- Creates the T wave of the EKG

Phase 4

- Resting membrane potential
- Fast Na^+, L-type Ca^{2+}, and rectifying K^+ channels (IK_R) close, but IK_1 channels remain open.

Action Potential (Nodal Cells)

Nodal tissue (SA and AV) lacks fast Na^+ channels. Thus, the upstroke of the action potential is mediated by a Ca^{2+} current rather than an Na^+ current. In addition, note that phases 1 and 2 are absent.

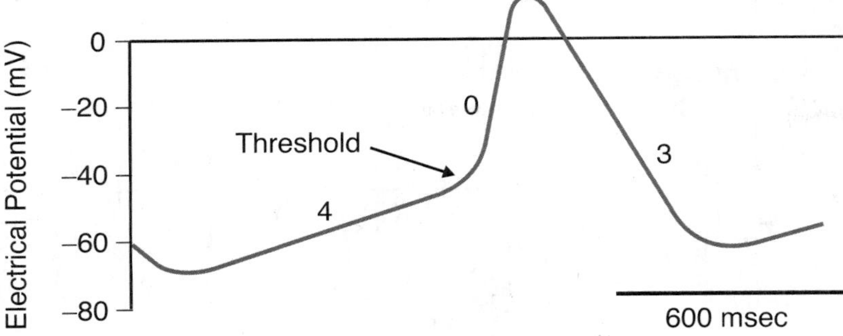

Figure II-3-2. SA Nodal (Pacemaker) Action Potential

Phase 4

- Resting membrane potential
- Given this tissue is specialized for automaticity (see above), these cells show a spontaneous depolarization at rest. This spontaneous depolarization is referred to as the "pacemaker" potential and results from:
  - **Inward Ca^{2+} current:** Primarily related to T-type Ca^{2+} channels. These differ from the L-type in that they open at a more negative membrane potential (~ -70 mV).
  - **Inward Na^{+} current:** This inward Na^{+} current is referred to as the "funny" current (I_f) and the channel involved is a hyperpolarization-activated cyclic nucleotide-gated (HCN) channel. HCN are non-selective monovalent cation channels and thus conduct both Na^{+} and K^{+}. However, opening of these channels evokes a sodium-mediated depolarization (similar to nicotinic receptors, see previous chapter). These channels open when the membrane repolarizes (negative membrane potential), and they close in response to the depolarization of the action potential.
  - **Outward K^{+} current:** There is a reduced outward K^{+} current as the cell repolarizes after the action potential. Reducing this current helps to produce the pacemaker potential.

Phase 0

- Upstroke of the action potential
- Mediated by opening of L-type (primarily) Ca^{2+} channels
- Note the time scale: the slope of phase 0 is not steep in nodal tissue like it is in ventricular myocytes or the upstroke of the action potential in nerves. This is part of the reason conduction velocity is slow in the AV node.

Phase 3

- Repolarization phase
- Mediated by voltage-gated K^{+} channels

CONTROL OF NODAL EXCITABILITY

Catecholamines

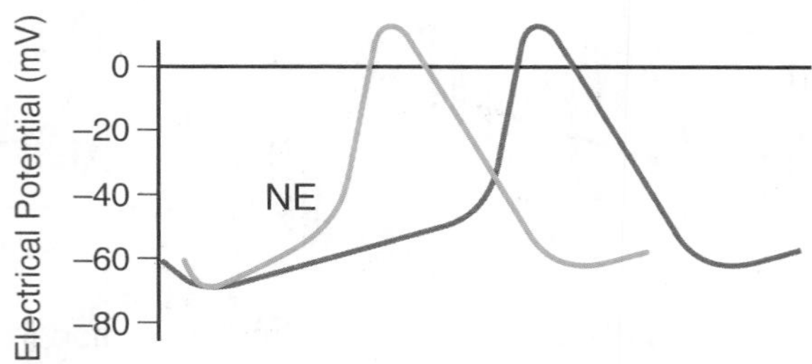

Figure II-3-3. Sympathetic Effects on SA Nodal Cells

- Norepinephrine (NE) from postganglionic sympathetic nerve terminals and circulating epinephrine (Epi)
- β-1 receptors; Gs—cAMP; stimulates opening of HCN and Ca^{2+} channels
- Increased slope of pacemaker potential (gets to threshold sooner)
- Functional effect
  - Positive chronotropy (SA node): increased HR
  - Positive dromotropy (AV node): increased conduction velocity through the AV node

Bridge to Pharmacology

Class II antiarrhythmics are the beta-blockers, while class IV antiarrhythmics are the Ca^{2+} channel blocks. These drugs reduce automaticity and conduction through the AV node and can be very efficacious in tachyarrhythmias.

Parasympathetic

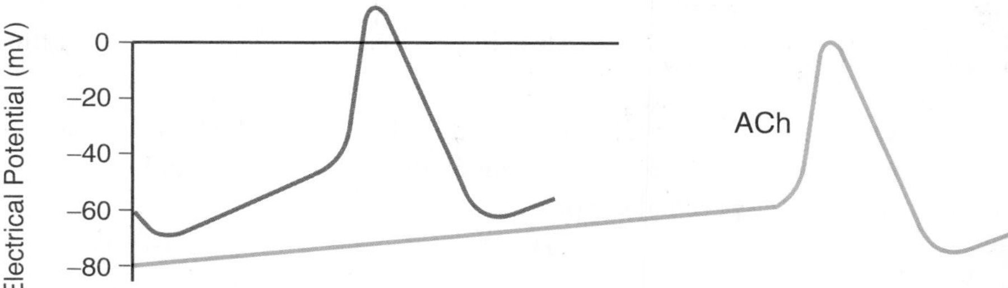

Figure II-3-4. Parasympathetic Effects on SA Nodal Cells

- Ach released from post-ganglionic fibers.
- M_2 receptor; Gi-Go; Opens K^+ channels and inhibits cAMP
- Hyperpolarizes; reduced slope of pacemaker potential
- Functional effect
  - Negative chronotropy (SA node): Decreased HR
  - Negative dromotropy (AV node): Decreased conduction velocity through the AV node

ELECTROCARDIOLOGY

The Electrocardiogram (EKG or ECG)

The normal pattern is demonstrated in Figure II-3-5.

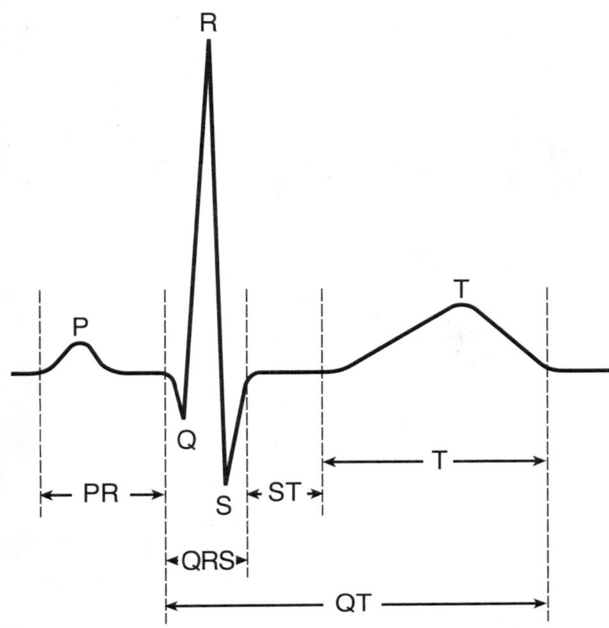

Figure II-3-5. Normal Pattern of an ECG

P wave: atrial depolarization

QRS complex: ventricular depolarization (40–100 msec)

R wave: first upward deflection after the P wave

S wave: first downward deflection after an R wave

T wave: ventricular repolarization

PR interval: start of the P wave to start of the QRS complex (120–200 msec); mostly due to conduction delay in the AV node

QT interval: start of the QRS complex to the end of the T wave; represents duration of the action potential (see Figure II-3-6)

ST segment: ventricles are depolarized during this segment; roughly corresponds to the plateau phase of the action potential

J point: end of the S wave; represents isoelectric point

Note: Height of waves is directly related to (a) mass of tissue, (b) rate of change in potential, and (c) orientation of the lead to the direction of current flow.

Figure II-3-6 further illustrates the alignment of the cardiac action potential and the ECG recording. To recap:

- Phase 0 produces the QRS complex.
- Phase 3 produces the T wave.
- The ST segment occurs during phase 2.
- The QT interval represents the duration of the action potential and this interval is inversely related to heart rate. For example, stimulation of sympathetics to the heart increases heart rate and reduces the duration of the action potential, thus decreasing the QT interval.

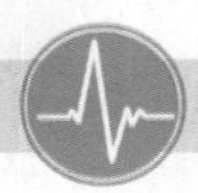

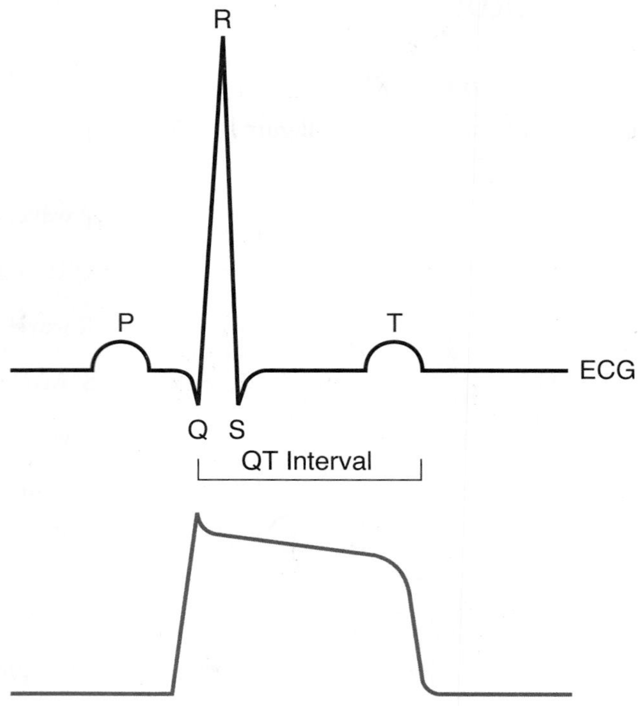

Figure II-3-6. Ventricular Action Potential Versus ECG

Standard Conventions

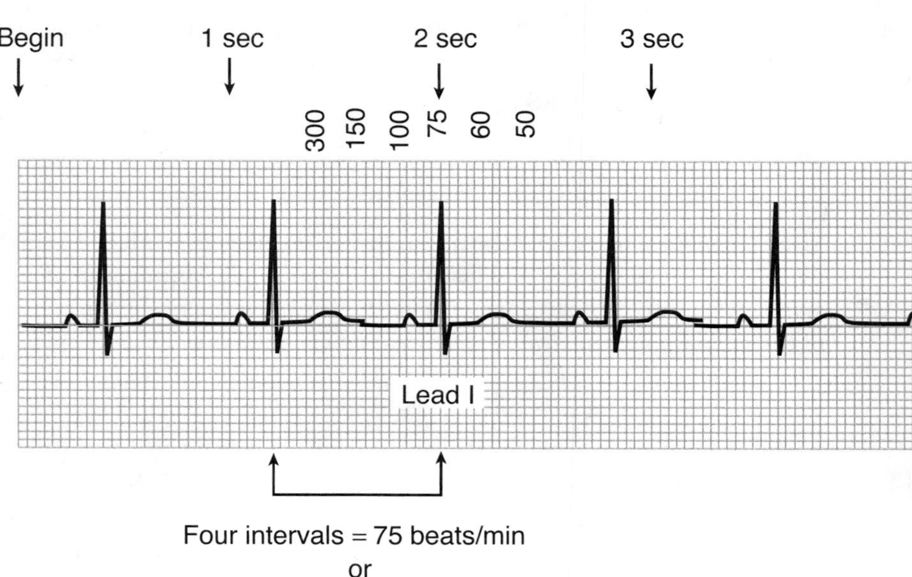

Figure II-3-7. Estimation of Heart Rate

Figure II-3-7 shows a normal ECG trace from a single lead. The ECG measures volts (Y-axis) per unit time (X-axis) and the scales are standardized. Note the heavier (darker) lines both horizontally and vertically. These represent "big" boxes, each of which is further subdivided into 5 "small" boxes.

- **Y-axis (volts): one big box = 0.5 mV**
  - Because there are 7 big boxes above the bottom line in Figure II-3-7, the total height is 3.5 mV.
- **X-axis (time): one big box = 0.2 sec (200 msec)**
  - Because there are 5 subdivisions within each big box, each small box is 0.04 sec (40 msec). As noted in Figure II-3-7, 5 big boxes equal one second.

Reading an ECG

The ECG is a powerful clinical tool and it takes years of training to become fully competent in detecting the many abnormalities it can detect. Thus, a detailed explanation is beyond the scope of this book. However, there are some arrhythmias and alterations that one should be able to recognize early in one's medical training. The following represents a step-wise approach that should allow the student to detect these alterations in the ECG.

Step 1: rate and rhythm

If provided, use the rhythm strip (lead II) that typically runs the length of the recording and is located on the bottom of the printout. We will use a single trace illustrated in Figure II-3-7.

- **Rhythm:** Qualitatively look at the trace and determine if there is a steady rhythm. This means the R waves occur regularly, i.e., the space between each is approximately the same. If so then there is a steady rhythm; if not then an unsteady rhythm.
- **Rate:** It is typically not necessary to determine the exact heart rate (HR); rather, simply determine if it is within the normal range (60–100 beats/min). The simplest way to do this is to find an R wave that is on a heavy (darker) vertical line, and note where the next R wave occurs with respect to the following count of subsequent heavy vertical lines (Illustrated in Figure II-3-7):

  1 = 300 beats/min

  2 = 150

  3 = 100

  4 = 75

  5 = 60

  6 = 50

  For example, if the subsequent R wave occurs at the second heavy line from the first R wave, then HR is 150 beats/min. If it occurs at the third heavy line from the first R wave, then HR is 100 beats/min, and so on. In Figure II-3-7, it occurs at the fourth heavy line, thus HR is 75 beats/min for this ECG.

If the subsequent R wave occurs between heavy lines, then the HR is between the values denoted for those lines. Even though it won't be a precise number, one can ascertain whether it is above or below the normal range.

Step 2: Waves

- Qualitatively examine the trace for the presence of P, QRS, and T. Can they be seen and do they look somewhat "normal"?

Step 3: PR interval

- Find the PR interval and determine if it is in the normal range (120–200 msecs). This normal range translates into 3-5 small boxes.
- Look at several cycles to see if the PR interval is consistent.

Step 4: Estimate the mean electrical axis (MEA)

- The MEA indicates the net direction (vector) of current flow during ventricular depolarization.
- Each lead can be represented by an angle, as is illustrated in Figure II-3-8. Although the MEA axis can be determined very precisely, it is not important to do so at this stage. Instead, we will simply define what quadrant (quadrant method) the MEA falls in using a very simplified approach.

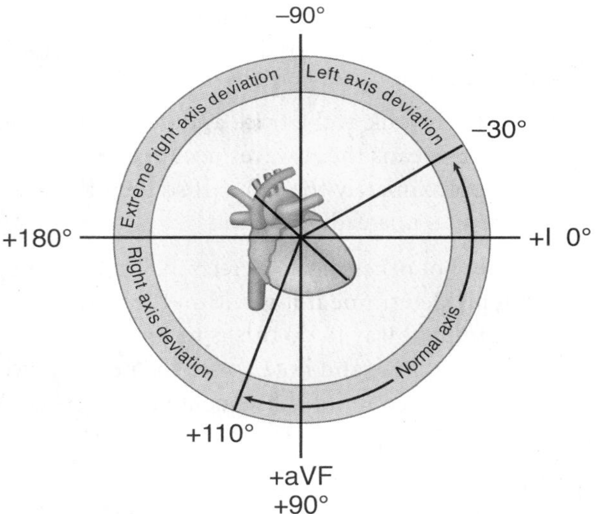

Figure II-3-8. Axis Ranges

Quadrant method

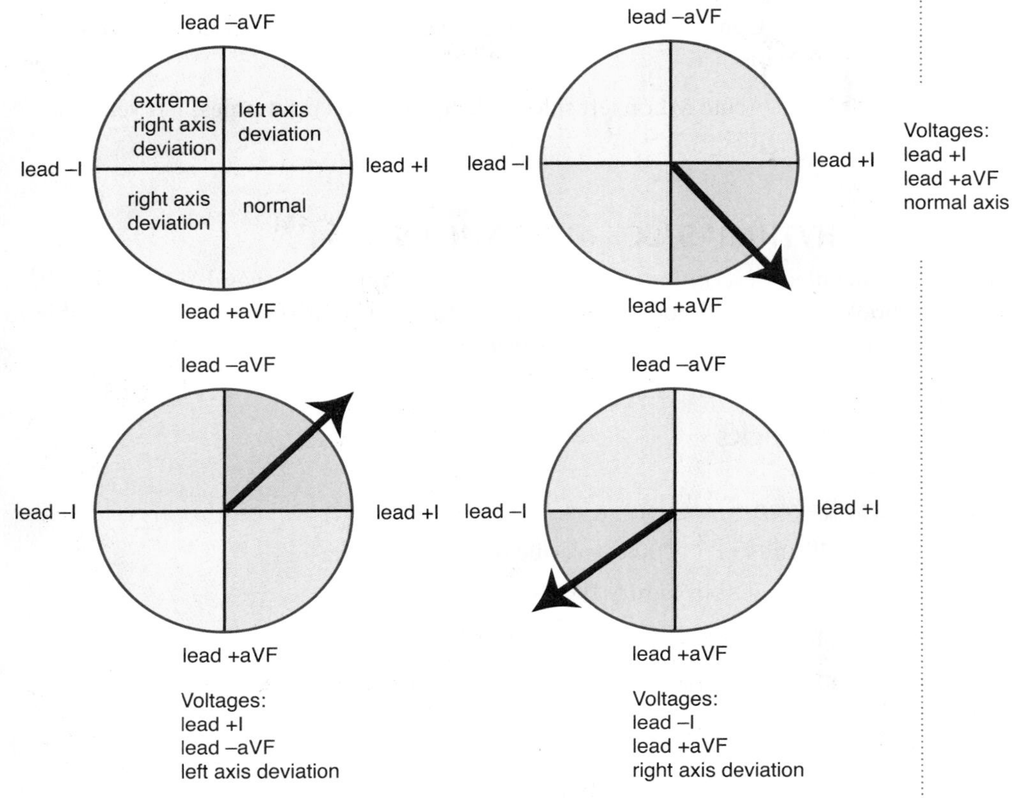

Figure II-3-9. Quadrant Method

- Determine the net QRS deflection (upward minus downward) in lead I and aVF. Using these 2 leads allows us to partition the mathematical grid into 4 basic quadrants (upper left panel of Figure II-3-9).
- If the net deflections for leads I and aVF are positive, then the MEA is between 0° and 90°, and is thus normal (upper right panel of Figure II-3-9). Note: The normal range for MEA is -30° and +110°. Even though the quadrant method is not precise, it is close enough at this juncture.
- If the net deflection is positive in lead I and negative in aVF, then the MEA is between 0° and -90°, and there is a left axis deviation (lower left panel of Figure II-3-9).
  - Causes of left axis deviation are:
    - Left heart enlargement, either left ventricular hypertrophy or dilation
    - Conduction defects in the left ventricle, except in the posterior bundle branch
    - Acute MI on right side tends to shift axis left unless right ventricle dilates
- If the net deflection is negative in lead I and positive in aVF, then the MEA is between 90° and 180°, and there is a right axis deviation (lower right panel of Figure II-3-9).

- Causes of right axis deviation are:
  - Right heart enlargement, hypertrophy, or dilation
  - Conduction defects of right ventricle or the posterior left bundle branch
  - Acute MI on left side tends to shift axis right unless left ventricle dilates

ARRHYTHMIAS/ECG ALTERATIONS

A detailed description of the various arrhythmias is beyond the scope of this book, but we will go through some of the ones that should be recognizable to students early in their medical education.

Heart Blocks

First-Degree

Long PR interval (>200 msec; one big box)

- Illustrated in Figure II-3-10
- Slowed conduction through the AV node
- Characteristics: rate and rhythm are typically normal

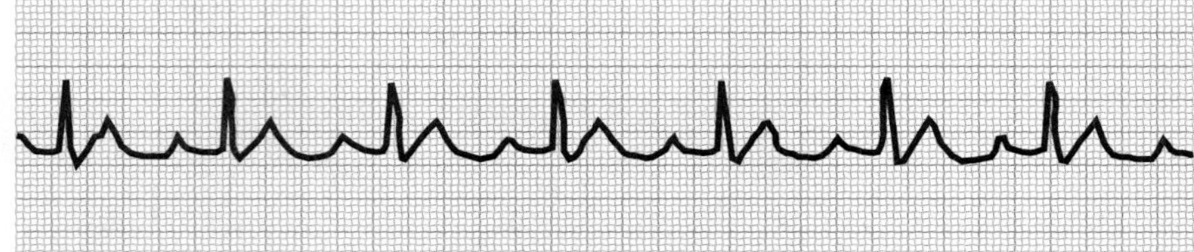

Figure II-3-10. First-Degree Heart Block

Second-Degree

Every QRS complex is preceded by a P wave, but not every P wave is followed by a QRS complex.

- Some impulses are not transmitted through the AV node.
- Two types:
  - **Mobitz type I (Wenckebach; Figure II-3-11):** Progressive prolongation of PR interval until a ventricular beat is missed and then the cycle begins again. This arrhythmia will have an unsteady rhythm.

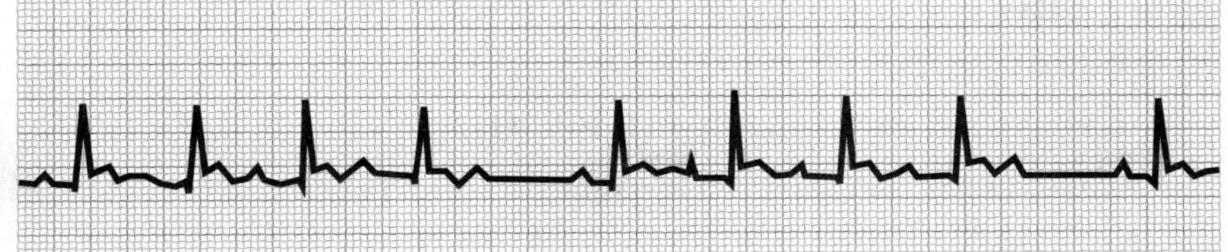

Figure II-3-11. Second-Degree Heart Block (Mobitz Type I)

- **Mobitz type II (Figure II-3-12):** The PR interval is consistent, i.e., it doesn't lengthen and this separates it from Wenckebach. The rhythm can be steady or unsteady depending upon block ratio (P to QRS ratio: 2:1, 3:1, 3:2, etc.).

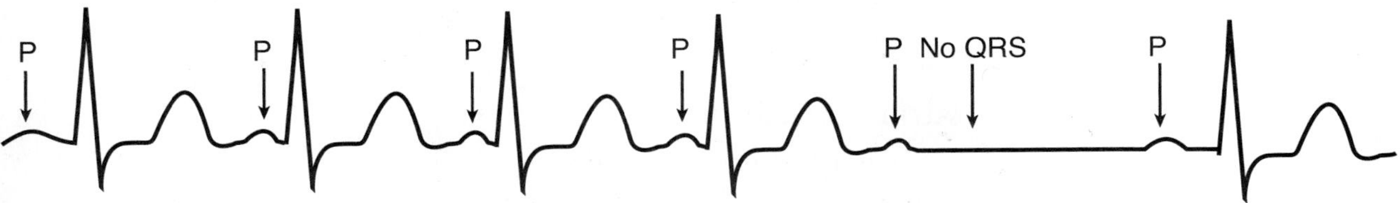

Figure II-3-12. Second-Degree Heart Block (Mobitz Type II)

Third-Degree (Complete)

Complete dissociation of P waves and QRS complexes (Figure II-3-13)

- Impulses are not transmitted through the AV node.
- Characteristics: steady rhythm (usually) and very slow ventricular HR (usually); no consistent PR interval because impulses are not transmitted through the AV node; rate for P waves is different than rate for R waves

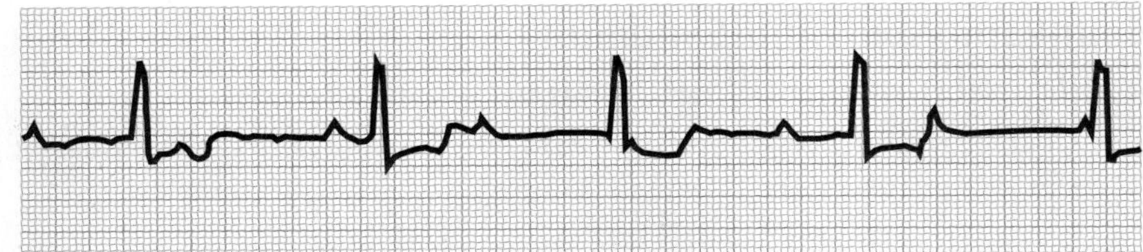

Figure II-3-13. Complete Heart Block

Atrial Flutter

Very fast atrial rate (>280 beats/min)

- Although fast, atrial conduction is still intact and coordinated.
- Characteristics: "saw-tooth" appearance of waves between QRS complexes; no discernible T waves; rhythm typically steady

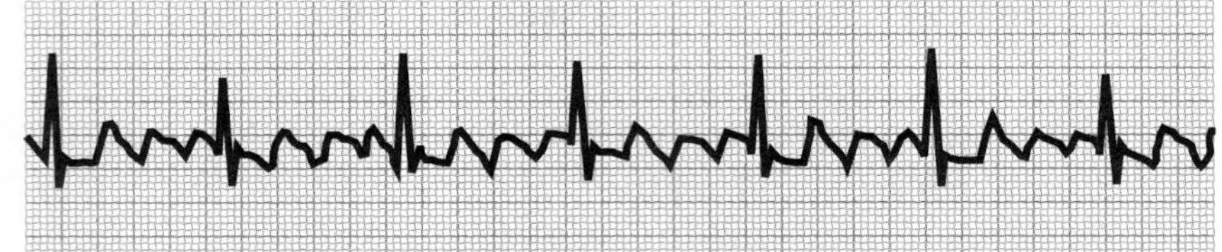

Figure II-3-14. Atrial Flutter

Atrial Fibrillation

Uncoordinated atrial conduction

- Lack of a coordinated conduction results in no atrial contraction
- Characteristics: unsteady rhythm (usually) and no discernible P waves

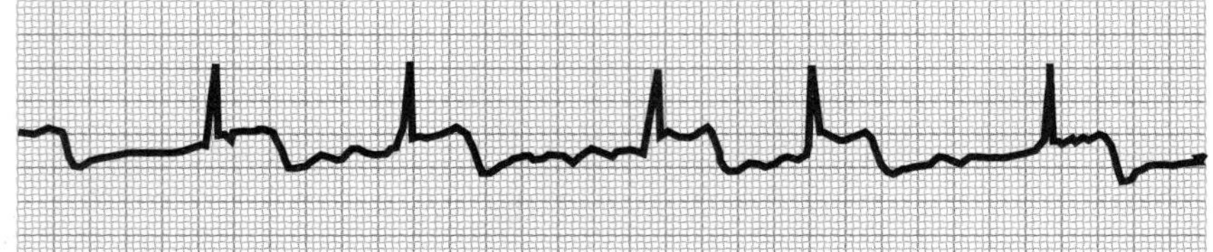

Figure II-3-15. Atrial Fibrillation

Wolff-Parkinson-White Syndrome

Accessory pathway (Bundle of Kent) between atria and ventricles

- Characteristics: short PR interval; steady rhythm and normal rate (usually); slurred upstroke of the R wave (delta wave); widened QRS complex
- The cardiac impulse can travel in retrograde fashion to the atria over the accessory pathway and initiate a reentrant tachycardia.

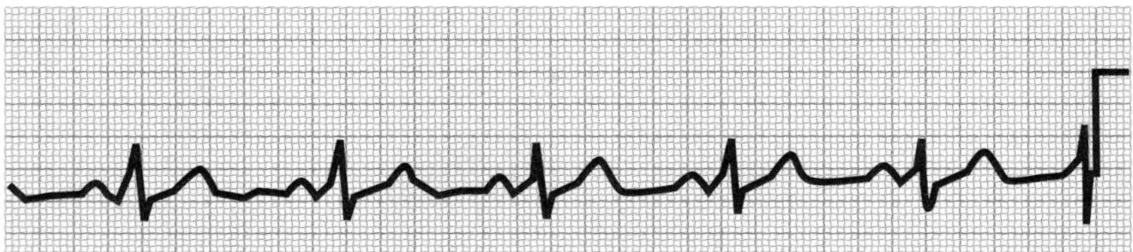

Figure II-3-16. Wolff-Parkinson-White Syndrome

Other Factors Changing the ECG

ST segment changes

- Elevated: Transmural infarct or Prinzmetal angina (coronary vasospasm)
- Depressed: Subendocardial ischemia or exertional (stable) angina

Potassium

- Hyperkalemia: Increases rate of repolarization, resulting in sharp-spiked T waves and a shortened QT interval.
- Hypokalemia: Decreases rate of repolarization, resulting in U waves and a prolonged QT interval.

Calcium

- Hypercalcemia: Decreases the QT interval
- Hypocalcemia: Increases the QT interval

Chapter Summary

- Different parts of the heart have cardiac tissue that is specialized for automaticity, conduction, and contraction.
- Myocytes and Purkinje cells have fast Na^+ channels, while nodal cells (SA and AV) lack these channels. Thus, the upstroke of the action potential (phase 0) is much faster in myocytes and Purkinje cells.
- There are 5 phases for cardiac action potentials from myocytes and Purkinje cells, but only 3 phases for nodal cells.
- The plateau phase (phase 2) is due to influx of calcium through L-type channels and potassium efflux via voltage-gated channels.
- Repolarization is due to open potassium channels.
- Nodal cells in the heart are characterized by an unstable phase 4 (resting membrane potential) that is primarily mediated by calcium and the sodium "funny" current.
- In SA nodal cells, sympathetics (β-1) increase the slope of the pacemaker potential and thus the intrinsic rate, whereas parasympathetics (M_2) hyperpolarize and decrease the intrinsic rate.
- The mean electrical axis of the heart is about 60°. It tends to move toward hypertrophied tissue and away from infarcted tissue.
- First-degree heart block is a slowed conduction through the AV node, second-degree heart block is the lack of transmission of some impulses through the AV node, and third-degree heart block is a total block at the AV node.
- There are 2 types of second-degree block: Wenckebach (Mobitz type I) and Mobitz type II.
- Atrial flutter is characterized by a steady rhythm and a "saw tooth" wave appearance between QRS complexes
- Atrial fibrillation is characterized by an unsteady rhythm and lack of discernible P waves.
- Wolff-Parkinson-White syndrome is characterized by an accessory pathway between the atria and ventricles. This shortens the PR interval and may produce a reentrant tachycardia.

SECTION III

Muscle

Excitation-Contraction Coupling 1

Learning Objectives

- ❑ Interpret scenarios on skeletal muscle structure-function relationships
- ❑ Interpret scenarios on regulation of cytosolic calcium
- ❑ Interpret scenarios on altering force in skeletal muscle
- ❑ Interpret scenarios on comparison of striated muscles (skeletal vs. cardiac)
- ❑ Interpret scenarios on smooth muscle function

SKELETAL MUSCLE STRUCTURE–FUNCTION RELATIONSHIPS

Ultrastructure of a Myofibril

- A muscle is made up of individual cells called muscle fibers.
- Longitudinally within the muscle fibers, there are bundles of myofibrils. A magnified portion is shown in the figure below.
- A myofibril can be subdivided into individual sarcomeres. A sarcomere is demarked by a Z lines.
- Sarcomeres are composed of filaments creating bands as illustrated below.
- Contraction causes no change in the length of the A band, a shortening of the I band, and a shortening in the H zone (band).
- Titin anchors myosin and is an important component of striated muscle's elasticity.

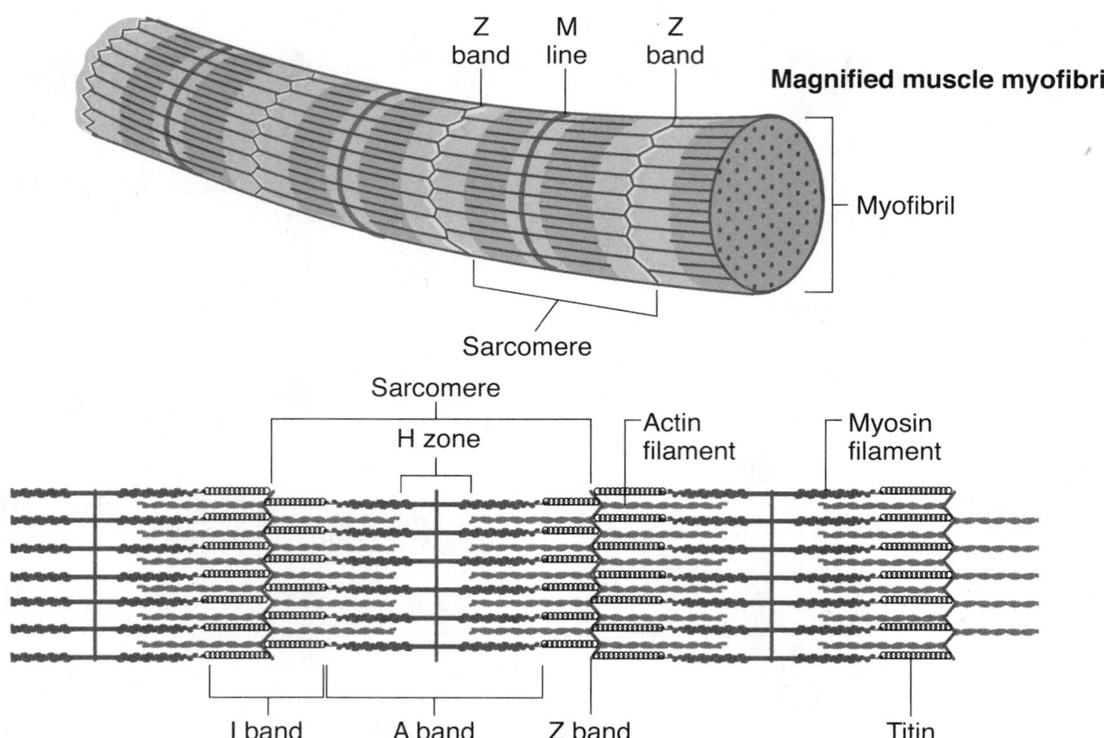

Figure III-1-1. Organization of Sarcomeres

Ultrastructure of the Sarcoplasmic Reticulum

The external and internal membrane system of a skeletal muscle cell is displayed below.

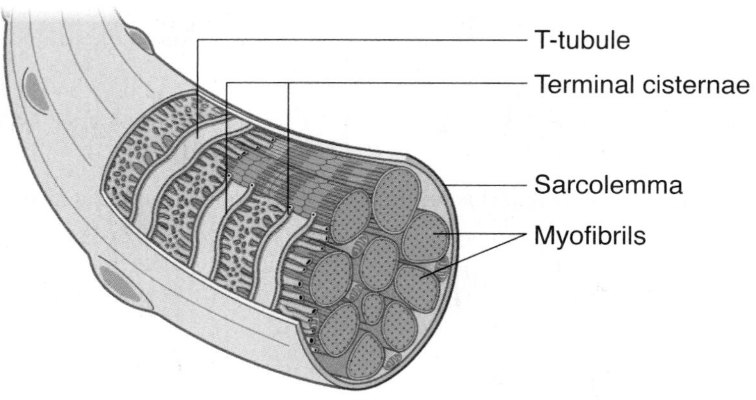

Figure III-1-2. Skeletal Muscle Cell Membranes

T-tubule membranes are extensions of the surface membrane; therefore, the interiors of the T tubules are part of the extracellular compartment.

Terminal cisternae: The sarcoplasmic reticulum is part of the internal membrane system, one function of which is to store calcium. In skeletal muscle, most of the calcium is stored in the terminal cisternae close to the T-tubule system.

Functional Proteins of the Sarcomere

Figure III-1-3 shows the relationships among the various proteins that make up the thin and thick filaments in striated muscle (skeletal and cardiac) and the changes that occur with contraction.

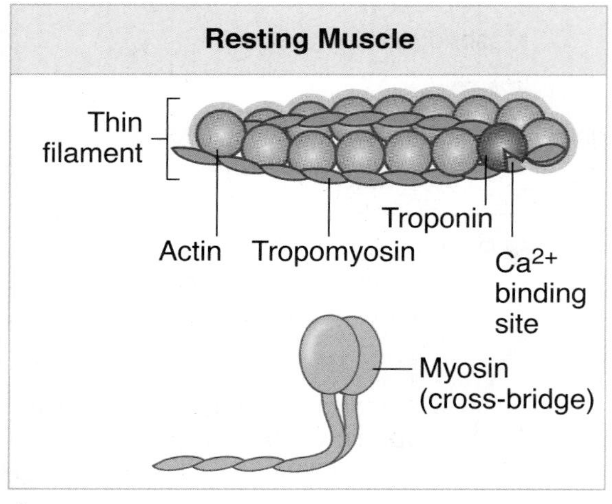

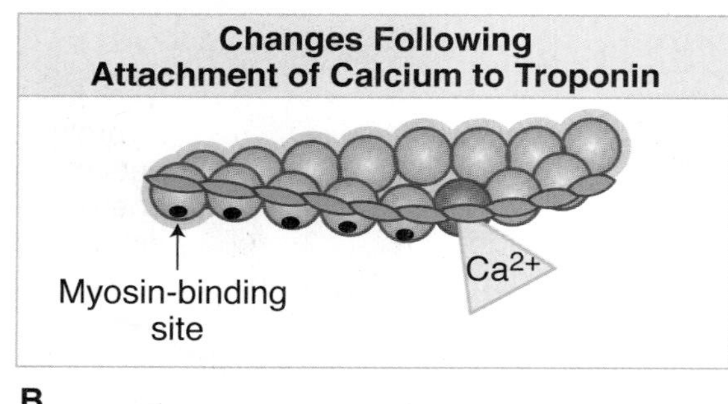

Figure III-1-3. Regulation of Actin by Troponin

Proteins of the thin filaments

- **Actin** is the structural protein of the thin filament. It possesses attachment sites for myosin.
- **Tropomyosin** blocks myosin binding sites on actin.
- **Troponin** is composed of 3 subunits: **troponin-T** (binds to tropomyosin), **troponin-I** (binds to actin and inhibits contraction), and **troponin-C** (binds to calcium).
  - Under resting conditions, no calcium is bound to the troponin, preventing actin and myosin from interacting.
  - When calcium binds to troponin-C, the troponin-tropomyosin complex moves, exposing actin's binding site for myosin. (Figure III-1-3 B)

Proteins of the thick filaments

Myosin has ATPase activity. The splitting of ATP puts myosin in a "high energy" state; it also increases myosin's affinity for actin.

- Once myosin binds to actin, the chemical energy is transferred to mechanical energy, causing myosin to pull the actin filament. This generates active tension in the muscle and is commonly referred to as "the power stroke."
- If the force generated by the power stroke is sufficient to move the load (see next chapter), then the muscle shortens (isotonic contraction).
- If the force generated is not sufficient to move the load (see next chapter), then the muscle doesn't shorten (isometric contraction).

Cross-Bridge Interactions (Chemical-Mechanical Transduction)

Figure III-1-4 illustrates the major steps involved in cross-bridge cycling in a contracting muscle.

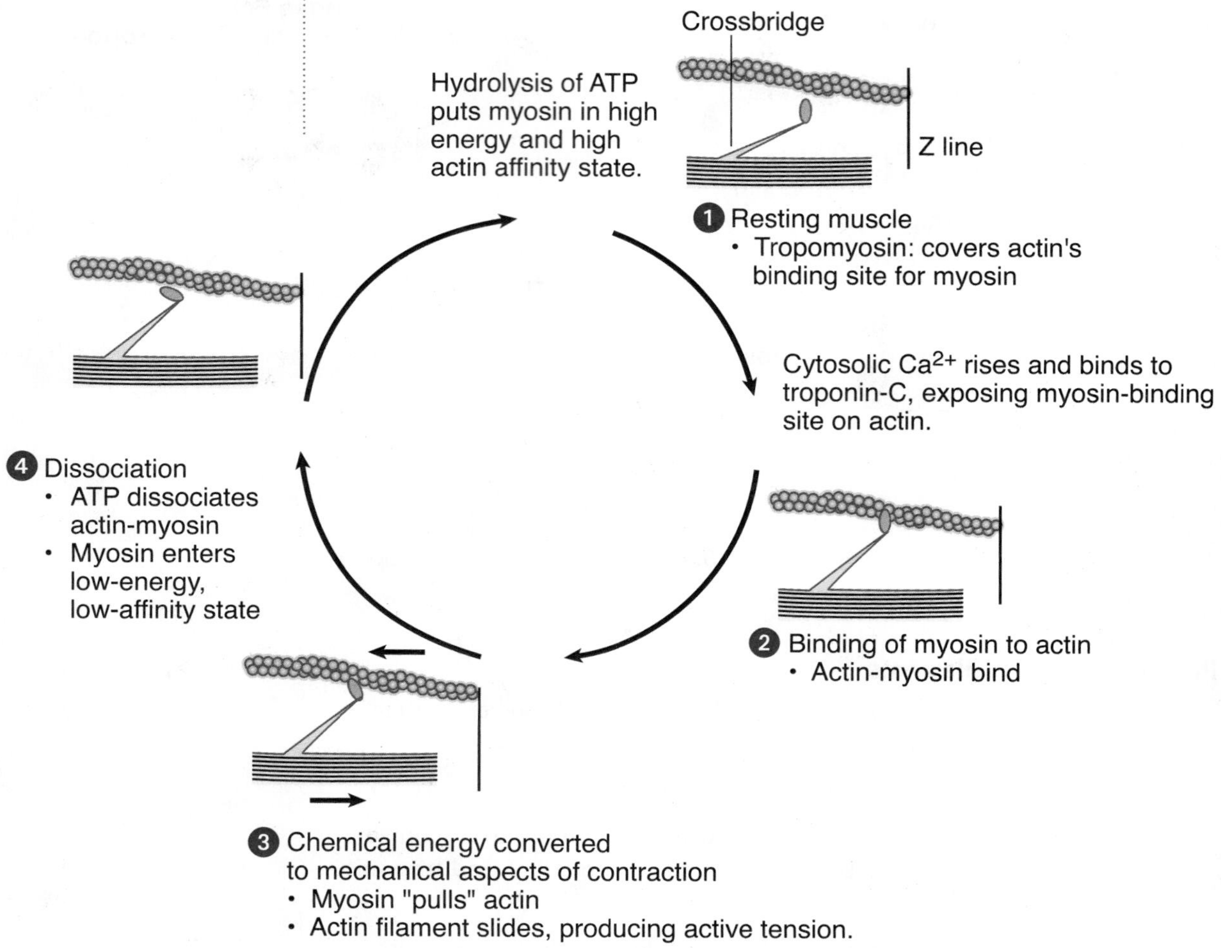

Figure III-1-4. Crossbridge Cycling During Contraction

- Cross-bridge cycling starts when free calcium is available and attaches to troponin, which in turn moves tropomyosin so that myosin binds to actin.
- Contraction is the continuous cycling of cross-bridges.
- ATP is not required to form the cross-bridge linking to actin but is required to break the link with actin.

- Cross-bridge cycling (contraction) continues until either of the following occurs:
  - Withdrawal of Ca^{2+}: cycling stops at position 1 (normal resting muscle)
  - ATP is depleted: cycling stops at position 3 (rigor mortis; this would not occur under physiologic conditions)

REGULATION OF CYTOSOLIC CALCIUM

The sarcoplasmic reticulum (SR) has a high concentration of Ca^{2+}. Thus, there is a strong electrochemical gradient for Ca^{2+} to diffuse from the SR into the cytosol. There are 2 key receptors involved in the flux of Ca^{2+} from the SR into the cytosol: dihydropyridine (DHP) and ryanodine (RyR).

Dihydropyridine (DHP)

- DHP is a voltage-gated Ca^{2+} channel located in the sarcolemmal membrane
- Although it is a voltage-gated Ca^{2+} channel, Ca^{2+} **does not** flux through this receptor in skeletal muscle. Rather, DHP functions as a voltage-sensor.
- When skeletal muscle is at rest, DHP blocks RyR (Figure III-1-5a).

Ryanodine Receptor (RyR)

- RyR is a calcium channel on the SR membrane.
- When the muscle is in the resting state, RyR is blocked by DHP (Fig III-1-5a). Thus, Ca^{2+} is prevented from diffusing into the cytosol.

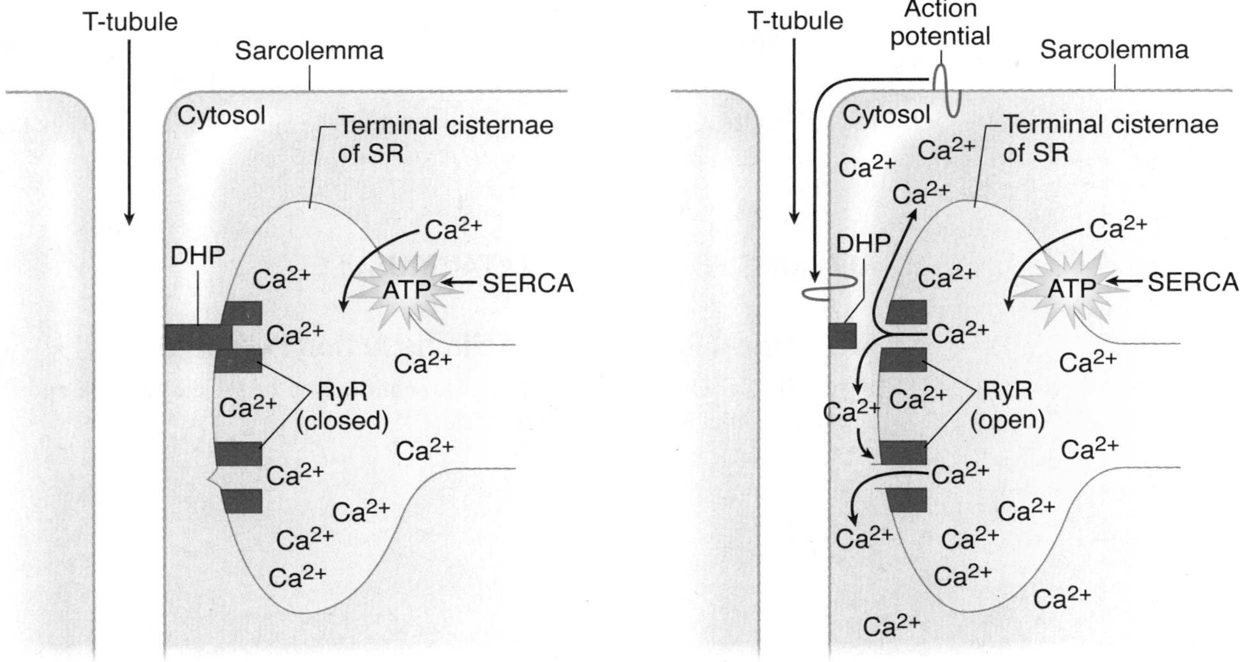

Figure III-1-5. Regulation of Ca^{2+} Release by Sarcoplasmic Reticulum

Sequence

1. Skeletal muscle action potential is initiated at the neuromuscular junction (see section II, chapter 2).
2. The action potential travels down the T-tubule.
3. The voltage change causes a conformation shift in DHP (voltage sensor), removing its block of RyR (Figure III-1-5b).
4. Removal of the DHP block allows Ca^{2+} to diffuse into the cytosol (follows its concentration gradient).
5. The rise in cytosolic Ca^{2+} opens more RyR channels (calcium-induced calcium release).
6. Ca^{2+} binds to troponin-C, which in turn initiates cross-bridge cycle, creating active tension.
7. Ca^{2+} is pumped back into the SR by a calcium ATPase on the SR membrane called sarcoplasmic endoplasmic reticulum calcium ATPase (SERCA).
8. The fall in cytosolic Ca^{2+} causes tropomyosin to once again cover actin's binding site for myosin and the muscle relaxes, provided of course ATP is available to dissociate actin and myosin.

Key Points

- Contraction-relaxation states are determined by cytosolic levels of Ca^{2+}.
- The source of the calcium that binds to the troponin-C in skeletal muscle is solely from the cell's sarcoplasmic reticulum. Thus, no extracellular Ca^{2+} is involved.
- Two ATPases are involved in contraction:
  - **Myosin ATPase** supplies the energy for the mechanical aspects of contraction by putting myosin in a high energy and affinity state.
  - **SERCA** pumps Ca^{2+} back into the SR to terminate the contraction, i.e., causes relaxation.

ALTERING FORCE IN SKELETAL MUSCLE

Mechanical Response to a Single Action Potential

Figure III-1-6 illustrates the mechanical contraction of skeletal muscle and the action potential on the same time scale.

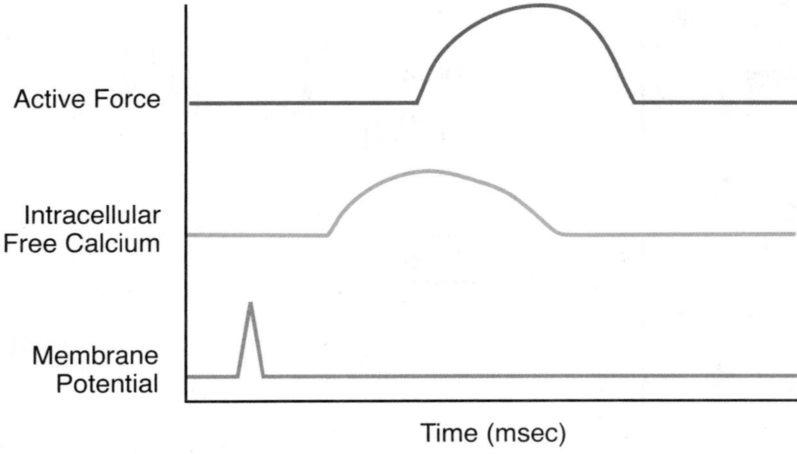

Figure III-1-6. The Time Course of Events During Contraction

- Note the sequence of events: action potential causes Ca^{2+} release.
- Release of Ca^{2+} evokes muscle contraction (twitch).
- Note that the muscle membrane has completely repolarized well before the start of force development.

Summation and Recruitment

Under normal circumstances, enough Ca^{2+} is released by a single muscle action potential to completely saturate all the troponin-C binding sites. This means all available cross-bridges are activated and thus force cannot be enhanced by increasing cytosolic Ca^{2+}. Instead, peak force in skeletal muscle is increased in 2 ways: summation and recruitment.

Summation

- Because the membrane has repolarized well before force development, multiple action potentials can be generated prior to force development.
- Each action potential causes a pulse of Ca^{2+} release.
- Each pulse of Ca^{2+} initiates cross-bridge cycling and because the muscle has not relaxed, the mechanical force adds onto (summates) the force from the previous action potential (Figure III-1-7).
- This summation can continue until the muscle tetanizes in which case there is sufficient free Ca^{2+} so that cross-bridge cycling is continuous.

Recruitment

- A single alpha motor neuron innervates multiple muscle fibers. The alpha motor neuron and all the fibers it innervates is called a motor-unit.
- Recruitment means activating more motor units, which in turn engage more muscle fibers, causing greater force production.

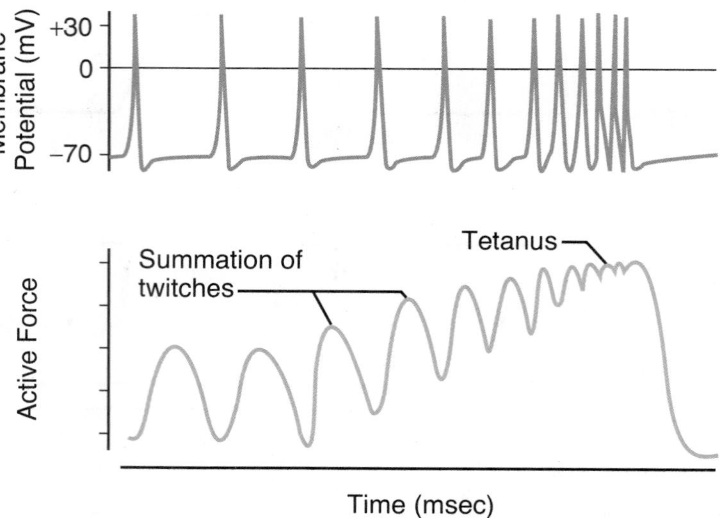

Figure III-1-7. Summation of Individual Twitches and Fusion into Tetanus

COMPARISON OF STRIATED MUSCLES (SKELETAL VS. CARDIAC)

Skeletal and cardiac muscle are both striated muscle and share many similarities. Nevertheless, there are important differences.

Similarities

- Both have the same functional proteins, i.e., actin, tropomyosin, troponin, myosin, and titin.
- A rise in cytosolic Ca^{2+} initiates cross-bridge cycling thereby producing active tension.
- ATP plays the same role.
- Both have SERCA.
- Both have RyR receptors on the SR and thus show calcium-induced calcium release.

Bridge to Pathology

Dysfunction in the titin protein has been associated with dilated and restrictive cardiomyopathies (see next section).

Differences

- Extracellular Ca^{2+} is involved in cardiac contractions, but not skeletal muscle. This extracellular Ca^{2+} causes calcium-induced calcium release in cardiac cells.
- Magnitude of SR Ca^{2+} release can be altered in cardiac (see section on cardiac mechanics), but not skeletal muscle.
- Cardiac cells are electrically coupled by gap junctions, which do not exist in skeletal muscle.
- Cardiac myocytes remove cytosolic Ca^{2+} by 2 mechanisms: SERCA and a Na^+—Ca^{2+} exchanger (3 Na^+ in, 1 Ca^{2+} out) on the sarcolemmal membrane. Skeletal muscle only utilizes SERCA.

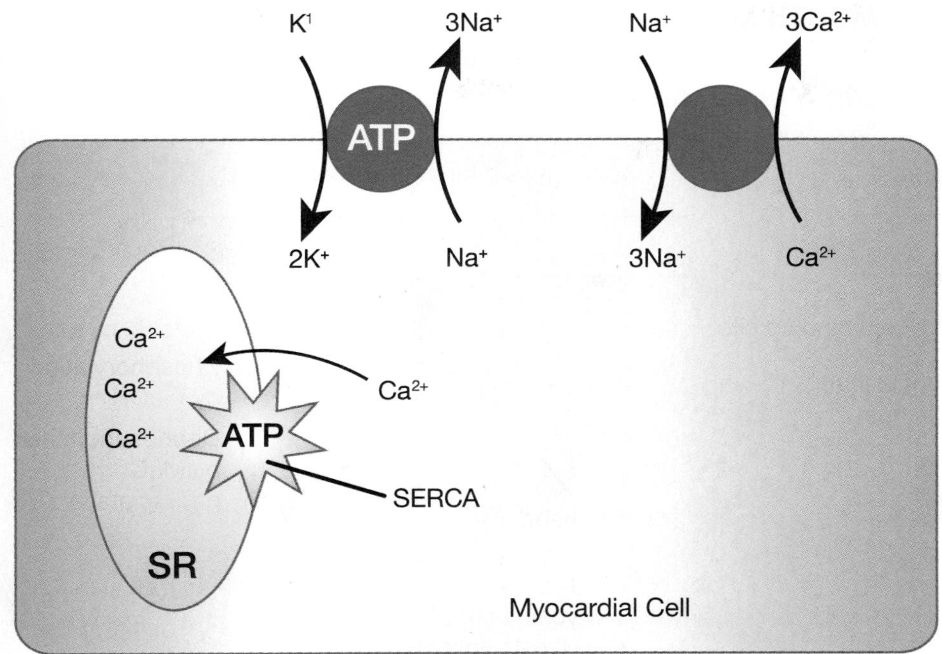

Figure III-1-8. Removal of Cytosolic Calcium in Myocardial Cells

- Cardiac cells have a prolonged action potential (Figure III-1-8). This figure illustrates that the twitch tension is already falling (muscle starting to relax) while the action potential is still in the absolute refractory period. Thus, a second action potential cannot be evoked before the mechanical event is almost completed. This approximately equal mechanical and electrical event prevents summation of the force and if the muscle can't summate, it can't tetanize.

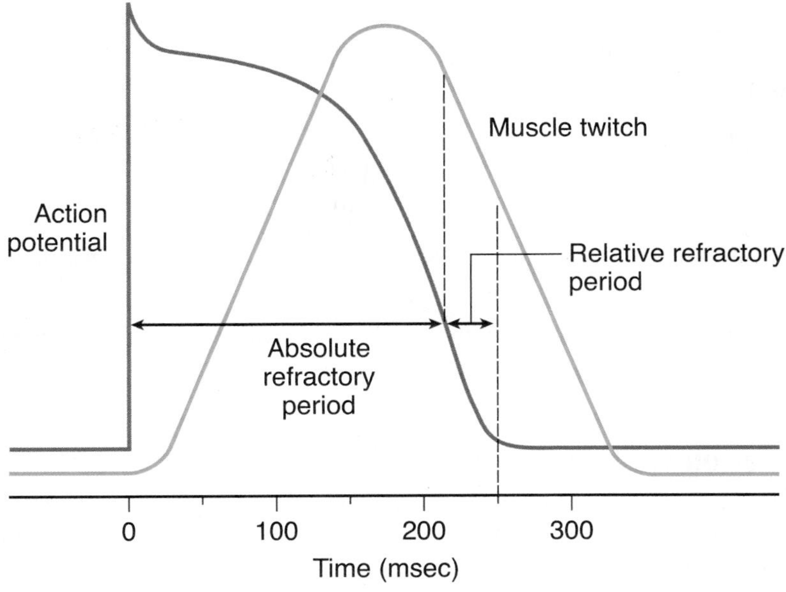

Figure III-1-9. Force and Refractory Periods

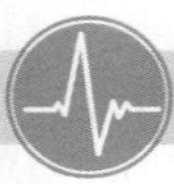

SMOOTH MUSCLE

Actin-Myosin Interaction

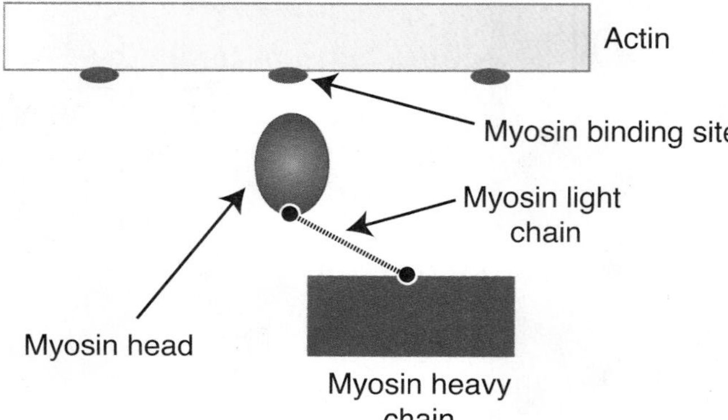

Figure III-1-10a. Relaxed Smooth Muscle

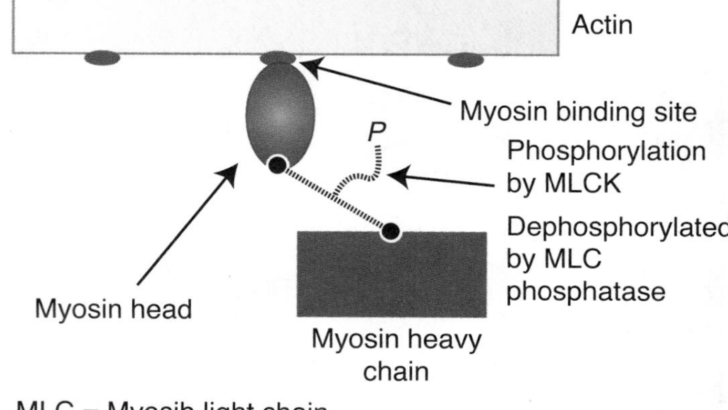

Figure III-1-10b. Contracted Smooth Muscle

- In contrast to striated muscle, smooth muscle lacks tropomyosin, troponin, and titin.
- Similar to striated muscle, the binding of actin and myosin produces tension.
- Phosphorylation of myosin light-chain (MLC) puts myosin in a high-affinity state for actin, causing binding and the production of tension. (Similar to striated muscle, energy comes from the presence of ATPase in the myosin head.)
- In the resting state, MLC is not phosphorylated and has very low affinity for actin. Thus they do not interact and smooth muscle is relaxed (Figure III-1-10a).
- On the other hand, phosphorylation of MLC puts myosin in a high-affinity state for actin, resulting in the binding of actin and myosin to produce a power stroke (Figure III-1-10b).
- MLC is phosphorylated by myosin light-chain kinase (MLCK) and dephosphorylated by MLC phosphatase.
- Similar to striated muscle, the trigger for contraction is increasing cytosolic calcium, which activates MLCK.

Regulation of Smooth Muscle

- Voltage-gated calcium channels (L-type) reside in the sarcolemma of smooth muscle. Depolarization opens these channels, resulting in calcium influx into the cytosol. This calcium triggers calcium release from the SR (calcium-induced calcium release, similar to cardiac muscle).
- Increasing IP3 also evokes calcium efflux from the SR. IP3 is increased by an agonist binding a Gq coupled receptor (e.g., the alpha-1 receptor).

- This cytosolic calcium binds to the protein calmodulin (CAM). This calcium-calmodulin complex activates MLCK, which in turn phosphorylates MLC.
- As indicated above, phosphorylation of MLC causes binding of actin and myosin, in turn eliciting a contraction of smooth muscle.
- Although not illustrated in Figure III-1-11, similar to striated muscle (see above), ATP dissociates actin and myosin. If MLC remains phosphorylated, then actin and myosin rebind to produce tension (similar to cross-bridge cycling described above for striated muscle).
- MLC phosphatase dephosphorylates myosin, reducing the affinity of myosin for actin, causing relaxation.
- When cytosolic calcium is high, MLCK dominates. When cytosolic calcium is low, MLC phosphatase dominates.
- Smooth muscle reduces cytosolic calcium via the same mechanisms described above for cardiac cells (Figure III-1-8).

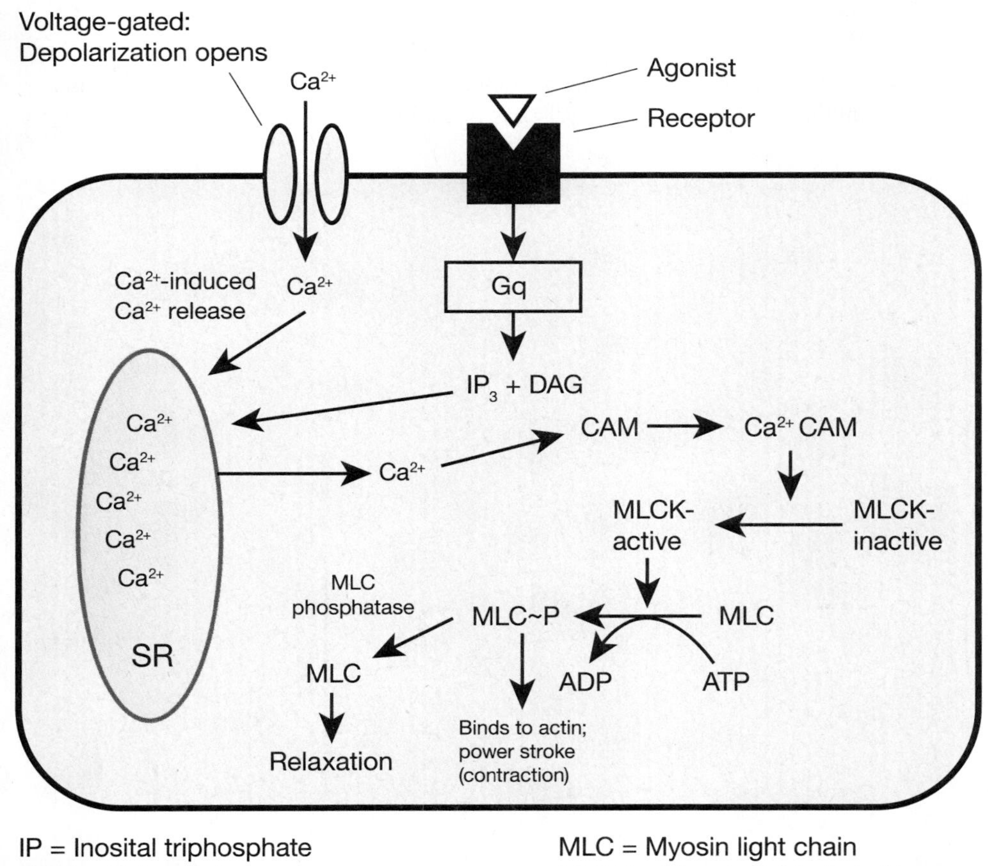

Figure III-1-11. Smooth Muscle Cell

Chapter Summary

- Actin is the structural protein of the thin filaments. The regulatory proteins are tropomyosin and troponin, the latter binding calcium. These proteins determine the availability of myosin binding sites on the thin filaments.
- In resting skeletal muscle, DHP prevents SR Ca^{2+} release by blocking RyR, which is a Ca^{2+} channel on the SR membrane. An action potential removes this block of RyR, allowing Ca^{2+} to flow into the cytosol, which in turn, initiates contraction and the development of active force.
- All Ca^{2+} for skeletal muscle contraction comes from the SR, while the rise in cytosolic Ca^{2+} comes from both the extracellular space and the SR in cardiac muscle.
- The hydrolysis of ATP by the myosin ATPase provides the energy for the mechanical aspects of contraction. ATP also serves to dissociate actin and myosin.
- Sustained saturation of the skeletal muscle cell with free calcium causes tetanus, which is simply the continuous cycling of all available cross-bridges. Cardiac muscle cannot be tetanized due to the long duration of its absolute refractory period.
- Smooth muscle contracts as a result of actin and myosin binding, but what initiates this cross-bridge cycling is phosphorylation of MLC.

Skeletal Muscle Mechanics 2

Learning Objectives

- ❑ Use knowledge of overview of muscle mechanics
- ❑ Interpret scenarios on length-tension curves
- ❑ Use knowledge of relationship between velocity and load
- ❑ Demonstrate understanding of properties of white vs. red muscle
- ❑ Solve problems concerning comparison of muscle types

OVERVIEW OF MUSCLE MECHANICS

Preload

Preload is the load on a muscle in a relaxed state, i.e., before it contracts. Applying preload to muscle does 2 things:

- Stretches the muscle: This in turn, stretches the sarcomere. **The greater the preload, the greater the stretch of the sarcomere.**
- Generates passive tension in the muscle: Muscle is elastic (see titin, previous chapter) and thus "resists" the stretch applied to it. Think of the "snap-back" that occurs when one stretches a rubber band. The force of this resistance is measured as passive tension. **The greater the preload, the greater the passive tension in the muscle.**

Afterload

Afterload is the load the muscle works against. If one wants to lift a 10 Kg weight, then this weight represents the afterload. Using the 10 kg weight example, 2 possibilities exist:

- If the muscle generates more than 10 kg of force, then the weight moves as the muscle shortens. This is an **isotonic contraction**.
- If the muscle is unable to generate more than 10 kg of force, then the muscle won't shorten. This is an **isometric contraction**.
- Types of tension
  - Passive: Produced by the preload
  - Active: Produced by cross-bridge cycling (described in previous chapter)
  - Total: The sum of active and passive tension

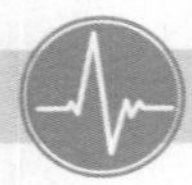

LENGTH–TENSION CURVES

Length–tension curves are important for understanding both skeletal and cardiac muscle function. The graphs that follow are all generated from skeletal muscle in vitro, but the information can be applied to both skeletal muscle and heart muscle in vivo.

Passive Tension Curve

The green line in Figure III-2-1 shows that muscle behaves like a rubber band. The elastic properties of the muscle resist this stretch and the resulting tension is recorded. There is a direct (non-linear) relationship between the degree of stretch and the passive tension created that resists this stretch.

Point A: No preload, thus no stretch and no passive tension

Point B: Preload of 1 g stretches muscle, thus increasing its resting length, resulting in ~1 g of passive tension

Point C: Preload of 5 g increases muscle stretch, producing a greater resting length and thus a greater passive tension.

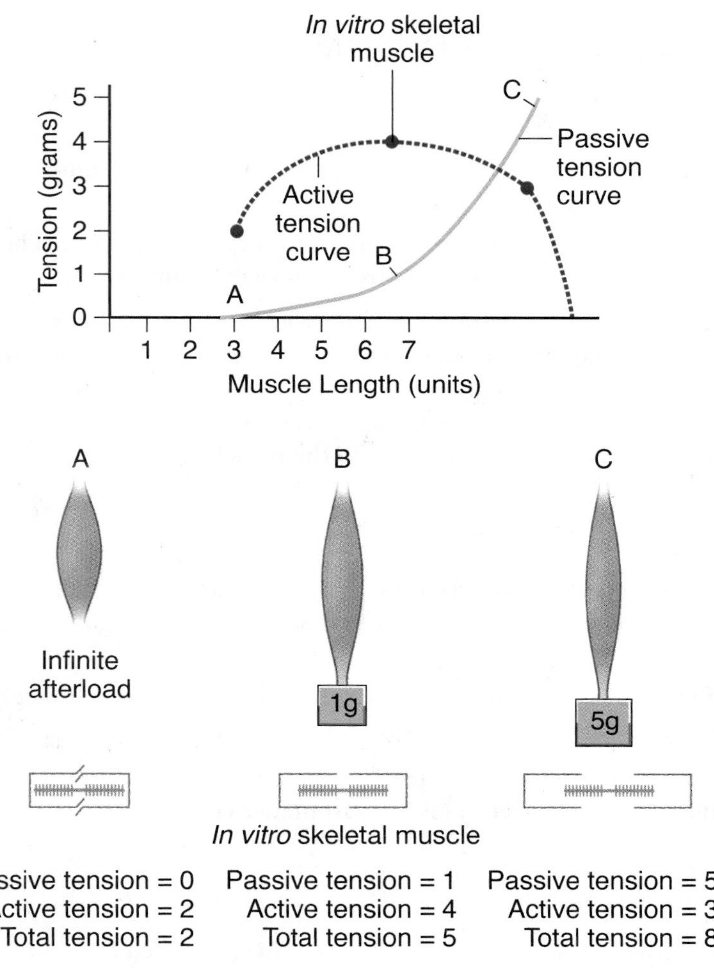

Figure III-2-1. Preload, Active and Passive Tension: The Length–Tension Relationship

Active Tension

The purple line in Figure III-2-1 shows the tension developed by stimulating the muscle to contract at the different preloads. In this example, the contraction is a **maximal isometric contraction**, i.e., the contraction produces tension, but the afterload is much greater than the tension the muscle develops and thus the muscle doesn't shorten. Recall that active tension represents the force generated by cross-bridge cycling. It is important to note the shape (bell-shaped) of the active tension curve.

- Preload of A: When there is no preload, the evoked muscle contraction develops ~2 g of active tension.
- Preload of B: At this preload, the active tension produced by stimulation of the muscle is greater, ~4 g.
- Preload of C: This preload results in less active tension than the previous preload. Thus, active tension increases as the muscle is stretched, up to a point. If stretched beyond this point, then active tension begins to fall.
- Optimal length (L_0): L_0 represents the muscle length (preload) that produces the greatest active tension. In Figure III-2-1, this occurs at the preload designated by B.

Explanation of Bell-shaped Active Tension Curve

Figure III-2-1 shows a simplified picture of a sarcomere. Actin is the thin brown line, while myosin is depicted in purple. The magnitude of active tension depends on the number of actin-myosin cross-bridges that can form (directly related).

- Preload A: actin filaments overlap
  - Thus, the force that can be exerted by myosin tugging the actin is compromised and the active tension is less.
- Preload B (L_0): all myosin heads can bind to actin, and there is separation of actin filaments
  - Thus, active tension generated is greatest here because there is optimal overlap of actin and myosin.
- Preload C: the stretch is so great that actin has been pulled away from some of the myosin filament, and thus fewer actin-myosin interactions are available, resulting in diminished active tension.
  - If taken to the extreme, greater stretch could pull actin such that no actin-myosin interactions can occur, and thus no active tension results (active tension curve intersects the X-axis). This is an experimental, rather than physiologic phenomenon.
- Total tension: sum of passive and active tension (bottom of Figure III-2-1)

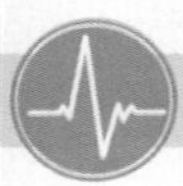

RELATIONSHIP BETWEEN VELOCITY AND LOAD

Figure III-2-2 shows that the maximum velocity of shortening (Vmax) occurs when there is no afterload on the muscle. Increasing afterload decreases velocity, and when afterload exceeds the maximum force generated by the muscle, shortening does not occur (isometric contraction).

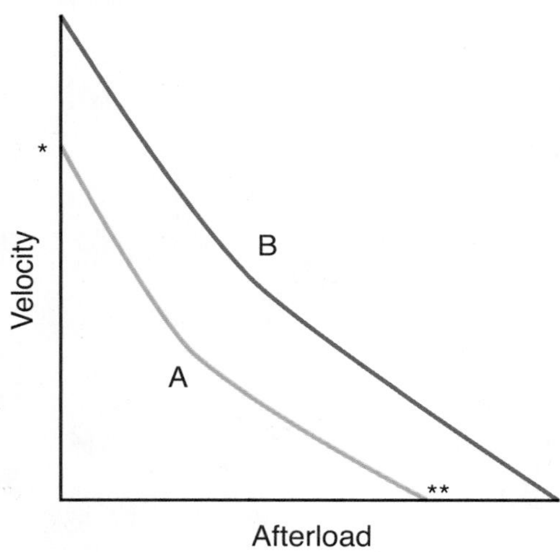

Figure III-2-2. Force–Velocity Curve

In Figure III-2-2:

*Maximum velocity (Vmax) is determined by the muscle's ATPase activity. It is the ATPase activity that determines a fast versus a slow muscle.

**Maximum force generated by a muscle. This occurs when summation is maximal (complete summation) and all motor units for the given muscle are fully recruited. The absolute amount of force is directly related to muscle mass and preload, with the greatest force occurring when the preload is at L_o.

Muscle A: a smaller, slower muscle (red muscle)

Muscle B: a larger, faster muscle (white muscle)

As load increases, the distance shortened during a single contraction decreases. So, with increased afterload, both the velocity of contraction and the distance decrease.

PROPERTIES OF WHITE VS. RED MUSCLE

White Muscle

Generally, this is the large (powerful) muscle that is utilized short-term, e.g., ocular muscles, leg muscles of a sprinter. Major characteristics are as follows:

- Large mass per motor unit
- High ATPase activity (fast muscle)
- High capacity for anaerobic glycolysis
- Low myoglobin

Red Muscle

Generally, this is the smaller (less powerful) muscle utilized long-term (endurance muscle), e.g., postural muscle. Major characteristics are as follows:

- Small mass per motor unit
- Lower ATPase activity (slower muscle)
- High capacity for aerobic metabolism (mitochondria)
- High myoglobin (imparts red color)

Chapter Summary

- Preload generates passive muscle tension and stretches the sarcomere.
- The degree of sarcomere stretch determines the maximum number of cycling cross-bridges that can result, and thus, the maximum active tension.
- In vivo, the preload of skeletal muscle is set by joint angles. When appropriately positioned to lift a load, the muscle is at L_o.
- White muscle is generally large and fast (high ATPase), whereas red muscle is smaller and slower (low ATPase).

SECTION IV

Cardiac Muscle Mechanics

Cardiac Muscle Mechanics 1

Learning Objectives

- ❑ Answer questions about systolic performance of the ventricle
- ❑ Explain information related to ventricular function curves
- ❑ Solve problems concerning chronic changes: systolic and diastolic dysfunction

SYSTOLIC PERFORMANCE OF THE VENTRICLE

Systolic performance actually means the overall force generated by the ventricular muscle during systole. The heart does 2 things in systole: pressurizes and ejects blood. An important factor influencing this systolic performance is the number of cross-bridges cycling during contraction.

The greater the number of cross-bridges cycling, the greater the force of contraction.

Systolic performance is determined by 3 independent variables:

- Preload
- Contractility
- Afterload

These 3 factors are summed together to determine the overall systolic performance of the ventricle. Recent work has demonstrated that they are not completely independent, but the generalizations made here will apply to the physiologic and clinical setting.

Preload

As in skeletal muscle, preload is the load on the muscle in the relaxed state.

More specifically, it is the load or prestretch on ventricular muscle at the end of diastole.

Preload on ventricular muscle is not measured directly; rather, indices are utilized.

The best indices of preload on ventricular muscle are those measured directly in the ventricles. Indices of left ventricular preload:

- Left ventricular end-diastolic volume (LVEDV)
- Left ventricular end-diastolic pressure (LVEDP)

Possibly somewhat less reliable indices of left ventricular preload are those measured in the venous system.

- Central venous pressure (CVP)
- Pulmonary capillary wedge pressure (PCWP)
- Right atrial pressure (RAP)

Pulmonary wedge pressure, sometimes called pulmonary capillary wedge pressure, is measured from the tip of a Swan-Ganz catheter, which, after passing through the right heart, has been wedged in a small pulmonary artery. The tip is pointing downstream toward the pulmonary capillaries, and the pressure measured at the tip is probably very close to pulmonary capillary pressure. Since the vessel is occluded and assuming minimal flow, the pressure is probably also very close to left atrial pressure as well. A rise in pulmonary capillary wedge pressure is evidence of an increase in preload on the left ventricle. In some cases, such as in mitral stenosis, it is not a good index of left ventricular preload.

Along similar lines, measurement of systemic central venous pressure is used as an index of preload.

Preload factor in systolic performance (Frank-Starling mechanism)

The preload effect can be explained on the basis of a change in sarcomere length. This is illustrated in Figure IV-1-1.

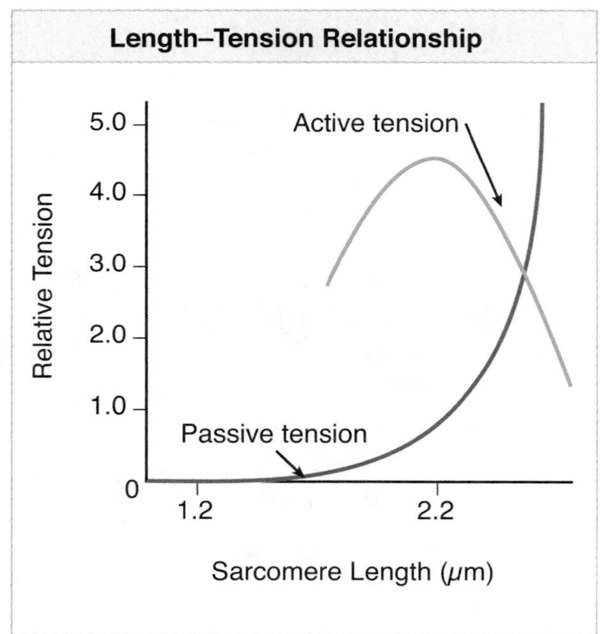

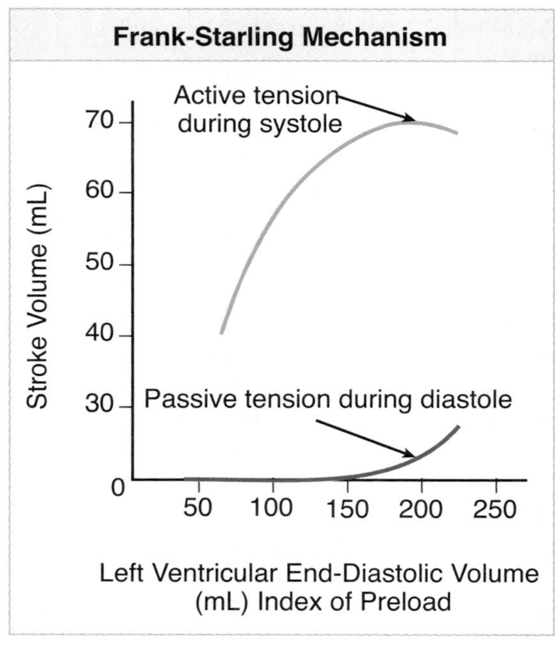

Figure IV-1-1. Length–Tension Relationships in Skeletal and Cardiac Muscle

The resting length of skeletal muscle *in vivo* is at a sarcomere length close to the optimum for maximal cross-bridge linking between actin and myosin during contraction (L_o).

Heart muscle at the end of diastole is below this point. Thus, in a normal heart, increased preload increases sarcomere length toward the optimum actin-myosin overlap. This results in more cross-linking and a more forceful contraction during systole.

Contractility (Inotropic State)

An acceptable definition of *contractility* would be a change in performance at a given preload and afterload. Thus, contractility is a change in the force of contraction at any given sarcomere length.

- Acute changes in contractility are due to changes in the intracellular dynamics of calcium.
- Drugs that increase contractility usually provide more calcium and at a faster rate to the contractile machinery.
- More calcium increases the availability of cross-link sites on the actin, increasing cross-linking and the force of contraction during systole.
- Calcium dynamics do not explain chronic losses in contractility, which in most cases are due to overall myocyte dysfunction.

Indices of contractility

Increased *dp/dt* (change in pressure vs. change in time) = rate of pressure development during isovolumetric contraction. Contractility affects the rate at which the ventricular muscle develops active tension, which is expressed as pressure in the ventricle during isovolumetric contraction.

Increased ejection fraction (stroke volume/end-diastolic volume). Ejection fraction can now be estimated fairly easily by a noninvasive technique and is currently a common clinical index of contractility. There is no ideal index of contractility. Ejection fraction is influenced by afterload, but in most cases an increase in contractility is accompanied by an increase in ejection fraction. Note that ejection fraction simply indicates the percentage of blood ejected from the ventricle; it does not by itself give information about preload or stroke volume.

When contractility increases, there are changes in addition to an increased force of contraction. This is illustrated in Figure IV-1-2. The solid line represents left ventricular pressure before (and the dashed line after) an increase in contractility via increased sympathetic stimulation. The numbers refer to the descriptions after the figure.

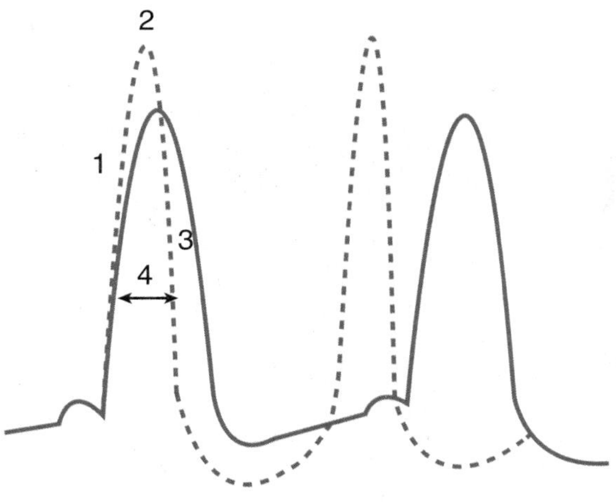

Figure IV-1-2. Effects of Increased Contractility

The overall changes induced by increased contractility can be summarized as follows:

1. Increased *dp/dt*: increased slope, thus increased rate of pressure development
2. Increased peak left ventricular pressure due to a more forceful contraction
3. Increased rate of relaxation due to increased rate of calcium sequestration
4. Decreased systolic interval due to effects #1 and #3

Both an increased preload and an increased contractility are accompanied by an increased peak left ventricular pressure, but only with an increase in contractility is there a decrease in the systolic interval.

Whereas contractility affects systolic interval, heart rate determines diastolic interval.Thus, increased sympathetic activity to the heart produces the following:

- Systolic interval decreased: contractility effect
- Diastolic interval decreased: heart rate effect

A high heart rate (pacemaker-induced) produces a small increase in contractility (Bowditch effect). Because Ca^{2+} enters the cell more rapidly than it is sequestered by the sarcoplasmic reticulum, intracellular Ca^{2+} increases. The increased contractility helps compensate for the reduced filling time associated with high heart rates.

Afterload

Afterload is defined as the "load" that the heart must eject blood against. Exactly what constitutes afterload to the heart is the subject of much debate. Probably, the best "marker" of afterload is systemic vascular resistance (SVR), also called total peripheral resistance (TPR). However, TPR is not routinely calculated clinically and thus arterial pressure (diastolic, mean, or systolic) is often used as the index of afterload.

Afterload is increased in 3 main situations:

1. When aortic pressure is increased (elevated mean arterial pressure); for example, when hypertension increases the afterload, the left ventricle has to work harder to overcome the elevated arterial pressures.
2. When systemic vascular resistance is increased, resulting in increased resistance and decreased compliance
3. In aortic stenosis, resulting in pressure overload of the left ventricle

In general, when afterload increases, there an initial fall in stroke volume.

VENTRICULAR FUNCTION CURVES

Ventricular function curves are an excellent graphical depiction of the effects of preload versus contractility and afterload (Figure IV-1-3).

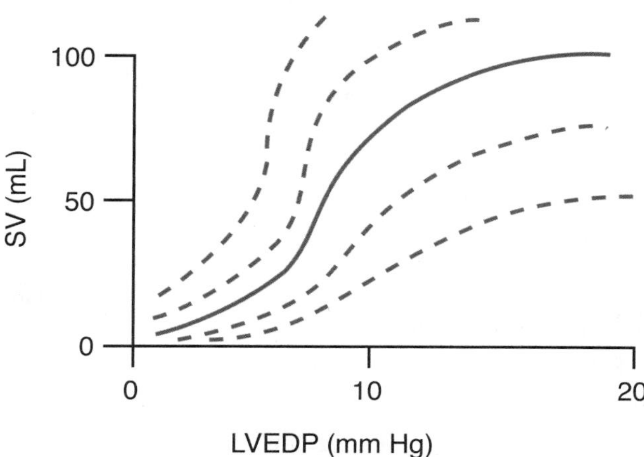

Figure IV-1-3. Family of Frank-Starling Curves

Changes in afterload and contractility shift the curve up or down, left or right.

There is no single Frank-Starling curve on which the ventricle operates. There is actually a family of curves, each of which is defined by the afterload and the inotropic state of the heart:

- Increasing afterload and decreasing contractility shift the curve down and to the right.
- Decreasing afterload and increasing contractility shift the curve up and to the left.

Application of Ventricular Function Curves

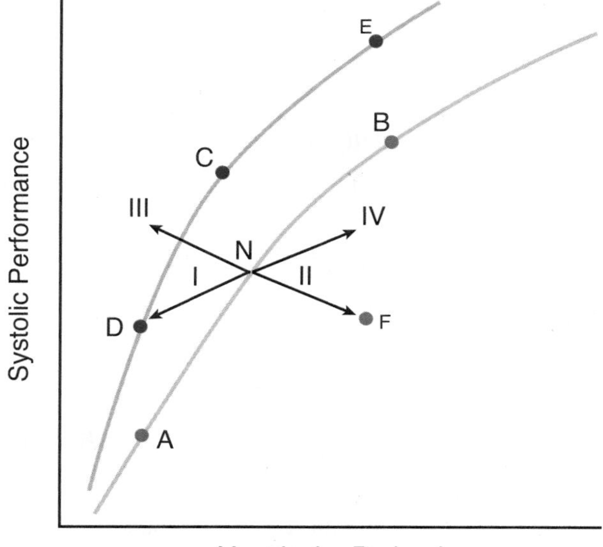

Figure IV-1-4. Ventricular Function Vectors

y axis: index of systolic performance, e.g., stroke work, stroke volume, cardiac output; all are indices of the force of ventricular contraction

x axis: index of ventricular preload, e.g., ventricular end-diastolic volume or pressure, RAP, or CVP

A ventricular function curve is the rise in ventricular performance as preload increases (Frank-Starling curve). Thus:

- All points on a ventricular function curve have the same contractility.
- All curves have an ascending limb, a peak point, and possibly a descending limb.
- The pericardium normally prevents the large increases in preload necessary to reach the peak of a cardiac function curve.

Starting at N, which represents a normal, resting individual:

- A = decreased performance due to a reduction in preload
- B = increased performance due to an increased preload

Starting at N, point C represents an increased performance due to an increase in contractility or a reduction in afterload.

- Any point above a ventricular function curve means increased contractility, or an acute decrease in afterload.
- Any point below a ventricular function curve means decreased contractility, or an acute increase in afterload..

Points C, D, and E represent different levels of performance due to changes in preload only (Frank-Starling mechanism); all 3 points have the same contractility.

Vector I: consequences of a loss in preload, e.g., hemorrhage, venodilators (nitroglycerin)

- Performance decreases because of a loss in preload.
- The loss of venous return and preload reduces cardiac output and blood pressure, and via the carotid sinus, reflex sympathetic stimulation to the heart increases.
- The increased contractility partially compensates for the loss of preload.
- When there is a loss of either preload or contractility that compromises performance, the other factor usually increases to return performance toward normal. However, the compensatory mechanism is usually incomplete.

Vector II: consequences of a loss in contractility, e.g., congestive heart failure

- Performance decreases because of a loss in contractility.
- A decrease in contractility decreases ejection fraction, which increases preload.
- The increased preload partially compensates for the loss of contractility.
- An acute increase in afterload, e.g., peripheral vasoconstriction, produces the same change.

Vector III: consequences of an acute increase in contractility

- Performance increases.
- The increased contractility increases ejection fraction.
- The increased ejection fraction decreases preload.
- An acute decrease in afterload, e.g., peripheral vasodilation, produces the same shift in the curve.

Vector IV: consequences of an acute increase in preload, e.g., volume loading in the individual going from the upright to the supine position.

- Increased venous return increases preload, which increases performance and cardiac output.

- Increasing cardiac output raises blood pressure, and via the carotid sinus reflex, sympathetic stimulation to the heart decreases.
- The decreased sympathetic stimulation reduces contractility.

All of the preceding sequences assume no dramatic change in heart rate, which could reduce or eliminate some of the expected changes. Whenever there is a change in sympathetic stimulation to the heart, there is a change in both contractility and heart rate.

Ventricular Volumes

End-diastolic volume (EDV): volume of blood in the ventricle at the end of diastole

End-systolic volume (ESV): volume of blood in the ventricle at the end of systole

Stroke volume (SV): volume of blood ejected by the ventricle per beat

$$SV = EDV - ESV$$

Ejection Fraction (EF): EF = SV/EDV
(should be greater than 55% in a normal heart)

CHRONIC CHANGES: SYSTOLIC AND DIASTOLIC DYSFUNCTION

Systolic dysfunction can be defined as an abnormal reduction in ventricular emptying due to impaired contractility or excessive afterload.

Diastolic dysfunction is a decrease in ventricular compliance during the filling phase of the cardiac cycle due to either changes in tissue stiffness or impaired ventricular relaxation. The consequence is a diminished Frank-Starling mechanism.

Pressure Overload

- Examples of a pressure overload on the left ventricle include hypertension and aortic stenosis.
- Initially, there is no decrease in cardiac output or an increase in preload since the cardiac function curve shifts to the left (increased performance due to increased contractility).
- Chronically, in an attempt to normalize wall tension (actually internal wall stress), the ventricle develops a concentric hypertrophy. There is a dramatic increase in wall thickness and a decrease in chamber diameter.
- The consequence of concentric hypertrophy (new sarcomes laid down in parallel, i.e., the myofibril thickens) is a decrease in ventricular compliance and diastolic dysfunction, followed eventually by a systolic dysfunction and ventricular failure.

Volume Overload

- Examples of a volume overload on the left ventricle include mitral and aortic insufficiency and patent ductus arteriosus.
- Fairly well tolerated if developed slowly. A large acute volume overload less well tolerated and can precipitate heart failure.
- Due to the LaPlace relationship, a dilated left ventricle must develop a greater wall tension to produce the same ventricular pressures.

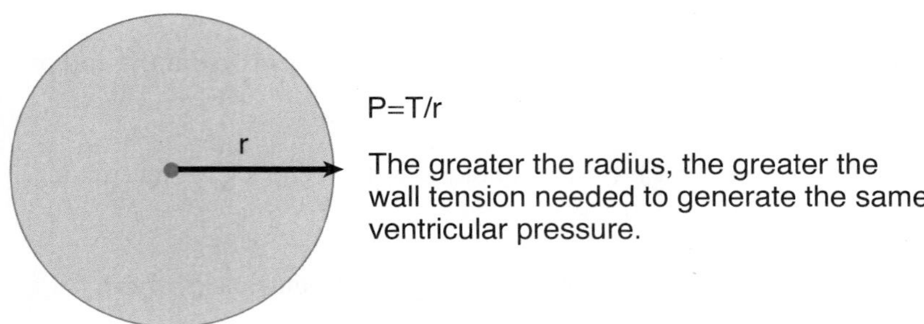

r
P=T/r
The greater the radius, the greater the wall tension needed to generate the same ventricular pressure.

Figure IV-1-5

- Chronically, in an attempt to normalize wall tension (actually external wall stress), the ventricle develops an eccentric hypertrophy (new sarcomeres laid down end-to-end, i.e., the myofibril lengthens). As cardiac volumes increase, there is a modest increase in wall thickness that does not reduce chamber size.
- Compliance of the ventricle is not compromised and diastolic function is maintained.
- Eventual failure is usually a consequence of systolic dysfunction.

Cardiomyopathy

- Cardiac failure or more specifically congestive failure is a syndrome with many etiologies.
- Cardiomyopathy is a failure of the myocardium where the underlying cause originates within the myocyte.
- Excluded would be valvular heart disease, afterload problems, and coronary heart disease.
- There are 3 basic types of cardiomyopathy:
  - Dilated cardiomyopathy
  - Restrictive cardiomyopathy
  - Hypertrophic cardiomyopathy

Dilated cardiomyopathy

- Ventricular dilation with only a modest hypertrophy that is less than appropriate for the degree of dilation
- It can occur for the left heart, right heart, or can include both.
- Diastolic function remains intact and helps compensate for the chamber dilation.

- Compensation also includes increased sympathetic stimulation to the myocardium.
- Systolic dysfunction despite compensations via Frank-Starling and increased contractility
- Further dilation over time and mitral and tricuspid failure enhance systolic dysfunction with eventual complete failure.

Restrictive cardiomyopathy

- Decreased ventricular compliance with diastolic dysfunction and a decrease in ventricular cavity size
- Increased filling pressures lead to left- and right-sided congestion.
- Ventricular hypertrophy may or may not be present.
- Systolic maintained close to normal

Hypertrophic cardiomyopathy

- Septal or left ventricular hypertrophy is unrelated to a pressure overload.
- Diastolic dysfunction due to increased muscle stiffness and impaired relaxation
- Is a subtype of hypertrophic cardiomyopathy, often resulting in a restriction of the ventricular outflow tract (idiopathic hypertrophic subaortic stenosis) and pulmonary congestion. Currently this is referred to clinically as hypertrophic obstructive cardiomyopathy (HOCM).
- Hypertrophy may be related to septal fiber disarray.

Chapter Summary

- Ventricular performance is determined by the amount of preload, the level of contractility, and afterload.
- Acutely, the preload effect determines sarcomere length, and the contractility effect by the availability of calcium.
- The best indices of preload are ventricular end-diastolic volume and pressure, and indices of contractility include the rate of pressure development during isovolumetric contraction, systolic interval, and ejection fraction. The ejection fraction (SV/EDV) in normal individuals should usually be greater than 55%.
- Both preload and contractility alter the force of ventricular contraction, but only contractility has a significant effect on systolic interval (decreasing it).
- A loss of preload or contractility produces an increase in the other factor, which functions to minimize the loss in ventricular performance.
- Afterload on the ventricle represents the overall force the ventricular muscle must develop to pump the blood out of the ventricle. A close approximation for the left ventricle is the resistance of the arterioles (TPR).
- Systolic dysfunction is an abnormal reduction in ventricular emptying due to impaired contractility or excessive afterload.
- Diastolic dysfunction is a decrease in muscle compliance and a diminished Frank-Starling mechanism.
- A pressure overloaded ventricle causes a concentric hypertrophy, diastolic dysfunction, and eventually a systolic dysfunction.
- A volume overloaded ventricle causes an eccentric hypertrophy. Diastolic function is usually maintained with failure, which is the result of a systolic dysfunction.
- Cardiomyopathy is a failure of the myocardium where the underlying cause originates within the myocyte.

SECTION V

Peripheral Circulation

General Aspects of the Cardiovascular System

1

Learning Objectives

- ❑ Demonstrate understanding of overview of the cardiovascular system
- ❑ Demonstrate understanding of systemic arterial pressure regulation
- ❑ Demonstrate understanding of hemodynamics
- ❑ Demonstrate understanding of wall tension
- ❑ Use knowledge of vessel compliance
- ❑ Use knowledge of determinants of cardiac output
- ❑ Solve problems concerning the effect of gravity
- ❑ Answer questions about characteristics of systemic arteries

OVERVIEW OF THE CARDIOVASCULAR SYSTEM

Figure V-1-1 illustrates the general organization of the cardiovascular system.

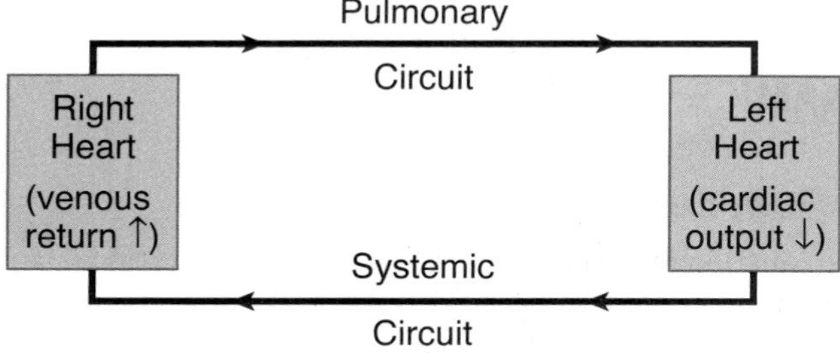

Figure V-1-1. Overview of Circulatory System

The cardiovascular system consists of two pumps (left and right ventricles) and two circuits (pulmonary and systemic) connected in series.

- When circuits are connected in series, flow must be equal in the two circuits.
- Cardiac output is the output of either the left or right ventricle, and because of the series system, they are equal.
- The chemical composition of pulmonary venous blood is very close to the chemical composition of systemic arterial blood
- Systemic mixed venous blood entering the right atrium has the same composition as pulmonary arterial blood.

In a Nutshell

The function of the heart is to transport blood and deliver oxygen in order to maintain adequate tissue perfusion. It also removes waste products, e.g., CO_2 created by tissue metabolism.

Because the heart is a "demand pump" that pumps out whatever blood comes back into it from the venous system, it is effectively the amount of blood returning to the heart that determines how much blood the heart pumps out.

Structure–Function Relationships of the Systemic Circuit

Figure V-1-2 shows that the systemic circuit is a branching circuit. It begins as a large single vessel, the aorta, and branches extensively into progressively smaller vessels until the capillaries are reached. The reverse then takes place in the venous circuit.

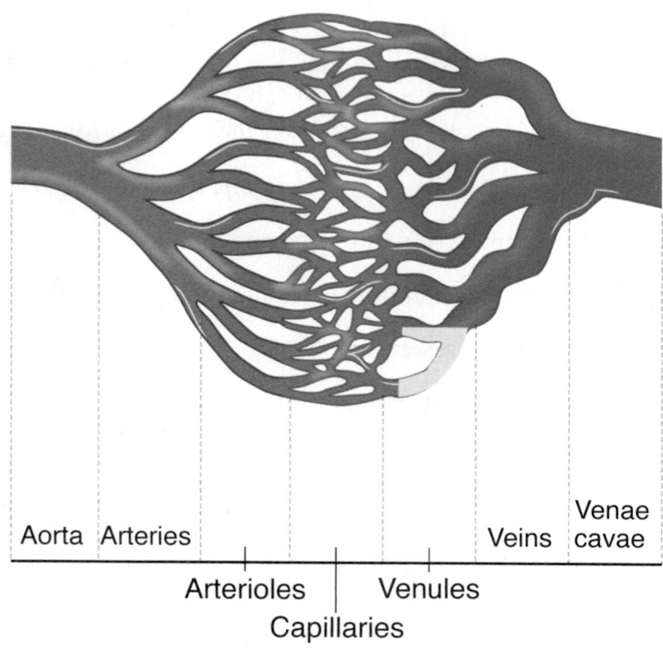

Figure V-1-2. Organization of the Systemic Vessels

HEMODYNAMICS

Pressure, Flow, Resistance

The Poiseuille equation represents the relationship of flow, pressure, and resistance.

$$Q = \frac{P_1 - P_2}{R}$$

Q: flow (mL/min)

P_1: upstream pressure (pressure head) for segment or circuit (mm Hg)

P_2: pressure at the end of the segment or circuit (mm Hg)

R: resistance of vessels between P_1 and P_2 (mm Hg/mL/min)

It can be applied to a single vessel (Figure V-1-3), an organ, or an entire circuit.

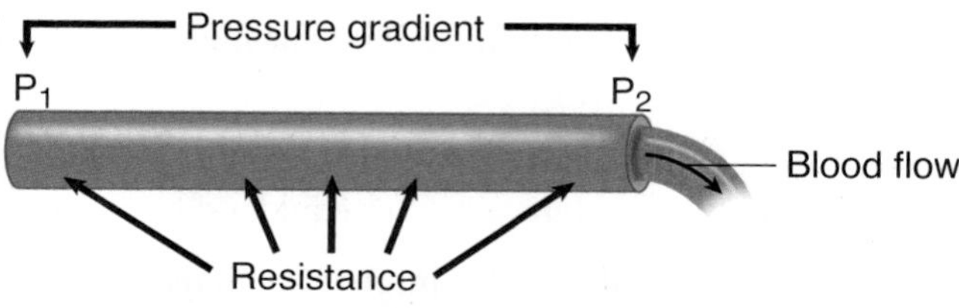

Figure V-1-3. Poiseuille Equation Applied to Single Vessel

The flow to an organ such as the kidney, for example, could be calculated as mean arterial pressure minus renal venous pressure divided by the resistance of all vessels in the renal circuit.

Determinants of resistance

$$\text{Resistance} = \frac{P_1 - P_2}{Q}$$

$$\text{Units of Resistance} = \frac{\text{mm Hg}}{\text{mL/min}} = \frac{\text{pressure}}{\text{volume/time}}$$

The resistance of a vessel is determined by 3 major variables: $R \propto \frac{\nu L}{r^4}$

Vessel radius (r) is the most important factor determining resistance. If resistance changes, then the following occurs:

- Increased resistance decreases blood flow, increases upstream pressure, and decreases downstream pressure.
- Decreased resistance increases blood flow, decreases upstream pressure and increases downstream pressure.
- The pressure "drop" (difference between upstream and downstream) is directly related to the resistance. There is a big pressure drop when resistance is a high and minimal pressure drop when resistance is a low.

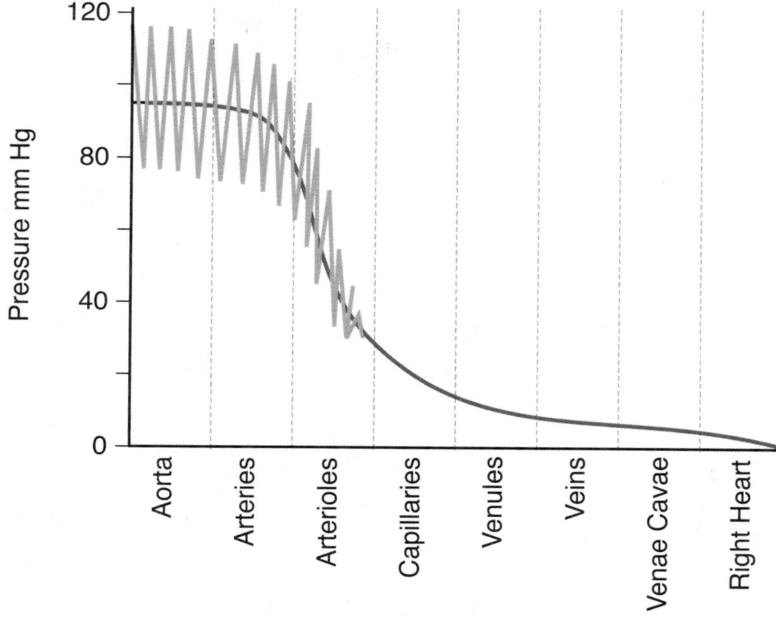

Figure V-1-4. Systemic System Pressures

Whole body application of resistance

- Figure V-1-4 shows, in a horizontal subject, the phasic and mean pressures from the aorta to the vena cava.
- Mean arterial pressure (MAP) is measured in the aorta and is about 93 mm Hg (time weighted average because more time is spent in diastole). This represents the pressure head (upstream pressure) for the systemic circulation.
- The pressure dissipates as the blood flows down the circulatory tree because of resistance. The amount of pressure lost in a particular segment is proportional to the resistance of that segment.
- There is a small pressure drop in the major arteries (low-resistance segment); the largest drop is across the arterioles (highest resistance segment), and another small pressure drop occurs in the major veins (low-resistance segment).
- Dilation of arterioles decreases arteriolar resistance, which increases flow, decreases upstream pressure (MAP), and increases downstream pressure (capillary pressure).
- Likewise, constriction of arterioles increases arteriolar resistance, which in turn decreases flow, increases upstream pressure (MAP), and decreases downstream pressure (capillary pressure).
- Since blood flows from high pressure to low pressure, the sequence of the vessels in any system or part of a system will also be the sequence of pressures, from highest to lowest.

Note

What is the hematocrit?

Answer: If a blood sample from an adult is centrifuged in a graduated test tube, the relative volume of packed red cells is termed the *hematocrit*. For a normal adult this volume is about 40–45% of the total, meaning the red cells occupy about 40–45% of the blood in the body. The white blood cells are less dense than the red blood cells and form a thin layer (the so-called buffy coat). This is why the hematocrit is a major determinant of blood viscosity.

Blood viscosity (ν) is a property of a fluid that is a measure of the fluid's internal resistance to flow:

- The greater the viscosity, the greater the resistance.
- The prime determinant of blood viscosity is the hematocrit. Figure V-1-5 shows how viscosity varies with hematocrit.

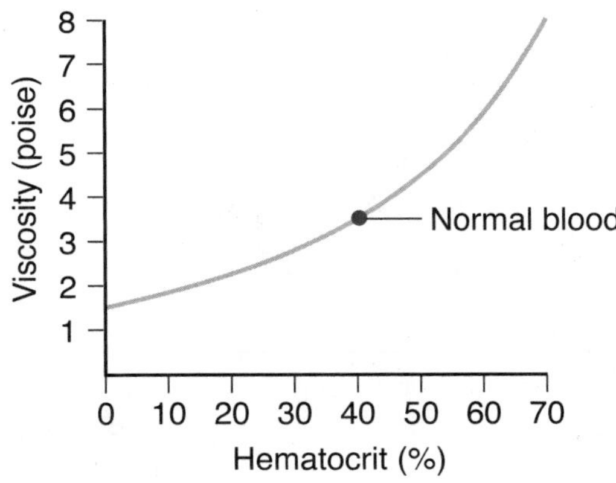

Figure V-1-5. Effect of Hematocrit on Blood Viscosity

Anemia decreases viscosity. Polycythemia increases viscosity.

Vessel length (L)

The greater the length, the greater the resistance.

- If the length doubles, the resistance doubles.
- If the length decreases by half, the resistance decreases by half.
- Vessel length is constant; therefore, changes in length are not a physiologic factor in regulation of resistance, pressure, or flow.

Velocity

Velocity refers to the rate at which blood travels through a blood vessel. Although velocity is directly related to blood flow, it is different in that it refers to a rate, e.g., cm/sec. Mean linear velocity is equal to flow divided by the cross-sectional area (CSA). Thus, velocity is directly related to flow, but if CSA changes, then velocity is affected. The important functional applications of this are:

- CSA is high in capillaries, but low in the aorta.
- Velocity is therefore high in the aorta and low in the capillaries.
- The functional consequence of this is that low velocity in the capillaries optimizes exchange.
- The potential pathology of this is that because the aorta has high velocity and a large diameter, turbulent blood flow can occur here (see below).

Laminar versus Turbulent Flow

There can be two types of flow in a system: laminar and turbulent.

Characteristics of laminar flow:

- As shown in Figure V-1-6, laminar flow is flow in layers.
- Laminar flow occurs throughout the normal cardiovascular system, excluding flow in the heart.
- The layer with the highest velocity is in the center of the tube.

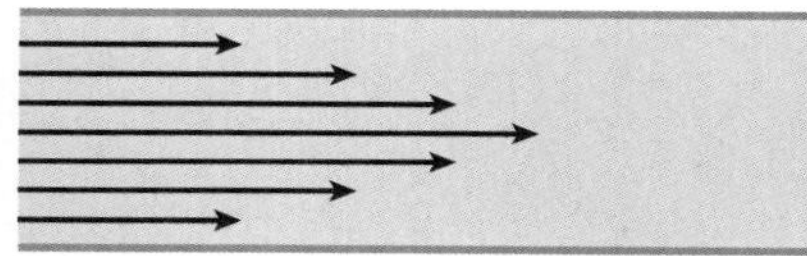

Figure V-1-6. Laminar Flow

Characteristics of turbulent flow:

As shown in Figure V-1-7, turbulent flow is nonlayered flow.

- It creates murmurs. These are heard as bruits in vessels with severe stenosis.
- It produces more resistance than laminar flow.

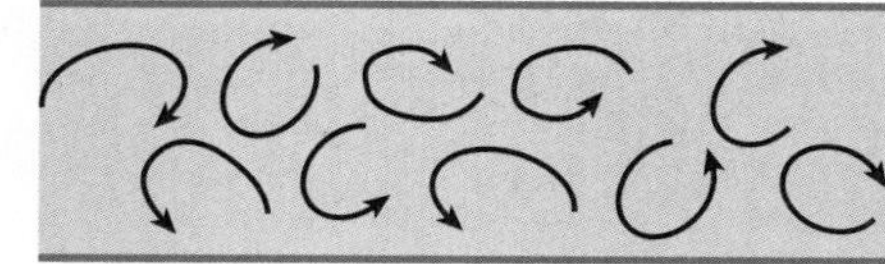

Figure V-1-7. Turbulent Flow

Relation of Reynold's number to laminar and turbulent flow

$$\textbf{Reynold's number} = \frac{\textbf{(diameter) (velocity) (density)}}{\textbf{viscosity}}$$

>2,000: turbulent flow
<2,000: laminar flow

The number inducing turbulence is not absolute. For example, atherosclerosis reduces the Reynold's number at which turbulence begins to develop in the systemic arteries. In addition, thrombi are more likely to develop with turbulent flow than in a laminar flow system.

The following promote the development of turbulent flow (i.e., increase Reynolds' number):

- Increasing tube diameter
- Increasing velocity
- Decreasing blood viscosity, e.g., anemia (cardiac flow murmer)

The vessel in the systemic circuit that is closest to the development of turbulent flow is the aorta. It is a large-diameter vessel with high velocity. This is where turbulence should appear first in anemia.

The following also promote turbulence:

- Vessel branching
- Narrow orifice (severe stenosis)—due to very high velocity of flow

During inspiration and expiration, turbulent flow occurs in the large airways of the conducting zone.

Series Versus Parallel Circuits

- If resistors are in series, then the total resistance is the sum of each individual resistor.

  RT = R1 + R2 + R3...

- If resistors are in parallel, then the total resistance is added as reciprocals of each resistor.

  1/RT = 1/R1 + 1/R2 + 1/R3...

- Thus, total resistance is less in parallel circuits compared to series circuits.
- The application of this concept is that blood flow to the various organ beds of the systemic circulation is the result of parallel branches off of the aorta.
  - Because they are parallel branches, the total resistance of the systemic circulation is less than if the organs were in series bloodflow-wise.

SHORT-TERM REGULATION OF SYSTEMIC ARTERIAL PRESSURE

Arterial Baroreceptors

The baroreceptor reflex is the short-term regulation of blood pressure. The renin-angiotensin-aldosterone system is the long-term regulation of blood pressure. Figure V-1-18 illustrates the main features of the baroreceptor reflex.

Clinical Correlate

Increasing vagal outflow to the heart can be beneficial for patients with supraventricular tachycardia. Because it increases baroreceptor afferent activity, carotid massage is one maneuver that increases vagal outflow to the heart.

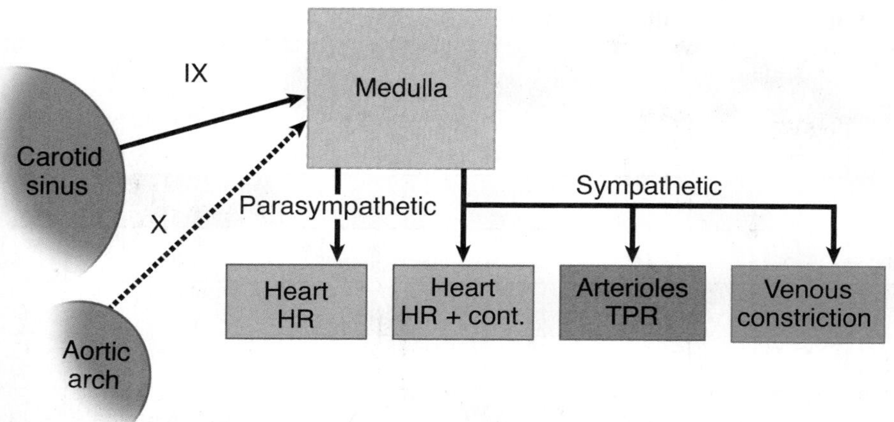

Figure V-1-8. Baroreflexes

$$\text{MAP} = \text{CO} \times \text{TPR}$$

Key points regarding arterial baroreceptors:

- Mechanoreceptors imbedded in the walls of the aortic arch and carotid sinus that are stimulated by a rise in intravascular pressure.
- Afferent activity is relayed to the medulla via cranial nerves IX (carotid sinus) and X (aortic arch).
- Baroreceptor activity exists at the person's resting arterial blood pressure.
- Afferent activity stimulates the parasympathetic nervous system and inhibits the sympathetic nervous system.
- A fall in arterial blood pressure evokes a reflex decrease in parasympathetic activity and increase in sympathetic activity. This is a negative feedback system to bring blood pressure back to its original level.
- A rise in arterial blood pressure evokes a reflex increase in parasympathetic activity and fall in sympathetic activity. This is a negative feedback system to bring blood pressure back to its original level.
- Activation of arterial baroreceptors inhibits the secretion of ADH.

Table V-1-1. Reflex Changes for Specific Maneuvers

Condition	Afferent Activity	Parasympathetic Activity	Sympathetic Activity	BP	HR
BP increase	↑	↑	↓		
BP decrease	↓	↓	↑		
Carotid occlusion	↓	↓	↑	↑	↑
Carotid massage	↑	↑	↓	↓	↓
Cut afferents	↓	↓	↑	↑	↑
Lying to stand Orthostatic hypotension Fluid loss	↓	↓	↑	↑ toward normal	↑
Volume load Weightlessness	↑	↑	↓	↓ toward normal	↓

Cardiopulmonary Mechanoreceptors (Baroreceptors)

- Mechanoreceptors imbedded in the walls of the heart (all 4 chambers), great veins where they empty into the right atrium, and the pulmonary artery.
- Afferent activity is relayed to the medulla via cranial nerve X (vagus).
- Because this region is highly compliant, volume changes are the primary stimulus.
- A reduction in volume in the heart and/or the vessels leading to the heart evokes a reflex increase in SNS activity and a decrease in PNS activity.
- A rise in volume in the heart and/or the vessels leading to the heart evokes a reflex decrease in SNS activity and an increase in PNS activity.
- Similar to arterial baroreceptors, this represents a negative feedback regulation of arterial blood pressure. Further, like arterial baroreceptors, activation of these receptors inhibits ADH release.

Application of Hemodynamics to the Systemic Circulation

Figure V-1-9 is a simplified model of the circulation that we can use to examine whole-body cardiovascular regulation. Blood flows from the aorta to the large arteries that supply the various organs. Within each organ, there are muscular arterioles that serve as the primary site of resistance (see above). The sum of these resistors (added as reciprocals because of the parallel arrangement) is TPR/SVR. This represents afterload to the heart (see previous chapter).

There are 2 functional consequences related to the fact arterioles serve as the primary site of resistance:

- They regulate blood flow to the capillaries (site of exchange with the tissue).
- They regulate upstream pressure, which is mean arterial pressure (MAP).

Tissues need nutrient delivery and thus have mechanisms to regulate the tone of arterioles (intrinsic regulation, discussed in the next chapter). However, from a whole body perspective it is imperative to maintain an adequate MAP because this is the pressure head (upstream pressure) for the entire body (extrinsic regulation).

Given the above, consider arterioles to effectively function as faucets. The tissues need to regulate the faucet to ensure adequate nutrient delivery (intrinsic regulation). On the other hand, these arterioles need a sufficient tone to maintain MAP (extrinsic regulation). If all the faucets were fully opened simultaneously then upstream pressure (MAP) plummets, in turn compromising blood flow to all the organs. Thus, a balance must exist with respect to the level of arteriolar tone ("how tight the faucet is") so there is enough flow to meet the metabolic demands without compromising MAP.

A variety of extrinsic mechanisms exist to regulate arterioles and thus maintain an adequate MAP. Factors that cause vasocontriction, resulting in increased MAP and reduced flow to the capillary include:

- Norepinephrine (NE) released from sympathetic postganglionic neurons
  - NE binds alpha-1 receptors to activate Gq which increases cytosolic calcium in smooth muscle cells, in turn causing vasoconstriction. The sympathetic nervous system is the dominant regulator of vascular tone and has a tonic effect on skeletal muscle and cutaneous vessels at rest. During times of stress, it can exert its effects on the splanchnic and renal circulations as well.
- Epinephrine (EPI) released from the adrenal medulla also activates alpha-1 receptors.
- Ang II via the AT1 receptor (Gq)
- Arginine vasopressin (AVP), also known as anti-diuretic hormone (ADH), via the V1 receptor (Gq)

Vasodilation of arterioles results in a drop in MAP with an increased flow to capillaries (provided MAP doesn't fall too much). Vasodilatory mechanisms include:

- Decreased sympathetic activity
  - Reduced NE release decreases alpha-1 vasoconstriction.
- EPI stimulates vascular beta-2 receptors (Gs–cAMP)
- Nitric oxide (NO)
  - Tonically released from vascular endothelium and activates soluble guanylyl cyclase to increase smooth muscle cGMP.
- A variety of compounds produced by tissue metabolism, e.g., adenosine, CO_2, K^+, and H^+

Bridge to Pharmacology

Drugs that mimic NE cause the same cardiovascular effects that NE produces. These include alpha-1 agonists, NE releasers, and NE reuptake inhibitors.

Bridge to Pharmacology

Drugs that block NE's vascular effects (alpha blockers), prevent NE release, liberate NO, activate beta-2 receptors, block calcium entry into smooth muscle cells, and/or open smooth muscle potassium channels mimic the vasodilatory effects indicated.

Bridge to Pathology

Sepsis, anaphylaxis, and neurogenic shock are examples of uncontrolled vasodilation in the periphery, leading to diminished MAP.

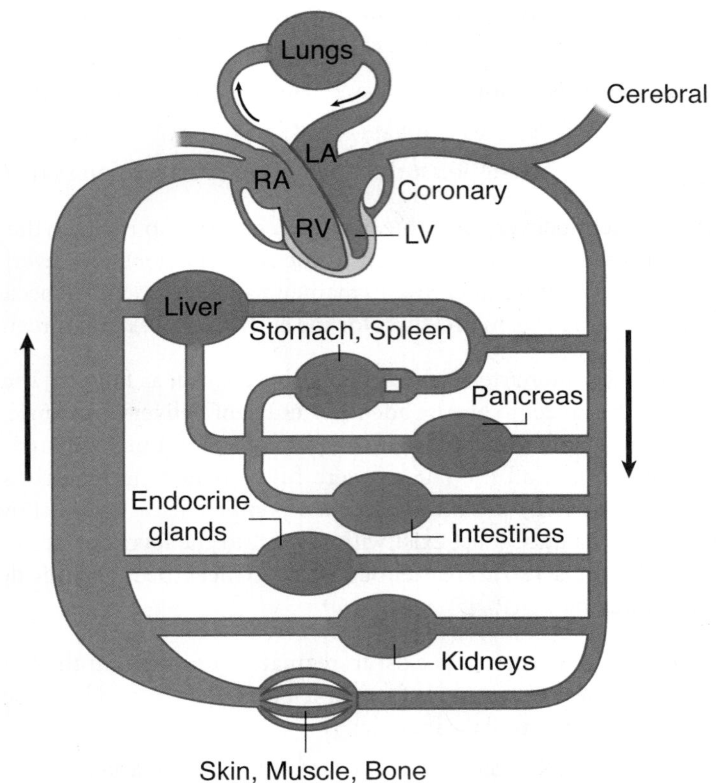

Figure V-1-9. Systemic Circuit

T: wall tension

P: pressure

r: radius

WALL TENSION

LaPlace relationship:

$$T \propto Pr$$

The aorta is the artery with the greatest wall tension (greatest pressure and radius).

Development of an Arterial Aneurysm

Figure V-1-10 shows a developing arterial aneurysm. The pressures at points A, B, and C will be approximately the same.

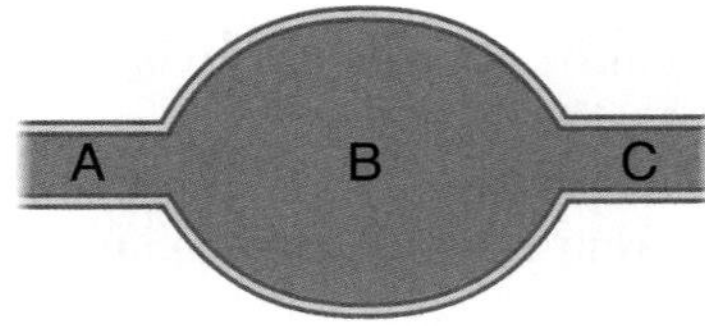

Figure V-1-10. Aortic Enlargement

- Thus, because the aneurysm has a greater radius, its wall tension is greater than that of the surrounding normal vessel segments.
- Also, as the aneurysm enlarges, wall tension increases and the vessel is more likely to burst. Examples are subarachnoid hemorrhage, aortic aneurysm, and diverticulitis.
- Another type of aneurysm is referred to as a dissecting aneurysm. In systemic arterial disease, the high velocity in the aorta may damage the endothelial lining, allowing blood to flow between and dissect the layers of the aorta. This weakens the aortic wall and is considered a life-threatening condition.
- This principle also is important in dilated heart failure, in which the increased chamber size places greater tension on the failing ventricle. This further reduces its performance (see In a Nutshell).

In a Nutshell

Heart with a dilated left ventricle vs. normal heart

If the aortic pressure is the same in both hearts, following the **law of LaPlace** the dilated heart must create greater tension to overcome the same aortic pressure and eject blood, because its internal diameter and volume are greater. Thus, the dilated heart exerts greater total tension on the myocytes (see also Section IV, Volume Overload).

VESSEL COMPLIANCE

$$C = \frac{\Delta V}{\Delta P}$$

Compliance of a vessel can be calculated, but the resulting number is, for all practical purposes, meaningless. It is much more important to simply have a good concept of compliance and understand the differences in compliance among the vessels that make up the cardiovascular system.

- Compliance is essentially how easily a vessel is stretched. If a vessel is easily stretched, it is considered very compliant. The opposite is non-compliant or stiff.
- Elasticity is the inverse of compliance. A vessel that has high elasticity (a large tendency to rebound from a stretch) has low compliance.

Systemic Veins

Systemic veins are about 20 times more compliant than systemic arteries.

- Veins also contain about 70% of the systemic blood volume and thus represent the major blood reservoir.
- If blood is in the veins, then it is not available for the heart to pump and is thus not contributing to the circulating blood volume.

In short: When considering whole-body hemodynamics, compliance resides in the venous system. One must not forget the functional implications of arterial compliance, particularly with respect to arterial pressures (see below), but for the circulation as a whole, compliance is in the venous system.

Venous Return

To understand vascular function and thus ultimately the regulation of cardiac output, one can "split" the circulation into 2 components (Figure V-1-11):

- Cardiac output (CO): flow of blood exiting the heart (down arrow on the arterial side).

- Venous return (VR): flow of blood returning to the heart (up arrow on the venous side). Because this is the flow of blood to the heart, it determines preload for the ventricles (assuming normal ventricular function).

Because the circulation is a closed system, these flows are intertwined and must be the same when one examines it "over time" or at steady-state. In addition, each flow is "dependent" on the other. For example:

- If CO fell to zero, then ultimately VR would become zero.
- If one were to stop VR, there would ultimately be no CO.

These are extreme examples to illustrate the point that altering one ultimately alters the other and a variety of factors can transiently or permanently alter each of the variables, resulting in the other variable being impacted to the same degree. In Section IV, chapter 1, we discussed ventricular function, which plays a pivotal role in CO. In this section, we discuss the regulation of VR. **VR represents vascular function** and thus understanding its regulation sets the stage for understanding CO regulation.

VR is the flow of blood back to the heart and it determines preload. Since it is a flow, it must follow the hemodynamic principles described above, i.e., it is directly proportional to the pressure gradient and inversely related to the resistance.

- **Right atrial pressure (RAP):** blood is flowing to the right atrium, thus RAP is the downstream pressure.
- **Mean systemic filling pressure (Psf):** represents the upstream pressure (pressure head) for VR.

Note

Engaging the muscle pump also increases Psf.

Mean systemic filling pressure (Psf): Although not a "theoretical" pressure (as per numerous experiments, Psf is typically ~7 mm Hg prior to endogenous compensations), this is not a pressure that can be conveniently measured, particularly in a patient. However, because it is the pressure when no flow exists, it is primarily determined by volume and compliance (see Vessel Compliance above):

- Blood volume: There is a direct relation between blood volume and Psf. The greater the blood volume, the higher the Psf and vice versa.
- Venous compliance: There is an inverse relation between venous compliance and Psf. The more compliant the veins, the lower the Psf and vice versa.

Because Psf is the pressure head (upstream pressure) driving VR, then VR is directly related to Psf. If all other factors are unchanged, it follows that:

- An increase in blood volume increases VR.
- A decrease in blood volume decreases VR.
- A decrease in venous compliance (sympathetic stimulation; muscle pump) increases VR.
- An increase in venous compliance (sympathetic inhibition; venodilators; alpha block) decreases VR.

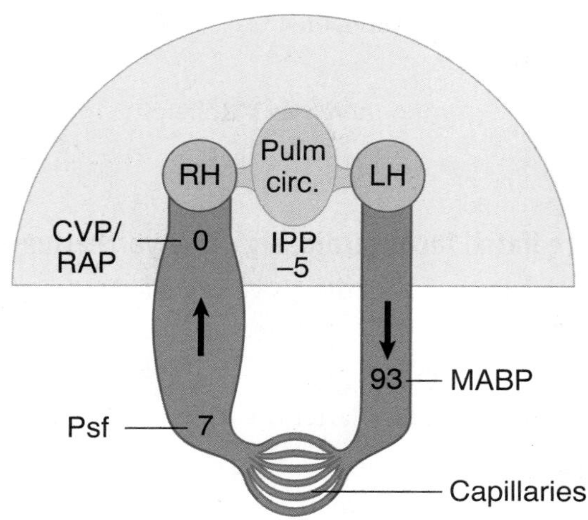

Figure V-1-11. Pressure Gradients in the Circulatory System

CVP:	central venous pressure
IPP:	intrapleural pressure
LH:	left heart
MABP:	mean arterial blood pressure
Psf:	mean systemic filling pressure
RH:	right heart
RAP:	right atrial pressure

DETERMINANTS OF CARDIAC OUTPUT

Because VR plays an important role in determining CO, we can now discuss the regulation of CO. The key point to remember is that **steady-state CO** is the interplay between **ventricular function** (see ventricular function curves in the previous chapter) and **vascular function**, which is defined by VR curves. The 4 determinants are as follows:

- Heart rate
- Contractility
- Afterload
- Preload (determined by VR)

The latter 3 factors can be combined on CO/VR curves, which are illustrated and discussed later. Let's first start with heart rate.

Heart Rate (HR)

CO = HR × SV (stroke volume)

Although HR and CO are directly related, the effect of changes in HR on CO is complicated because the other variable, SV must be considered (Figure V-1-12). High heart rates decrease filling time for the ventricles, and thus can decrease SV. In short, the effect of HR on CO depends upon the cause of the rise in HR.

Endogenously mediated tachycardia, e.g., exercise

In exercise, the rise in HR increases CO. Although filling time is reduced, a variety of changes occur that prevent SV from falling. These are:

- Sympathetic stimulation to the heart increases contractility. This helps maintain stroke volume. In addition, this decreases the systolic interval (see previous chapter) thus preserving some of the diastolic filling time.
- Sympathetic stimulation increases conduction velocity in the heart, thereby increasing the rate of transmission of the electrical impulse.

- Sympathetic stimulation venoconstricts, which helps preserve VR (see above) and ventricular filling.
- The skeletal muscle pump increases VR, helping to maintain ventricular filling.

Pathologically mediated tachycardia, e.g., tachyarrhythmias

- The sudden increase in HR curtails ventricular filling resulting in a fall in CO (Figure V-1-12).
- Although the fall in CO decreases MAP and activates the sympathetic nervous system, this occurs "after the fact" and is thus unable to compensate.
- There is no muscle pump to increase VR.

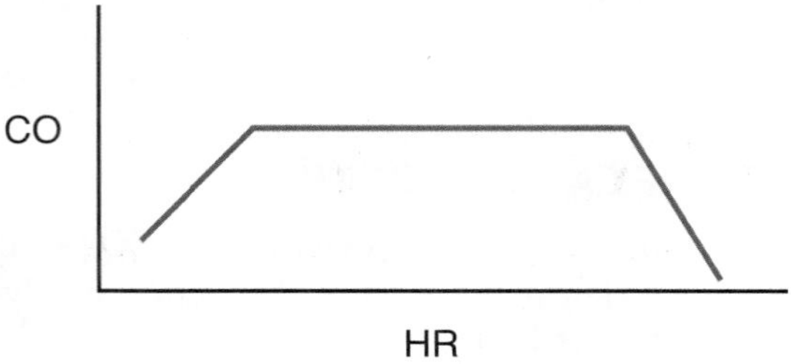

Figure V-1-12

Contractility

Contractility was discussed in depth in Chapter 1 of Section IV. There is a direct relation between contractility and ventricular output, thus there is typically a direct relation between contractility and CO.

Afterload

Afterload is the load the heart works against and the best marker of afterload is TPR. This was also discussed in Chapter 1 of Section IV. There is an inverse relation between afterload and ventricular output, thus there is generally an inverse relation between afterload and CO.

Preload

As discussed in Chapter 1 of Section IV, there is a direct relation between preload and ventricular output (Frank-Starling). Presuming there is no change in contractility or afterload, increasing preload increases CO and vice versa.

Cardiac Output (CO)/Venous Return (VR) Curves

CO/VR curves (Figure V-1-13) depict the interplay between ventricular and vascular function indicated in the venous return section above. Steady-state CO is determined by this interplay.

Ventricular function (solid line of Figure V-1-13)

- X-axis is RAP, a marker of preload.
- Y-axis is CO.
- Thus, this curve is the same as depicted in Figures IV-1-3 and IV-1-4 and it defines ventricular function.
- This curve shows that RAP has a positive impact on CO (Frank-Starling mechanism)

Vascular function (dashed line of Figure V-1-13)

- X-axis is RAP, the downstream pressure for VR.
- Y-axis is VR.
- The curve shows that as RAP increases, VR decreases. This is because RAP is the downstream pressure for VR. As RAP increases, the pressure gradient for VR falls, which in turn decreases VR. Thus, RAP has a negative impact on VR.
- X-intercept for the VR curve is Psf (point B on the graph). This is the pressure in the circulation when there is no flow (see section on venous return). Psf is the pressure head (upstream pressure) for VR. Thus, when RAP = Psf, flow (VR) is zero.

Steady-state CO

- The intersection of the ventricular and vascular function curves determines steady-state CO (point A in Figure V-1-13). In other words, point A represents the interplay between ventricular and vascular function.
- Discounting HR, the only way steady-state CO can change is if ventricular function, or vascular function, or both change.

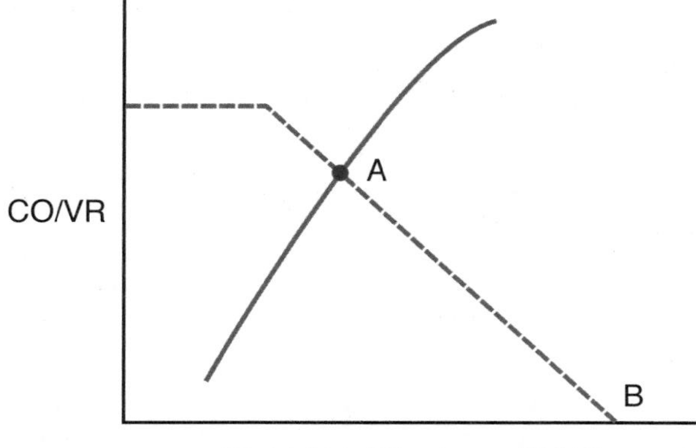

Figure V-1-13

A = steady-state cardiac output

All individuals operate at the intersection of the ventricular function and venous return curves.

B = mean systemic filling pressure (Psf)

This is directly related to vascular volume and inversely related to venous compliance.

Resistance

- The primary site of resistance for the circulation is the arterioles.
- If arterioles vasodilate (decreased resistance), VR increases (line A of Figure V-1-14). Recall that VR is a flow, and thus decreasing resistance increases flow. Note that this vasodilation provides more VR (move up the Frank-Starling curve).

  Although not depicted in the graph, vasodilation decreases afterload and thus shifts the ventricular function curve up and to the left (see Figures IV-1-3 & 4 for review). In short, arteriolar vasodilation enhances both ventricular and vascular function.
- If arterioles vasoconstrict (increased resistance), VR falls (line B of Figure V-1-14). Note that this vasoconstriction reduces VR, and steady-state CO falls as one moves down the Frank-Starling curve.

  Although not depicted in the graph, vasoconstriction increases afterload, shifting the ventricular function curve down and to the right (see Figures IV-1-3 & 4 for review). Thus, arteriolar vasoconstriction reduces both ventricular and vascular function.

Psf

- As indicated above (venous return section), Psf is directly related to blood volume and inversely related to venous compliance.
- Increasing vascular volume (infusion; activation of RAAS) or decreasing venous compliance (sympathetic stimulation; muscle pump; exercise; lying down) increases Psf, causing a right shift in the VR curve (line C of Figure V-1-14). Thus, either of these changes enhances filling of the ventricles (move up the Frank-Starling curve) and CO.
- Decreasing vascular volume (hemorrhage; burn trauma; vomiting; diarrhea) or increasing venous compliance (inhibit sympathetics; alpha block; venodilators; standing upright) decreases Psf, causing a left shift in the VR curve (line D of Figure V-1-14). Thus, either of these changes reduces filling of the ventricles (move down the Frank-Starling curve) and CO.

A = arteriolar dilation

B = arteriolar constriction

C = increased vascular volume; decreased venous compliance

D = decreased vascular volume; increased venous compliance

Solid circles represent starting CO.

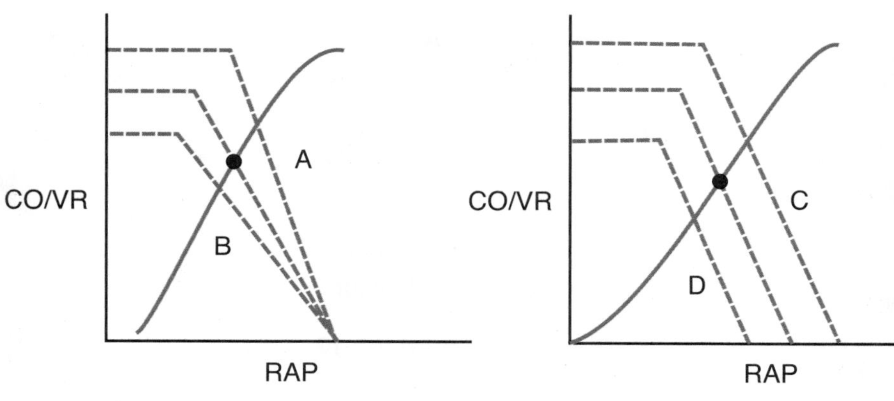

Figure V-1-14

THE EFFECT OF GRAVITY

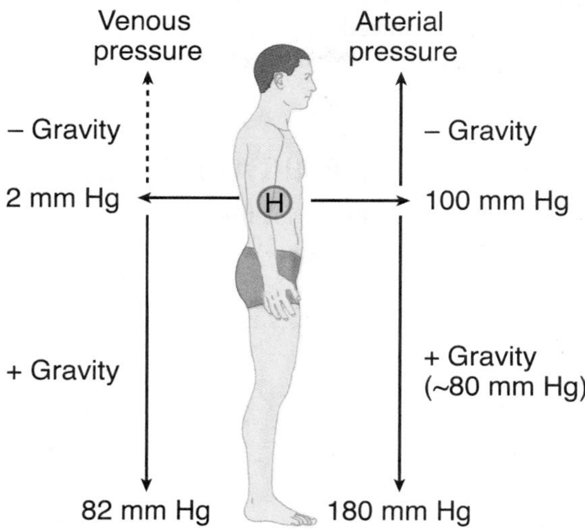

Figure V-1-15. Effect of Gravity

Below heart level, there are equal increases in systemic arterial and venous pressures (assuming no muscular action). Thus, the pressure difference between arteries and veins does not change.

Because veins are very compliant vessels, the higher pressures in the dependent veins mean a significant pooling of blood, a volume that is not contributing to cardiac output. Although venous compliance doesn't "technically" increase, gravity's impact is functionally the same as an increase in venous compliance.

When a person goes from supine to an upright posture, the following important changes take place:

- Pressure in the dependent veins increases.
- Blood volume in the dependent veins increases.
- VR decreases.
- If no compensations occurred, then MAP would fall because of the diminished SV.

The initial compensation arises from cardiopulmonary mechanoreceptors (described previously in this chapter), which, because their stretch is reduced, activate the SNS and inhibit the PNS.

The reflex activation of the sympathetic nervous system causes:

- Arteriolar vasoconstriction (TPR increases)
- Increase in HR
- Venoconstriction

If MAP falls, then the arterial baroreceptors also participate in the reflex changes.

Above heart level, systemic arterial pressure progressively decreases. Because venous pressure at heart level is close to zero, venous pressure quickly becomes subatmospheric (negative).

In a Nutshell

The Effect of Gravity

Case 1. When placing a central line in the internal jugular or subclavian vein of a patient in the medical intensive care unit, place the patient in the Trendelenburg position, in which the deep veins of the upper extremity are below the level of the heart. This position makes the venous pressure less negative, thus reducing the risk of forming an "air embolus," in which the needle forms a connection between the positive atmospheric pressure and the negative vein.

Case 2. To take an accurate blood pressure (BP) reading, place the sphygmomanometer *at the level of the heart*. If the cuff is above the level of the heart, the reading will be falsely low; conversely, if the cuff is below the level of the heart, the reading will be falsely high.

Bridge to Pathology/Pharmacology

The inability to maintain MAP when standing upright is called orthostatic intolerance. In this condition, the fall in MAP reduces cerebral blood flow, causing the patient to feel dizzy or light-headed. This can lead to a syncope event. One of the more common causes for this is reduced vascular volume. The low volume reduces VR and the added fall in VR (due to venous pooling) overwhelms the compensatory mechanisms. Other factors that can lead to orthostatic intolerance are venodilators, poor ventricular function such as heart failure or cardiac transplant, and dysautonomias.

Surface veins above the heart cannot maintain a significant pressure below atmospheric and will collapse; however, deep veins and those inside the cranium supported by the tissue can maintain a pressure that is significantly below atmospheric. A consequence of the preceding is that a severed or punctured vein above heart level has the potential for introducing air into the system.

CHARACTERISTICS OF SYSTEMIC ARTERIES

The following figure shows a pressure pulse for a major systemic artery.

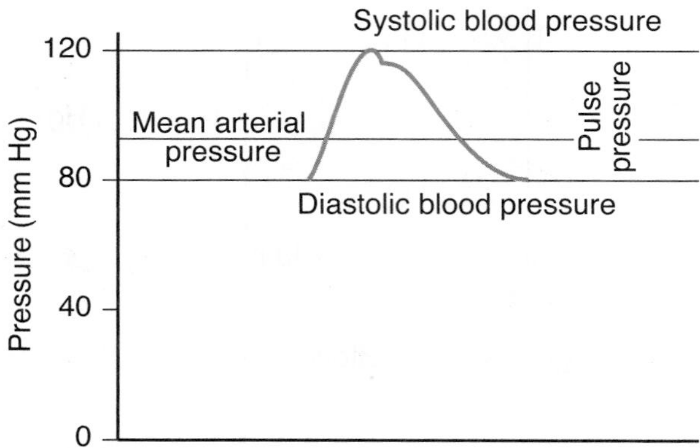

Figure V-1-16. Pulse Pressure and Mean Pressure

Pulse pressure equals systolic minus diastolic, so here, pulse pressure is 120 – 80 = 40 mm Hg.

Factors Affecting Systolic Pressure

- Systolic blood pressure is the highest pressure in the systemic arteries during the cardiac cycle.
- The main factor determining systolic blood pressure on a beat-to-beat basis is stroke volume.
- An increase in stroke volume increases systolic blood pressure and a decrease in stroke volume decreases systolic blood pressure.
- Systolic blood pressure is also directly related to ventricular contractility. In addition, the rate of pressure change in the aorta is directly related to contractility. Thus, if contractility increases, then the rate of pressure and the absolute level of aortic pressure increases, and vice-versa.
- In chronic conditions, a decrease in the compliance of the systemic arteries (age-related arteriosclerosis) also increases systolic blood pressure.

Factors Affecting Diastolic Pressure

- Diastolic blood pressure (DBP) is directly related to the volume of blood left in the aorta at the end of diastole.
- One important factor determining DBP is total peripheral resistance (TPR).
- Dilation of the arterioles decreases DBP and constriction of the arterioles increases DBP.

- HR is the second key factor influencing diastolic pressure and they are directly related: increased HR increases DBP, while decreased HR decreases DBP.
- DBP is also directly related to SV, but this is typically not a major factor.

Factors Affecting Pulse Pressure

The following increase (widen) pulse pressure:

- An increase in stroke volume (systolic increases more than diastolic)
- A decrease in vessel compliance (systolic increases and diastolic decreases)

The aorta is the most compliant artery in the arterial system. Peripheral arteries are more muscular and less compliant. Based on the preceding information, in Figure V-1-17 the pressure record on the left best represents the aorta, whereas the one on the right best represents the femoral artery.

Note

Theoretically, the **systemic pulse pressure** can be conceptualized as being proportional to stroke volume, or the amount of blood ejected from the left ventricle during systole, and inversely proportional to the compliance of the aorta.

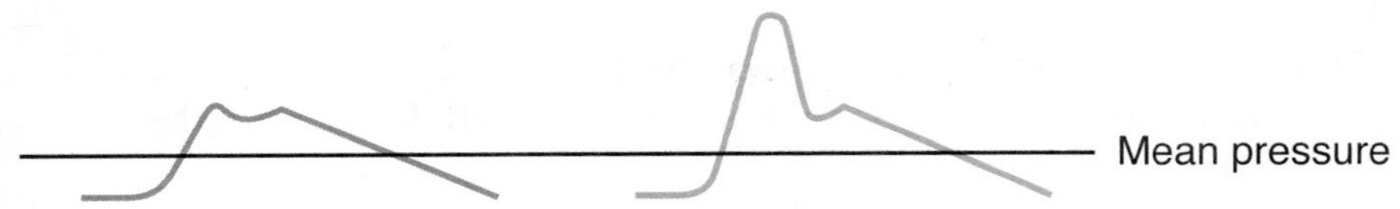

Figure V-1-17. Compliance and Pulse Pressure

The figure demonstrates that a compliant artery has a small pulse pressure and that a stiff artery has a large pulse pressure. Also, pulse pressure increases with age because compliance is decreasing. This can produce isolated systolic hypertension, in which mean pressure is normal because the elevated systolic pressure is associated with a reduced diastolic pressure.

Factors Affecting Mean Pressure

Mean pressure is pressure averaged over time. It is not the arithmetic mean and is closer to diastolic pressure than to systolic pressure.

Mean pressure can be approximated by the following formulas:

For a blood pressure of 120/80 mm Hg:

Mean pressure = diastolic + 1/3 pulse pressure

80 + 1/3(40) = 93 mm Hg

= 2/3 diastolic pressure + 1/3 systolic pressure

2/3(80) + 1/3(120) = 93 mm Hg

Any formula that calculates mean pressure must give a value between systolic and diastolic but closer to diastolic than systolic.

Factors that affect mean pressure (application of hemodynamics discussed above):

Q = cardiac output

P_1 = aortic pressure (mean arterial pressure)

P_2 = pressure at the entrance of the right atrium

R = resistance of all vessels in the systemic circuit. This is referred to as total peripheral resistance (TPR).

MAP: mean arterial pressure

CO: cardiac output

TPR: total peripheral resistance

Because the major component of TPR is the arterioles, TPR can be considered an index of arteriolar resistance.

Because P_1 is a very large number (93 mm Hg) and P_2 is a very small one (~0 mm Hg), that doesn't change dramatically in most situations, we can simplify the equation if we approximate P_2 as zero. Then:

$$CO = \frac{MAP}{TPR} \quad \text{or} \quad \mathbf{MAP = CO \times TPR}$$

This equation simply states that:

- Mean arterial pressure (MAP) is determined by only 2 variables: cardiac output and TPR.
- CO is the circulating volume. The blood stored in the systemic veins and the pulmonary circuit would not be included in this volume.
- TPR is the resistance of all vessels in the systemic circuit. By far the largest component is the resistance in the arterioles.
- However, if venous or right atrial pressure (RAP) is severely increased, it must be taken into account when estimating TPR. In this case, the formula is:

$$\mathbf{(MAP - RAP) = CO \times TPR}$$

$$\text{or rearranged to solve for resistance: } TPR = \frac{(MAP - RAP)}{CO}$$

Chapter Summary

- The cardiovascular system consists of two circuits and two pumps connected in series.
- Systemic pressure decreases slightly through the arteries, decreases markedly through the arterioles, and then decreases only slightly more through the major veins. The loss of pressure is determined by regional resistance.
- The cross-sectional area increases from a minimum in the aorta to a maximum in the capillaries. Velocity of the blood is inversely related to a region's cross-sectional area.
- The main blood reservoir is the systemic veins.
- Of the factors affecting a vessel's resistance, radius is the most important. The radius of the arterioles determines total peripheral resistance.
- The cardiovascular system is a laminar flow system. The factors that promote turbulence include decreased fluid viscosity, large-diameter tubes, increased fluid velocity, and vessel branching.
- Psf is the pressure-head driving VR. It is directly related to blood volume and inversely related to venous compliance.
- If ventricular function is normal, VR determines preload.
- CO is determined by HR, contractility, afterload, and preload. It is the interplay of ventricular and vascular function.
- Ventricular function curves describe ventricular function, while VR curves illustrate vascular function.
- Structures connected in series produce high resistance, and flow is dependent and equal at all points.
- Mean arterial pressure is determined only by the circulating blood volume (cardiac output) and the resistance of the arterioles.
- Vessel wall tension is directly proportional to pressure and radius.
- The aorta is the most compliant artery, but veins are more compliant than arteries.
- Gravity causes the pooling of blood in the dependent veins. This blood does not contribute to cardiac output.
- The baroreceptor and cardiopulmonary reflexes alter parasympathetic and sympathetic outflow to minimize acute changes in blood pressure.

Regulation of Blood Flow and Pressure

2

Learning Objectives

- ❑ Demonstrate understanding of Fick principle of blood flow
- ❑ Interpret scenarios on blood flow regulation
- ❑ Explain information related to blood flow to the various organs
- ❑ Demonstrate understanding of fetal circulation
- ❑ Explain information related to cardiovascular stress: exercise

FICK PRINCIPLE OF BLOOD FLOW

The Fick principle can be utilized to calculate the blood flow through an organ.

Calculation of flow through the pulmonary circuit provides a measure of the CO.

- $\textbf{Flow} = \dfrac{\textbf{uptake}}{\textbf{A} - \textbf{V}}$

Required data are: oxygen consumption of the organ

A – V oxygen content (concentration) difference across the organ (not PO_2)

Pulmonary venous (systemic arterial) oxygen content	= 20 vol%
	= 20 volumes O_2 per 100 volumes blood
	= 20 mL O_2 per 100 mL blood
	= 0.2 mL O_2 per mL blood

If pulmonary vessel data are not available, you may substitute arterial oxygen content for pulmonary venous blood and use venous oxygen content in place of pulmonary artery values.

Figure V-2-1 illustrates the situation in a normal resting individual.

In a Nutshell

Fick Principle

- First devised as a technique for measuring cardiac output (CO)
- Can calculate oxygen consumption (VO_2)

  $VO_2 = CO \times (CaO_2 - CvO_2)$

  CaO_2 = total arterial oxygen content

  (Hgb × 1.36 × SaO2) + PaO2 × 0.0031

These values are obtained from an ABG.

  CvO_2 = total venous oxygen content

  (Hgb × 1.36 × SvO2) + PvO2 × 0.0031

These values are obtained from a central venous or Swan-Ganz catheter, which samples blood from the pulmonary artery.

- The ($CaO_2 - CvO_2$) and CO are the two main factors that allow variation in the body's total oxygen consumption.

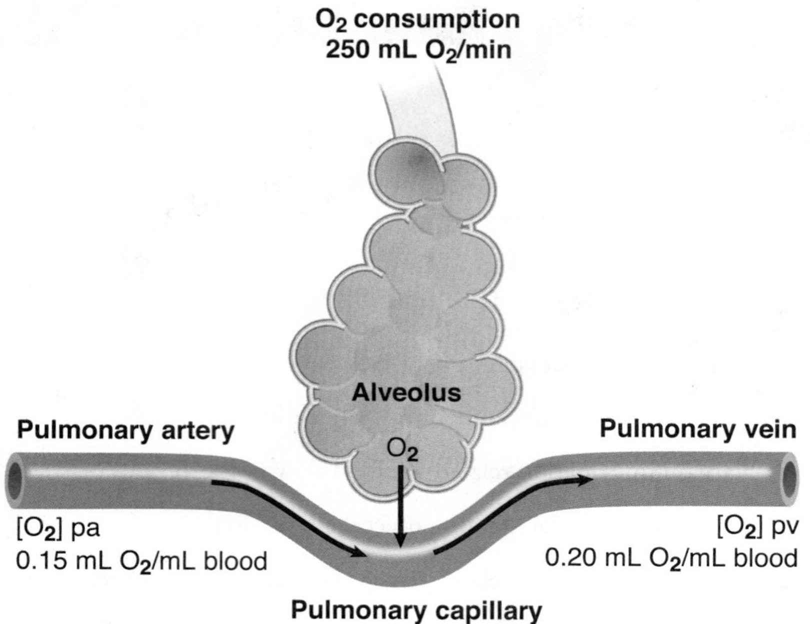

Figure V-2-1. Alveolar Oxygen Uptake

$$Q(\text{flow}) = \frac{\text{oxygen consumption}}{[O_2]\text{pv} - [O_2]\text{pa}}$$

$$= \frac{250 \text{ mL/min}}{0.20 \text{ mL/mL} - 0.15 \text{ mL/mL}} = 5{,}000 \text{ mL/min}$$

$$\text{Cardiac index} = \frac{\text{cardiac output}}{\text{body surface area}}$$

This would normalize the value for body size.

Application of the Fick Principle

Rearranging the Fick Principle to O_2 consumption = Q × (CaO_2 – CvO_2) can be applied to important concepts regarding homeostatic mechanisms and pathologic alterations (Figure V-2-2). CaO_2 – CvO_2 represents the extraction of O_2 by the tissue.

O_2 consumption

- O_2 consumption is dependent upon flow and the extraction of O_2.
- If tissue O_2 consumption increases, then flow or extraction or both must increase.
- The rise in flow in response to a rise in tissue O_2 consumption is the result of increased production of vasodilator metabolites (see metabolic mechanism below).
- In short, this change in flow and extraction represents homeostatic mechanisms designed to ensure adequate O_2 availability and thus sufficient ATP production.

O_2 delivery

- O_2 delivery = Q × CaO_2
  - The "first part" of the Fick Principle indicates that delivery of O_2 to the tissue is dependent upon Q and the total amount of O_2 in the blood (CaO_2).
- For any given tissue O_2 consumption, reduced delivery of O_2 results in increased lactic acid production and possible hypoxic/ischemic damage to tissues.
- For any given tissue O_2 consumption, if O_2 delivery decreases, then PvO_2 and SvO_2% fall.
- Clinical application
  - A fall in PvO_2 or SvO_2% indicates the patient's O_2 consumption increased and/or there was a fall in Q or CaO_2 or both.

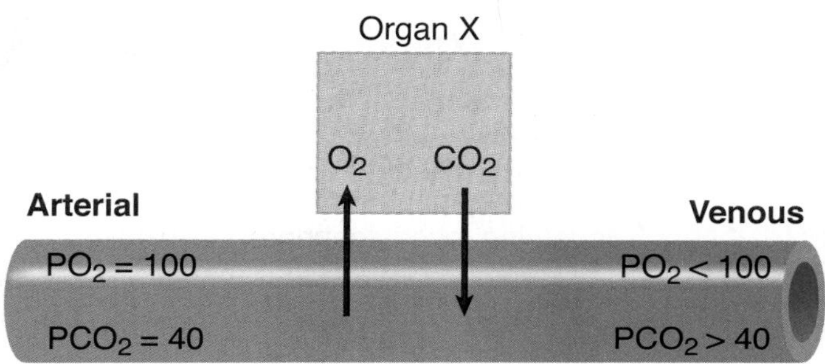

Figure V-2-2. Application of the Fick Principle

BLOOD FLOW REGULATION

Flow is regulated by constricting and dilating the smooth muscle surrounding the arterioles.

Intrinsic Regulation (Autoregulation)

The control mechanisms regulating the arteriolar smooth muscle are entirely within the organ itself.

- What is regulated is blood flow, not resistance. It is more correct to say that resistance is changed in order to regulate flow.
- No nerves or circulating substances are involved in autoregulation. Thus, the autonomic nervous system and circulating epinephrine have nothing to do with autoregulation.

There are 2 main mechanisms to explain autoregulation.

Metabolic mechanism

- Tissue produces a vasodilatory metabolite that regulates flow, e.g., adenosine, CO_2, H^+, and K^+.
- A dilation of the arterioles is produced when the concentration of these metabolites increases in the tissue. The arterioles constrict if the tissue concentration decreases.

Myogenic mechanism

- Increased perfusing pressure causes stretch of the arteriolar wall and the surrounding smooth muscle.
- Because an inherent property of the smooth muscle is to contract when stretched, the arteriole radius decreases, and flow does not increase significantly.

Major characteristics of an autoregulating tissue

Blood flow should be independent of blood pressure.

This phenomenon is demonstrated for a theoretically perfect autoregulating tissue in Figure V-2-3. The range of pressure over which flow remains nearly constant is the **autoregulatory range**.

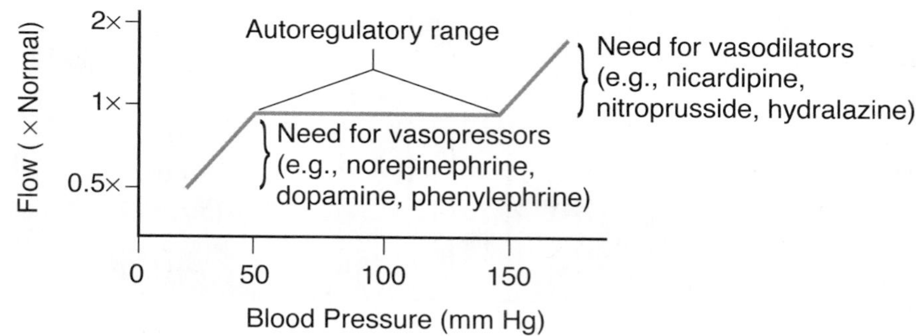

Figure V-2-3. Autoregulation

Blood flow in most cases is proportional to tissue metabolism.

Blood flow is independent of nervous reflexes (e.g., carotid sinus) or circulating humoral factors.

Autoregulating tissues include (tissues least affected by nervous reflexes):

- Cerebral circulation
- Coronary circulation
- Skeletal muscle vasculature during exercise

Extrinsic Regulation

These tissues are controlled by nervous and humoral factors originating outside the organ, e.g., resting skeletal muscle. Extrinsic mechanisms were covered in the previous chapter and thus will only be briefly reviewed here.

Figure V-2-4 illustrates an arteriole in skeletal muscle and the factors regulating flow under resting conditions.

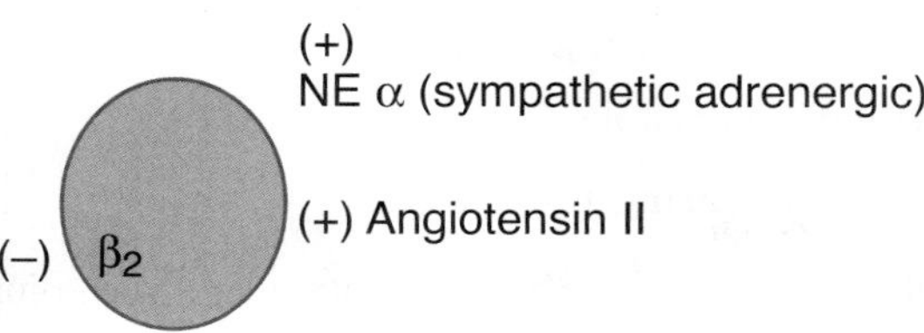

Figure V-2-4. Resting Skeletal Muscle Blood Flow

The key points for extrinsic regulation are:

- Norepinephrine (NE) released from sympathetic nerves has a tonic influence on arteriolar tone (α receptors) in resting skeletal muscle and skin vasculature in a thermo-neutral environment.
- In times of stress, sympathetic activation can evoke substantial vasoconstriction in the aforementioned tissues, but can also greatly affect renal and splanchnic circulations.
- Epinephrine can evoke vasodilation by binding to vascular β2 receptors.
- With the exception of the penis, the parasympathetic nervous system does not affect arteriolar tone.

Control of Resting versus Exercising Muscle

Resting muscle

Flow is controlled mainly by increasing or decreasing sympathetic α-adrenergic activity.

Exercising muscle

The elevated metabolism in exercising skeletal muscle demands an increase in blood flow (see application of the Fick principle above). In addition, the increased tissue O_2 consumption results in a fall the PvO_2 of blood leaving the working muscle. The primary mechanisms for increasing flow are:

- Production of vasodilator metabolites, e.g., adenosine, CO_2, H^+, and K^+ causes marked vasodilation. In addition, these metabolites diminish NE's ability to vasoconstrict the arterioles. Further, the increased endothelial shear-stress of the high flow liberates NO.
- Muscle pump

BLOOD FLOW TO THE VARIOUS ORGANS

Coronary Circulation

Coronary flow patterns

Characteristics of left coronary flow (flow to the left ventricular myocardium):

Left ventricular contraction causes severe mechanical compression of subendocardial vessels. Therefore:

> **Note**
>
> Be careful with drugs such as dobutamine, which can increase contractility through β_1 receptors but also can cause hypotension with some β_2 activation.

- Very little if any blood flow occurs during systole.
- Most of the blood flow is during diastole.
- Some subepicardial flow occurs during systole.

Characteristics of right coronary blood flow (flow to the right ventricular myocardium):

Right ventricular contraction causes modest mechanical compression of intramyocardial vessels. Therefore:

- Significant flow can occur during systole.
- The greatest flow under normal conditions is still during diastole.

Oxygenation

In the coronary circulation, the tissues extract almost all the oxygen they can from the blood, even under "basal" conditions. Therefore:

- The venous PO_2 is extremely low. It is the lowest venous PO_2 in a resting individual.
- Because the extraction of oxygen is almost maximal under resting conditions, increased oxygen delivery to the tissue can be accomplished only by increasing blood flow (Fick principle).
- In the coronary circulation, flow must match metabolism.
- Coronary blood flow is most closely related to cardiac tissue oxygen consumption and demand.

Pumping action

Coronary blood flow (mL/min) is determined by the pumping action, or **stroke work** times heart rate, of the heart.

Increased pumping action means increased metabolism, which increases the production of vasodilatory metabolites. In turn, coronary flow increases.

Increased pump function occurs with:

- An increase in any of the parameters that determine CO:
  - HR
  - Contractility
  - Afterload
  - Preload
- HR, contractility, and afterload (often called pressure work) are more metabolically costly than the work associated with preload (volume work).
- Thus, conditions in which HR, contractility, and/or afterload increase, e.g., hypertension, aortic stenosis, and exercise require a greater increase in flow compared to conditions that only increase volume work (supine, aortic regurgitation, volume loading).

Cerebral Circulation

Flow is proportional to arterial PCO_2. Under normal conditions, arterial PCO_2 is an important factor regulating cerebral blood flow.

- Hypoventilation increases arterial PCO_2, thus it increases cerebral blood flow.
- Hyperventilation decreases arterial PCO_2, thus it decreases cerebral blood flow.

As long as arterial PO_2 is normal or above normal, cerebral blood flow is regulated via arterial PCO_2. Therefore:

- If a normal person switches from breathing room air to 100% oxygen, there is no significant change in cerebral blood flow.
- However, a (large) decrease in arterial PO_2 increases cerebral blood flow; an example is high-altitude pulmonary edema (HAPE). Under these conditions, it is the low arterial PO_2 that is determining flow.
- Baroreceptor reflexes do not affect flow.

Intracranial pressure is an important pathophysiologic factor that can affect cerebral blood flow.

Cutaneous Circulation

- Almost entirely controlled via sympathetic adrenergic nerves
- Large venous plexus innervated by sympathetics
- A-V shunts innervated by sympathetics
- Sympathetic stimulation to the skin causes:
  - Constriction of arterioles and a decrease in blood flow, which is one reason why physicians use a central line to administer vasopressors to prevent distal necrosis
  - Constriction of the venous plexus and a decrease in blood volume in the skin
- Sympathetic activity to the skin varies mainly with the body's need for heat exchange with the environment.

Increased skin temperature directly causes vasodilation, which increases heat loss.

Temperature regulation

There are temperature-sensitive neurons in the anterior hypothalamus, whose firing rate reflects the temperature of the regional blood supply.

- Normal set point: oral 37°C (rectal + 0.5°C)
- Circadian rhythm: low point, morning; high point, evening

As illustrated in Figure V-2-5, the body does not lose the ability to regulate body temperature during a fever. It simply regulates body temperature at a higher set point.

Bridge to Anatomy

The **splanchnic circulation** is composed of the gastric small intestinal, colonic, pancreatic, hepatic, and splenic circulations, arranged in parallel with one another. The three major arteries that supply the splanchnic organs are the celiac, superior, and inferior mesenteric arteries.

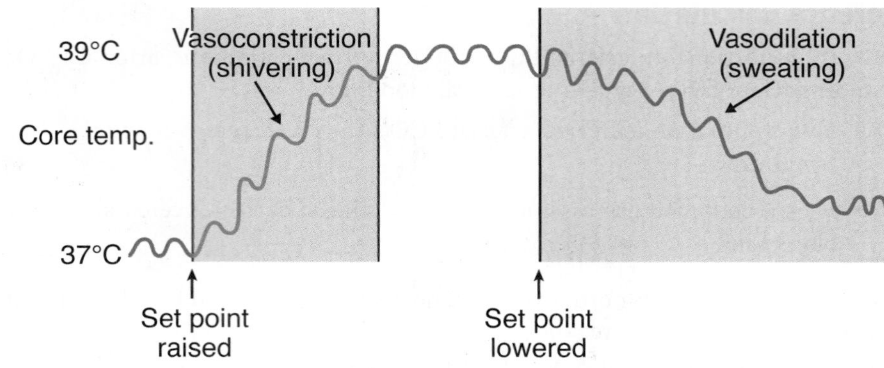

Figure V-2-5. Temperature Regulation

When a fever develops, body temperature rises toward the new higher set point. Under these conditions, heat-conserving and heat-generating mechanisms include:

- Shivering
- Cutaneous vasoconstriction

After a fever "breaks," the set point has returned to normal, and body temperature is decreasing. Heat-dissipating mechanisms include:

- Sweating (sympathetic cholinergics)
- Cutaneous vasodilation

Renal and Splanchnic Circulation

- A small change in blood pressure invokes an autoregulatory response to maintain renal and splanchnic blood flows.
- Thus, under normal conditions, the renal and splanchnic circulations demonstrate autoregulation.
- Situations in which there is a large increase in sympathetic activity (e.g., hypotension) usually cause vasoconstriction and a decrease in blood flow.
- Renal circulation is greatly overperfused in terms of nutrient requirements, thus the venous PO_2 is high.
- About 25% of the CO goes to the splanchnic circulation, thus it represents an important reservoir of blood in times of stress.
- Splanchnic blood flow increases dramatically when digesting a meal.

Pulmonary Circuit

Characteristics

- Low-pressure circuit, arterial = 15 mm Hg, venous = 5 mm Hg; small pressure drop indicates a low resistance.
- High flow, receives entire CO
- Very compliant circuit; both arteries and veins are compliant vessels
- Hypoxic vasoconstriction (low alveolar PO_2 causes local arteriolar vasoconstriction)

- Blood volume proportional to blood flow
  - Because of the very compliant nature of the pulmonary circuit, large changes in the output of the right ventricle are associated with only small changes in pulmonary pressures.

Pulmonary response to exercise

- A large increase in cardiac output means increased volume pumped into the circuit. This increases pulmonary intravascular pressures.
- Because of the compliant nature of the circuit, the pulmonary arterial system distends.
- In addition, there is recruitment of previously unperfused capillaries. Because of this recruitment and distension, the overall response is a large decrease in pulmonary vascular resistance (PVR).
- Consequently, when CO is high, e.g., during exercise, there is only a slight increase in pulmonary pressures.
  - Without this recruitment and distension, increasing CO would result in a very high pulmonary artery pressure.

Pulmonary response to hemorrhage

- A large decrease in CO reduces intravascular pulmonary pressures.
- Because these vessels have some elasticity, pulmonary vessels recoil. In addition, there is derecruitment of pulmonary capillaries, both of which contribute to a rise in PVR.
- Consequently, during hemorrhage, there is often only a slight decrease in pulmonary artery pressure.
- Vessel recoil also means less blood is stored in this circuit.

FETAL CIRCULATION

- The general features of the fetal circulatory system are shown in Figure V-2-6.
- The bolded numbers refer to the percent hemoglobin (%HbO_2) saturation.
- Of the fetal CO, 55% goes to the placenta.
- The umbilical vein and ductus venosus have highest %HbO_2 saturation (80%).
- When mixed with inferior vena caval blood (26% HbO_2), the %HbO_2 saturation of blood entering the right atrium is 67%.
- This blood is directed through the foramen ovale to the left atrium, left ventricle, and ascending aorta to perfuse the head and the forelimbs.
- Superior vena caval blood (40% HbO_2) is directed through the tricuspid valve into the right ventricle and pulmonary artery and shunted by the ductus arteriosus to the descending aorta. Shunting occurs because fetal pulmonary vascular resistance is very high, so 90% of the right ventricular output flows into the ductus arteriosus and only 10% to the lungs.
- The percent HbO_2 saturation of aortic blood is 60%.

- Fifty-five percent of the fetal CO goes through the placenta. At birth, the loss of the placental circulation increases systemic resistance. The subsequent rise in aortic blood pressure (as well as the fall in pulmonary arterial pressure caused by the expansion of the lungs) causes a reversal of flow in the ductus arteriosus, which leads to a large enough increase in left atrial pressure to close the foramen ovale.

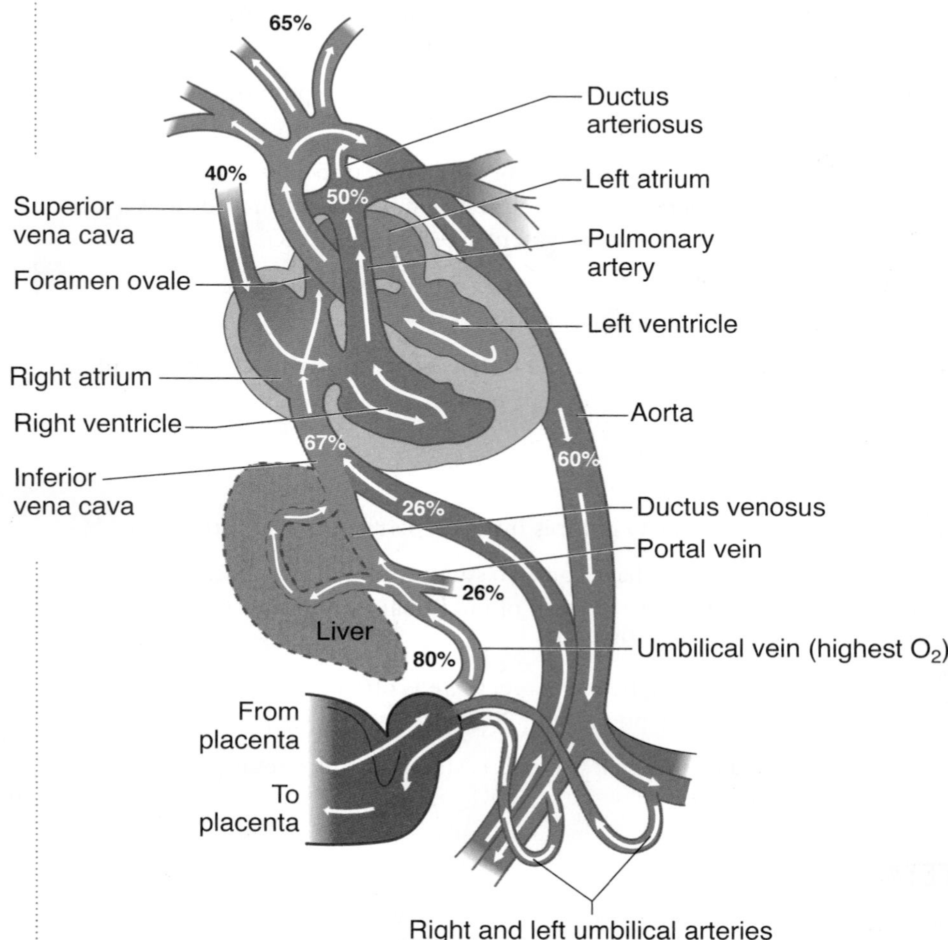

Figure V-2-6. Fetal Circulatory System

CARDIOVASCULAR STRESS: EXERCISE

The following assumes the person is in a steady state, performing moderate exercise at sea level.

Pulmonary Circuit

- Blood flow (CO): large increase
- Pulmonary arterial pressure: slight increase
- Pulmonary vascular resistance: large decrease
- Pulmonary blood volume: increase

- Number of perfused capillaries: increase
- Capillary surface area: increase, i.e., increased rate of gas exchange

Systemic Circuit

Arterial system

- PO_2: no significant change, hemoglobin still fully saturated
- PCO_2: until one approaches maximal O_2 consumption, there is no significant change; thus the increase in ventilation is proportional to the increase in metabolism
- pH: no change or a decrease due mainly to the production of lactic acid
- Mean arterial pressure: slight increase
- Body temperature: slight increase
- Vascular resistance (TPR): large decrease, dilation of skeletal muscle beds

Venous system

- PO_2: decrease
- PCO_2: increase

Regional Circulations

Exercising skeletal muscle

- Vascular resistance decreases.
- Blood flow increases.
- Capillary pressure increases.
- Capillary filtration increases.
- Lymph flow increases.
- As predicted by the Fick principle, oxygen extraction increases and venous PO_2 falls.

Cutaneous blood flow

Initial decrease, then an increase to dissipate heat

Coronary blood flow

Increase due to increased work of the heart

Cerebral blood flow

No significant change (arterial CO_2 remains unchanged)

Renal and GI blood flow

Both decrease

Physical conditioning

- Regular exercise increases maximal oxygen consumption ($\dot{V}O_2max$) by:
  - Increasing the ability to deliver oxygen to the active muscles. It does this by increasing the CO.
  - The resting conditioned heart has a lower heart rate but greater stroke volume (SV) than does the resting unconditioned heart.
  - At any level of exercise, stroke volume is elevated.
  - However, the maximal heart rate remains similar to that of untrained individuals.
- Regular exercise also increases the ability of muscles to utilize oxygen. There are:
  - An increased number of arterioles, which decreases resistance during exercise.
  - An increased capillary density, which increases the surface area and decreases diffusion distance.
  - An increased number of oxidative enzymes in the mitochondria.

Chapter Summary

- The Fick principle defines the relationship of O_2 uptake (consumption), flow, and O_2 extraction.
- The production of vasodilatory metabolites and the myogenic mechanism explains autoregulation of blood flow.
- Sympathetic noradrenergic nerves represent the main control in extrinsically regulated systemic tissues.
- Resting skeletal muscle exhibits extrinsic regulation, but exercising muscle autoregulates.
- Mechanical compression of the intramyocardial vessels restricts perfusion to the myocardium during systole.
- Because oxygen extraction is almost complete from the blood perfusing the myocardium, coronary flow must match myocardial metabolism.
- The main factor regulating cerebral blood flow is arterial carbon dioxide.
- The cutaneous circulation exhibits extrinsic regulation, and flow responds to the need for heat exchange with the environment.
- Normally, the kidney exhibits strong autoregulation but sympathetic noradrenergic nerves can vasoconstrict.
- The compliant nature of the pulmonary circuit minimizes changes in pulmonary pressures with large changes in cardiac output.

SECTION VI

Cardiac Cycle and Valvular Heart Disease

Cardiac Cycle and Valvular Heart Disease

1

Learning Objectives

- ❑ Interpret scenarios on normal cardiac cycle
- ❑ Interpret scenarios on pressure-volume loops
- ❑ Interpret scenarios on valvular dysfunction

NORMAL CARDIAC CYCLE

Figure VI-1-1 illustrates the most important features of the cardiac cycle.

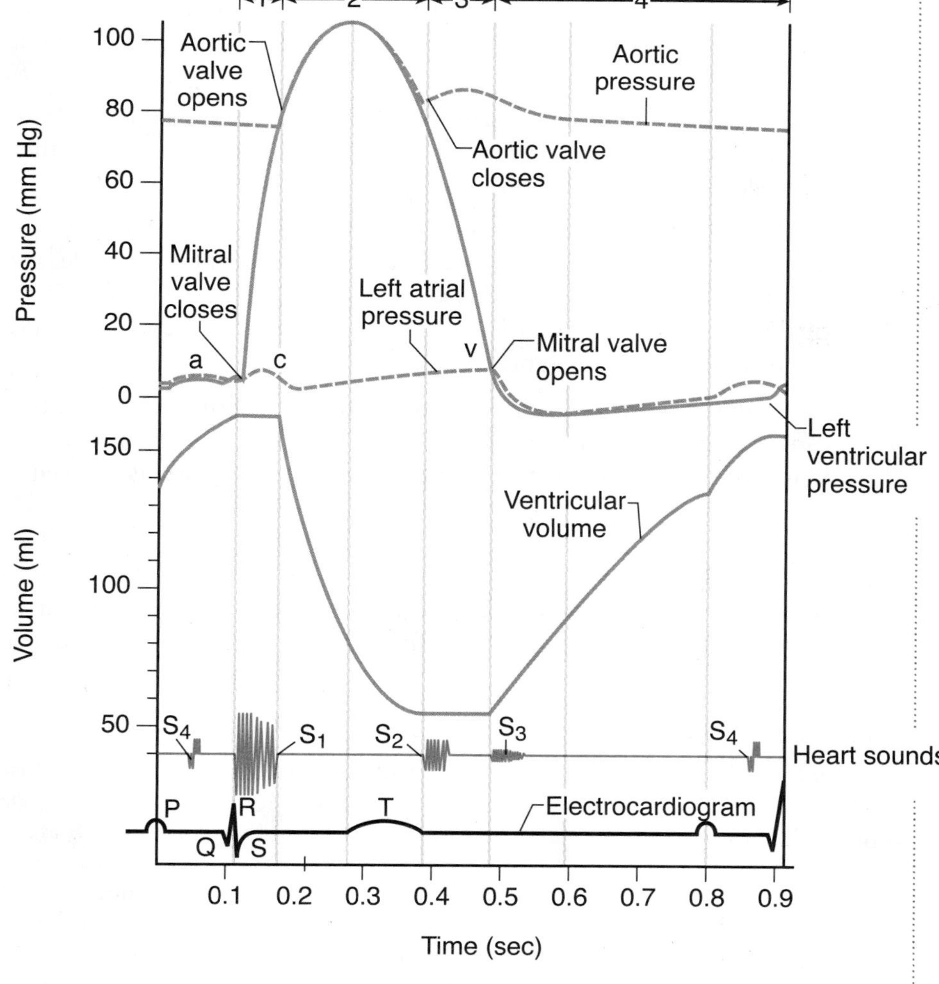

Figure VI-1-1. Cardiac Cycle

The most important aspects of Figure VI-1-1 are the following:

- → QRS → contraction of ventricle → rise in ventricular pressure above atrial pressure → closure of mitral valve
- It is always a pressure difference that causes the valves to open or close.
- Closure of the mitral valve terminates the ventricular filling phase and begins iso-volumetric contraction.
- Isovolumetric contraction—no change in ventricular volume, and both valves (mitral, aortic) closed. Ventricular pressure increases, and volume is equivalent to end-diastolic volume.
- Opening of the aortic valve terminates isovolumetric contraction and begins the ejection phase. The aortic valve opens because pressure in the ventricle slightly exceeds aortic pressure.
- Ejection Phase—ventricular volume decreases, but most rapidly in early stages. Ventricular and aortic pressures increase initially but decrease later in phase.
- Closure of the aortic valve terminates the ejection phase and begins isovolumetric relaxation. The aortic valve closes because pressure in the ventricle goes below aortic pressure. Closure of the aortic valve creates the dicrotic notch.
- Isovolumetric relaxation—no change in ventricular volume, and both valves (mitral, aortic) closed. Ventricular pressure decreases, and volume is equivalent to end-systolic volume.
- Opening of the mitral valve terminates isovolumetric relaxation and begins the filling phase. The mitral valve opens because pressure in the ventricle goes below atrial pressure.
- Filling Phase—the final relaxation of the ventricle occurs after the mitral valve opens and produces a rapid early filling of the ventricle. This rapid inflow will in some cases induce the third heart sound. The final increase in ventricular volume is due to atrial contraction, which is responsible for the fourth heart sound.
- In a young, healthy individual, atrial contraction doesn't provide significant filling of the ventricle. However, the contribution of atrial contraction becomes more important when ventricular compliance is reduced.

Heart Sounds

The systolic sounds are due to the sudden closure of the heart valves. Normally the valves on the left side of the heart close first. Valves on the right side open first.

Systolic sounds

S1: Produced by the closure of the mitral and tricuspid valves. The valves close with only a separation of about 0.01 seconds which the human ear can appreciate only as a single sound.

S2: Produced by the closure of the aortic (A2 component) and pulmonic valves (P2 component). They are heard as a single sound during expiration but during inspiration the increased output of the right heart causes a physiological splitting. The following figure illustrates several situations where splitting of the second heart sound may become audible.

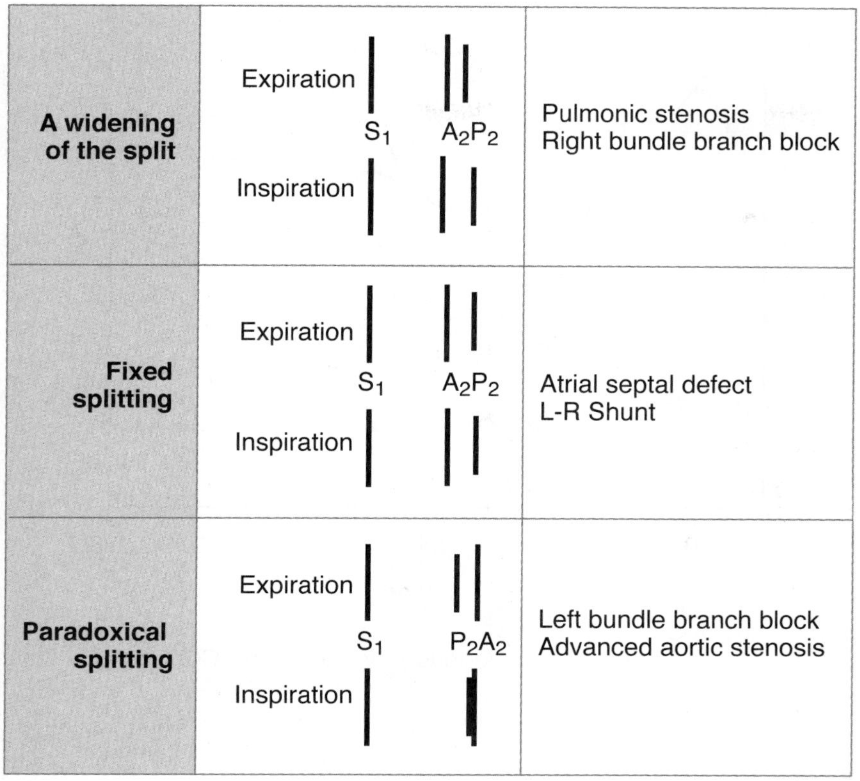

A widening of the split	Expiration / Inspiration; S_1 A_2P_2	Pulmonic stenosis Right bundle branch block
Fixed splitting	Expiration / Inspiration; S_1 A_2P_2	Atrial septal defect L-R Shunt
Paradoxical splitting	Expiration / Inspiration; S_1 P_2A_2	Left bundle branch block Advanced aortic stenosis

Figure VI-1-2. Abnormal Splitting of the Second Heart Sound (S_2)

S3: When it is present, occurs just after the opening of the AV valves during the rapid filling of the ventricle. It tends to be produced by the rapid expansion of a very compliant ventricle and is a normal finding in children and young adults. In older adults it occurs with volume overload and often is a sign of cardiac disease.

S4: Coincident with atrial contraction and is produced when the atrium contracts against a stiff ventricle. Examples include concentric hypertrophy, aortic stenosis, and myocardial infarction.

Venous Pulse

Figure VI-1-3 provides an example of a normal jugular venous pulse tracing. The jugular pulse is generated by changes on the right side of the heart. The pressures will generally vary with the respiratory cycle and are generally read at the end of expiration when intrapleural pressure is at its closest point to zero.

Clinical Correlate

Site of auscultation points:

- Aortic: Second intercostal space on the right side, about mid-clavicular line
- Pulmonic: Second intercostal space on the left side, about mid-clavicular line
- Tricuspid: Fifth intercostal space, just at the left sternal border
- Mitral: Sixth intercostal space on the left side, about mid-clavicular line

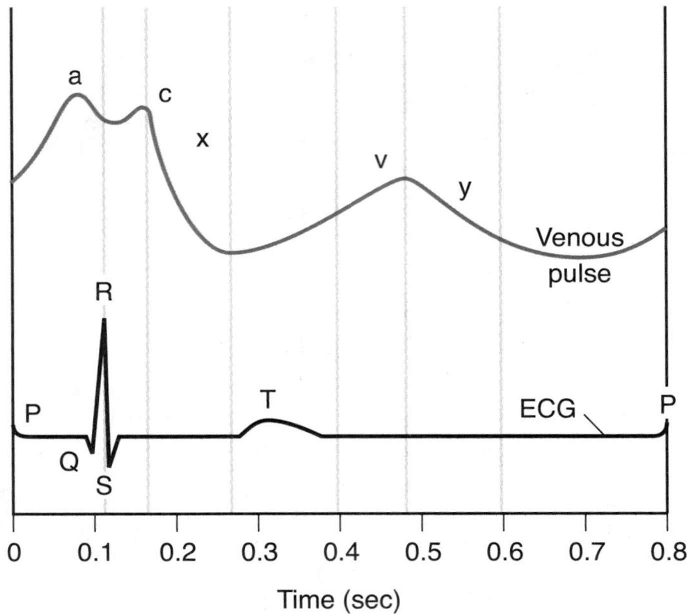

Figure VI-1-3. Venous Pulse and the ECG

a wave

- Highest deflection of the venous pulse and produced by the contraction of the right atrium
- Correlates with the PR interval (see figure)
- Is prominent in a stiff ventricle, pulmonic stenosis, and insufficiency
- Is absent in atrial fibrillation

c wave

- Mainly due to the bulging of the tricuspid valve into the atrium (rise in right atrial pressure)
- Occurs near the beginning of ventricular contraction (is coincident with right ventricular isovolumic contraction)
- Is often not seen during the recording of the venous pulse

x descent

- Produced by a decreasing atrial pressure during atrial relaxation
- Separated into two segments when the c wave is recorded
- Alterations occur with atrial fibrillation and tricuspid insufficiency

v wave

- Produced by the filling of the atrium during ventricular systole when the tricuspid valve is closed
- Corresponds to T wave of the EKG
- A prominent v wave would occur in tricuspid insufficiency and right heart failure

y descent

- Produced by the rapid emptying of the right atrium immediately after the opening of the tricuspid valve
- A more prominent wave in tricuspid insufficiency and a blunted wave in tricuspid stenosis.

Some abnormal venous pulses are shown in the following figure.

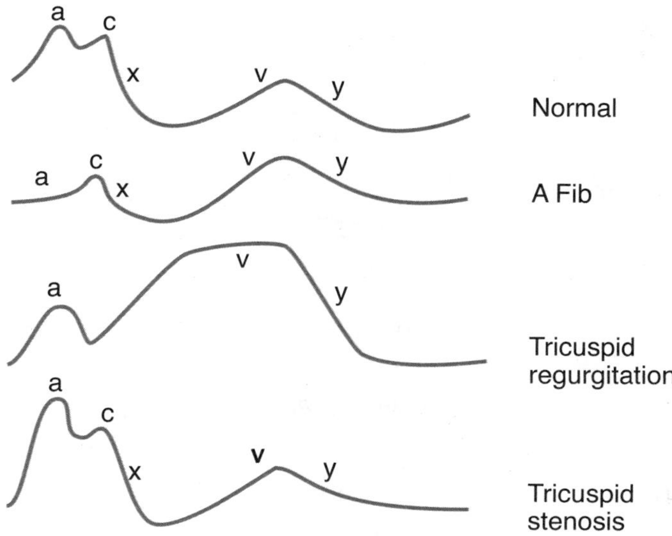

Figure VI-1-4. Normal Versus Abnormal Jugular Pulses

Similar recordings to the systemic venous pulse are obtained when recording pulmonary capillary wedge pressure. Left atrium mechanical events are transmitted in a retrograde manner, although they are somewhat damped and delayed. The figure below shows the pressure recording from the tip of a Swan-Ganz catheter inserted through a systemic vein through the right side of the heart into the pulmonary circulation and finally with the tip wedged in a small pulmonary artery. The pressure recorded at the tip of the catheter is referred to as pulmonary capillary wedge pressure and is close to left atrial pressure and is an index of preload on the left ventricle.

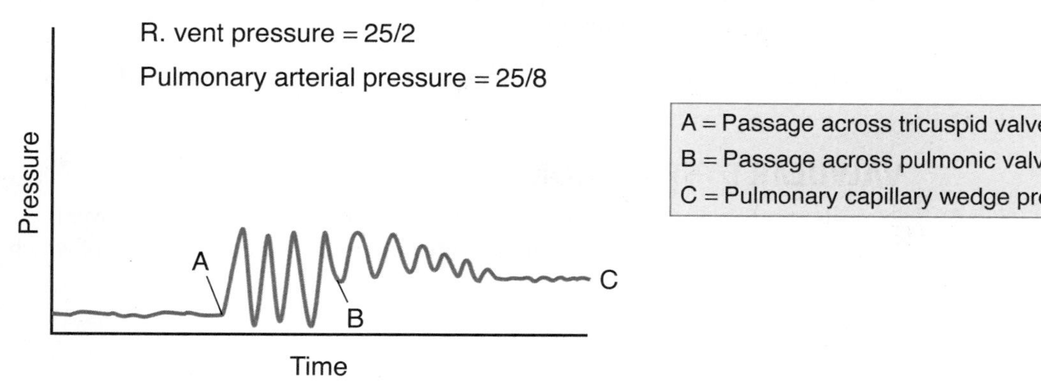

Figure VI-1-5. Swan-Ganz Catheterization

PRESSURE-VOLUME LOOPS

Figure VI-1-6 shows the major features of a left ventricular pressure–volume loop.

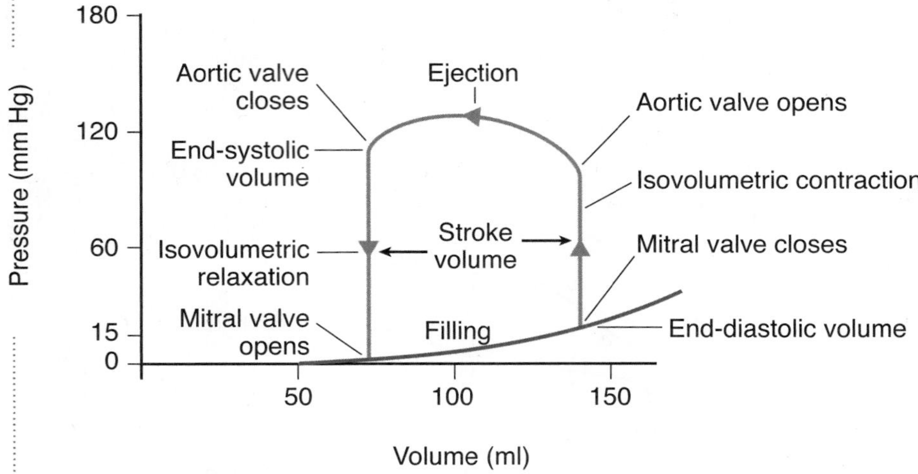

Figure VI-1-6. Left Ventricular Pressure–Volume Loop

- Most of the energy consumption occurs during isovolumetric contraction.
- Most of the work is performed during the ejection phase.

Mechanically Altered States

Aortic insufficiency: Increased preload, increased stroke volume, increased ventricular systolic pressure

- All the cardiac volumes are increased (EDV, ESV, SV)

Heart failure (decreased contractility): Decreased ventricular systolic pressure, increased preload, loop shifts to the right

Essential hypertension (aortic stenosis): Increased ventricular systolic pressure, little change in preload in the early stages

Increased contractility: Increased ventricular systolic pressure, decreased preload, increased ejection fraction, loop shifts to the left

Exercise: Increased ventricular systolic pressure, ejection fraction, and preload.

VALVULAR DYSFUNCTION

Stenosis of valves usually consists of chronic problems that develop slowly over time. Valvular insufficiency problems can be acute or chronic, the consequences of which can be quite different.

Aortic Stenosis

- Pathologic thickening and fusion of the valve leaflets that decreases the open valve area, creating a major resistance point in series with the systemic circuit.
- Large loss in pressure moving the blood through the narrow opening.
- Ventricular systolic pressure increases (increased afterload) to overcome the increased resistance of the aortic valve.
- Pressure overload of the left ventricle leads to a compensatory concentric hypertrophy (new sarcomeres laid down in parallel so that the myofibril thickens) which leads to decreased ventricular compliance (diastolic dysfunction) and coronary perfusion problems and eventually systolic dysfunction.
- Prominent "a" wave of the left atrium as the stiffer left ventricle becomes more dependent on atrial contraction for filling.
- Mean aortic pressure is maintained in the normal range in the early stages of the disorder. Arterial pressure rises slowly and the pulse pressure is reduced.
- There is a pressure gradient between the left ventricle and aorta during ejection.
- Systolic murmur that begins after S1 (midsystolic) which is crescendo-decrescendo in intensity.
- Slow closure of the aortic valve can cause a paradoxical splitting of the second heart sound (aortic valve closes after the pulmonic)

Note

Important considerations when thinking of valvular problems:

- A stenotic valve is a resistor and creates a murmur when the valve is open.
- A regurgitant valve allows backflow of blood and creates a murmur when the valve is normally closed.
- Pressure and volume "behind" the defective valve increases.
  - *Behind* refers to the direction of blood flow, e.g., the left ventricle is behind the aortic valve; the left atrium is behind the mitral valve, etc.

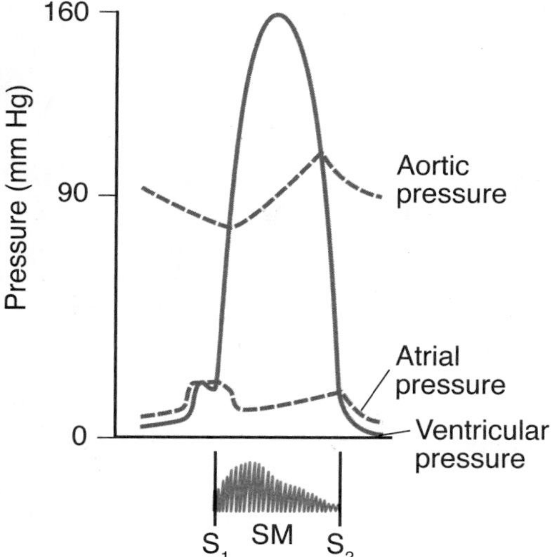

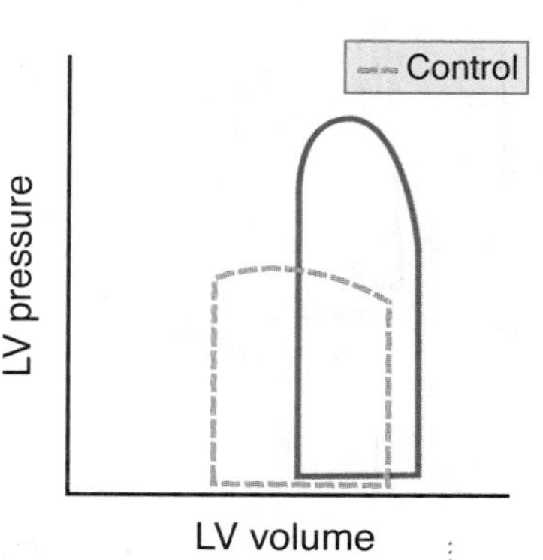

Figure VI-1-7. Aortic Stenosis

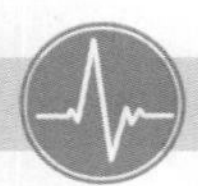

Aortic Insufficiency Regurgitation

The aortic valve does not close properly at the beginning of diastole. As a result, during diastole there is retrograde flow from the aorta into the ventricle.

- Acute insufficiency does not allow development of compensatory mechanisms, which can lead to pulmonary edema and circulatory collapse.
- Very large left ventricles are seen in aortic insufficiency. Large increase in LVEDV (increase preload) but close to normal end diastolic pressures. All the cardiac volumes are increased (EDV, ESV, SV).
- Ventricular failure raises pulmonary pressures and causes dyspnea.
- Increased preload causes increased stroke volume, which results in increased ventricular and aortic systolic pressures.
- Retrograde flow from the aorta to the left ventricle produces a low aortic diastolic pressure (the volume of blood left in the aorta at the end of diastole is rapidly reduced).
- There is no true isovolumetric relaxation and a reduced period of isovolumetric contraction.
- Aortic insufficiency is characterized by a large aortic pulse pressure and a low aortic diastolic pressure (hence the bounding pulse).
- Dilation of the ventricle produces a compensatory eccentric hypertrophy.

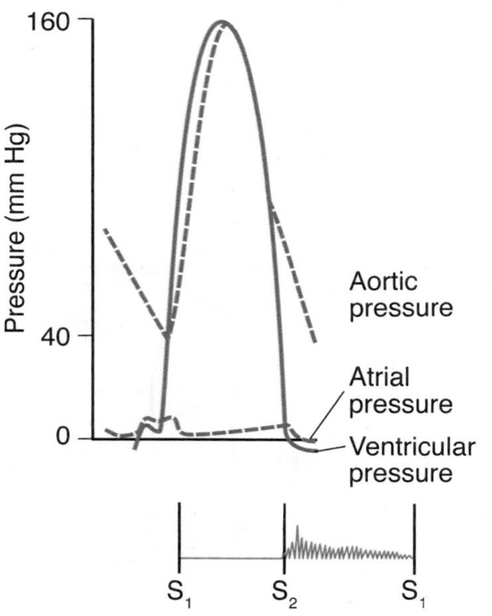

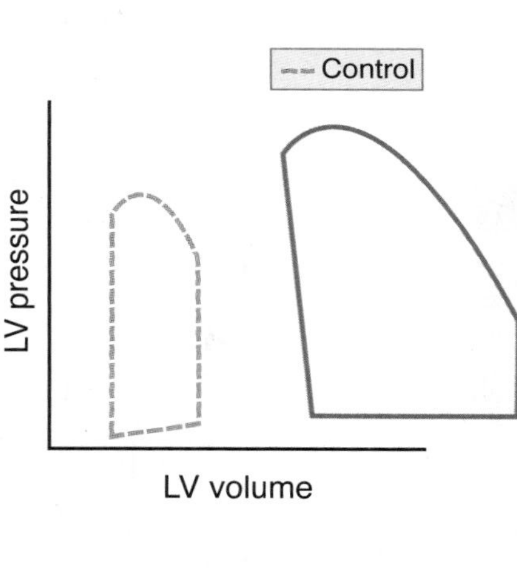

Figure VI-1-8. Aortic Insufficiency (Regurgitation) / (Diastolic Rumble ≈ Austin Flint Murmur)

Mitral Stenosis

- A narrow mitral valve impairs emptying of the left atrium (LA) into the left ventricle (LV) during diastole. This creates a pressure gradient between the atrium and ventricle during filling.
- Pressure and volume can be dramatically elevated in the left atrium, dilation of the left atrium over time, which is accelerated with atrial fibrillation.
- Thrombi appear in the enlarged left atrium
- Left atrial pressures are elevated throughout the cardiac cycle. Increased left atrial pressures transmitted to the pulmonary circulation and the right heart.
- Little change or a decrease in the size of the left ventricle. Systolic function normal.
- Diastolic murmur begins after S2 and is associated with altered atrial emptying; a late diastolic murmur and an exaggerated "a" wave are associated with atrial contraction.

Clinical Correlate

The opening snap (OS) to S2 interval is inversely related to left atrial pressure. A short OS:S2 interval is a reliable indicator of severe mitral stenosis.

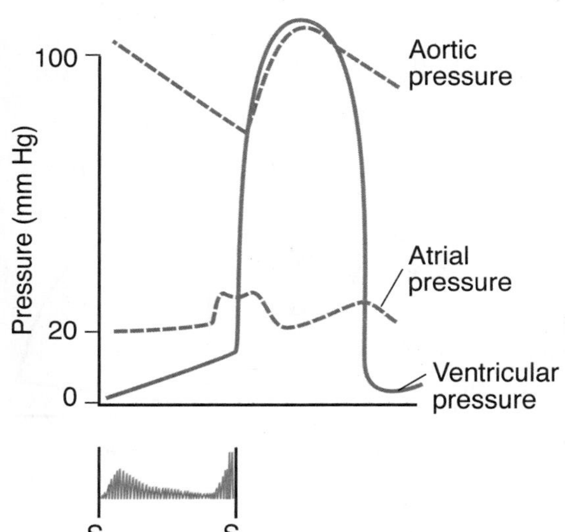

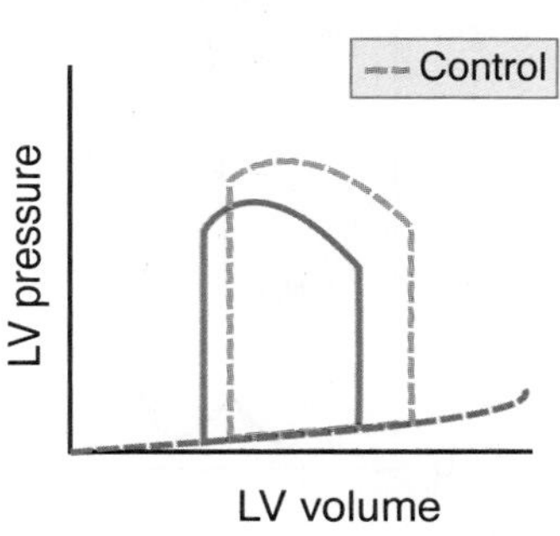

Figure VI-1-9. Mitral Stenosis

Mitral Insufficiency Regurgitation

- Acute mitral insufficiency can cause a sudden dramatic rise in pulmonary pressures and pulmonary edema.
- Can result from structural abnormalities in the valve itself, papillary muscles, chordae tendinae, or possibly a structural change in the mitral annulus.
- No true isovolumetric contraction. Regurgitation of blood from the left ventricle to the left atrium throughout ventricular systole.
- Atrial volumes and pressures increased but chronic dilation of the atrium prevents a dramatic rise in atrial pressures.
- Ventricular volumes and pressures are increased during diastole. Most patients develop chronic compensated left ventricular dilation and hypertrophy, then at some point the left ventricle cannot keep up with the demand and decompensated heart failure develops.
- Increased preload but with reduced afterload.
- Systolic murmur that begins at S1 (pansystolic).

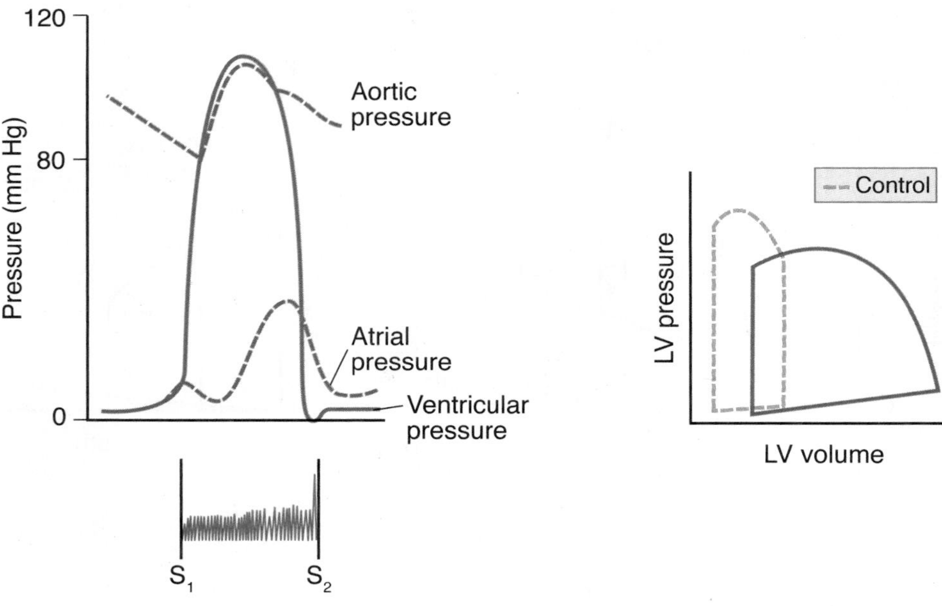

Figure VI-1-10. Mitral Insufficiency (Regurgitation)

Chapter Summary

- The cardiac cycle consists of isovolumetric contraction followed by the ejection phase followed by isovolumetric relaxation followed by the filling phase.
- The heart valves normally close on the left side before they close on the right.
- S1 the first systolic sound is due to the closure of the AV valves, and S2 the second systolic sound is due to the closure of the aortic and pulmonic valves.
- The diastolic sounds S3 and S4 are often not heard.
- An increased output of the right heart, as occurs during inspiration, produces an audible splitting of the second heart sound.
- The venous pulse recorded from a systemic vein reflects right heart events.
- A pressure–volume loop represents the changes in pressure and volume for a single cardiac cycle.
- Aortic stenosis increases afterload and produces a pressure gradient between the ventricle and aorta during ejection (midsystolic murmur).
- Aortic insufficiency increases preload and produces a retrograde flow from the aorta into the ventricle during isovolumetric relaxation (diastolic murmur begins at S2).
- Mitral stenosis increases left atrial volume and pressure, but ventricular volumes and pressures are normal or reduced (diastolic murmur begins after S2).
- Mitral insufficiency increases volumes and pressures in the atrium and ventricle (systolic murmur begins at S1).

SECTION VII

Respiration

Lung Mechanics 1

Learning Objectives

- ❑ Answer questions about overview of the respiratory system
- ❑ Interpret scenarios on lung volumes and capacities
- ❑ Solve problems concerning ventilation
- ❑ Use knowledge of lung mechanics
- ❑ Answer questions about cardiovascular changes with ventilation
- ❑ Solve problems concerning positive-pressure ventilation
- ❑ Answer questions about pneumothorax
- ❑ Use knowledge of lung compliance
- ❑ Interpret scenarios on airway resistance
- ❑ Explain information related to pulmonary function testing

OVERVIEW OF THE RESPIRATORY SYSTEM

The purpose of understanding lung mechanics is to view them in the big clinical picture of pulmonary function test (PFT) interpretation. The PFT is the key diagnostic test for the pulmonologist, just as the EKG is to the cardiologist. PFTs consist of three individual tests (covered in greater detail in the *Respiratory* section):

1. Measurements of static lung compartments (meaning lung volumes)
2. Airflow used to evaluate dynamic compliance using a spirometer
3. Alveolar membrane permeability using carbon monoxide as a marker of diffusion

LUNG VOLUMES AND CAPACITIES

Figure VII-1-1 shows graphically the relationships among the various lung volumes and capacities. Clinical measurements of specific volumes and capacities provide insights into lung function and the origin of disease processes. Those that provide the greatest information display an *.

The values for the volumes and capacities given below are typical for a 70 kg male.

Tidal volume (V_T): amount of air that enters or leaves the lung in a single respiratory cycle (500 mL)

Functional residual capacity (FRC): amount of gas in the lungs at the end of a passive expiration; the neutral or equilibrium point for the respiratory system (2,700 mL) ; it is a marker for lung compliance

Inspiratory capacity (IC): maximal volume of gas that can be inspired from FRC (4,000 mL)

Inspiratory reserve volume (IRV): additional amount of air that can be inhaled after a normal inspiration (3,500 mL)

Expiratory reserve volume (ERV): additional volume that can be expired after a passive expiration (1,500 mL)

Residual volume (RV): amount of air in the lung after a maximal expiration (1,200 mL)

Vital capacity (VC): maximal volume that can be expired after a maximal inspiration (5,500 mL)

Total lung capacity (TLC): amount of air in the lung after a maximal inspiration (6,700 mL)

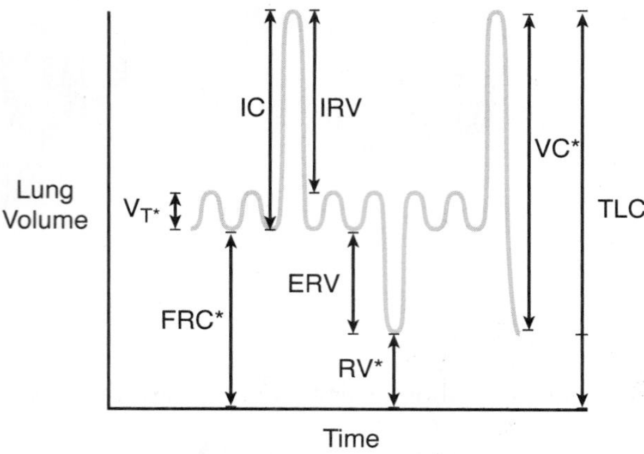

Figure VII-1-1. Lung Volumes and Capacities

A spirometer can measure only changes in lung volume. As such, it cannot measure the residual volume (RV) or any capacity containing RV. Thus, TLC and FRC cannot be measured using simple spirometry; an indirect method must be used. Three common indirect methods are helium dilution, nitrogen washout, and plethysmography.

VENTILATION

Total Ventilation

Total ventilation is also referred to as minute volume or minute ventilation. It is the total volume of air moved in or out (usually the volume expired) of the lungs per minute.

$$\dot{V}_E = V_T \times f$$

Normal resting values would be:

$V_T = 500$ mL

$f = 15$

500 mL × 15/min = 7,500 mL/min

> $\dot{V}_E$ = total ventilation
>
> V_T = tidal volume
>
> f = respiratory rate

Dead Space

Regions of the respiratory system that contain air but are not exchanging O_2 and CO_2 with blood are considered dead space.

Anatomic dead space

Airway regions that, because of inherent structure, are not capable of O_2 and CO_2 exchange with the blood. Anatomic dead space (anatV_D) includes the conducting zone, which ends at the level of the terminal bronchioles. Significant gas exchange (O_2 uptake and CO_2 removal) with the blood occurs only in the alveoli.

The size of the anatV_D in mL is approximately equal to a person's weight in pounds. Thus a 150-lb individual has an anatomic dead space of 150 mL.

In a Nutshell

What is the function of functional residual capacity (FRC)?

Answer: Breathing is cyclic, while blood flow through the pulmonary capillary bed is continuous. During the respiratory cycle, there are short periods of apneas at the end of inspiration and expiration when there is no ventilation but there is continuous blood flow. Without the FRC acting as a buffer for continued gas exchange during apneic periods, these conditions would in effect create an intrapulmonary shunt, inducing deoxygenated blood from the pulmonary capillaries to empty into the pulmonary veins.

Composition of the anatomic dead space and the respiratory zone

The respiratory zone is a very constant environment. Under resting conditions, rhythmic ventilation introduces a small volume into a much larger respiratory zone. Thus, the partial pressure of gases in the alveolar compartment changes very little during normal rhythmic ventilation.

Composition at the End of Expiration (Before Inspiration)

- At the end of an expiration, the anatV_D is filled with air that originated in the alveoli or respiratory zone.
- Thus, the composition of the air in the entire respiratory system is the same at this static point in the respiratory cycle.
- This also means that a sample of expired gas taken near the end of expiration (end tidal air) is representative of the respiratory zone.
- This situation is illustrated in Figure VII-1-2.

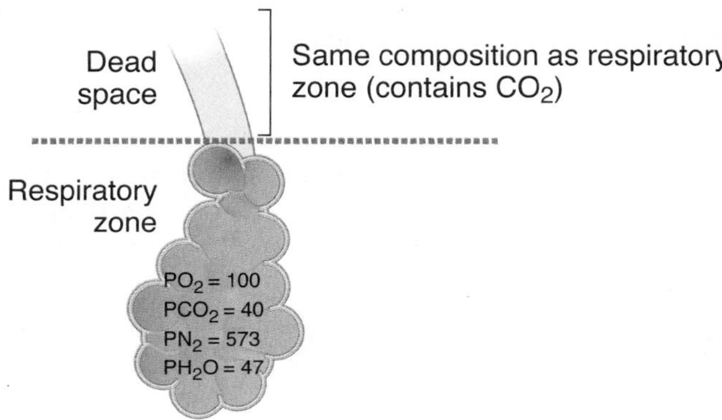

Figure VII-1-2. End of Expiration

Composition at the End of Inspiration (Before Expiration)

- The first 150 mL of air to reach the alveoli comes from the anatV_D.
- It is air that remained in the dead space at the end of the previous expiration and has the same composition as alveolar gas.
- After the first 150 mL enters the alveoli, room air is added to the respiratory zone.
- At the end of inspiration the anatV_D is filled with room air.
- The presence of the anatV_D implies the following: in order to get fresh air into the alveoli, one must always take a tidal volume larger than the volume of the anatV_D. This is illustrated in Figure VII-1-3.

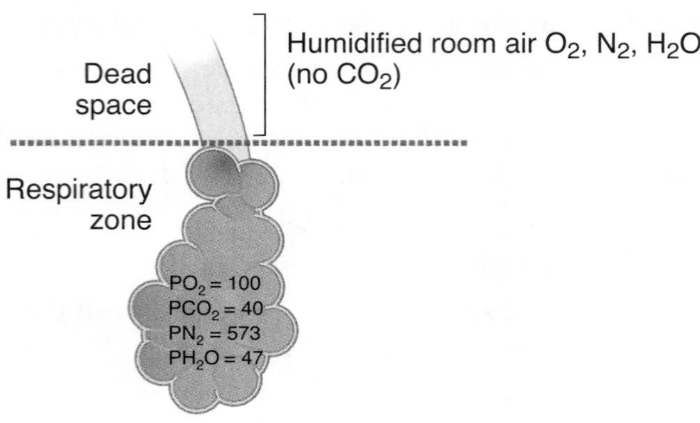

Figure VII-1-3. End of Inspiration

Alveolar dead space

Alveolar dead space ($alvV_D$) refers to alveoli containing air but without blood flow in the surrounding capillaries. An example is a pulmonary embolus.

Physiologic dead space

Physiologic dead space ($physioIV_D$) refers to the total dead space in the lung system ($anatV_D + alvV_D$). When the physiol V_D is greater than the $anatV_D$, it implies the presence of $alvV_D$, i.e., somewhere in the lung, alveoli are being ventilated but not perfused.

Total ventilation

$$V = VT\ (f)$$
$$= 500\ (15)$$
$$= 7{,}500\ mL/min$$

Minute ventilation ($\dot{V}$) is the total volume of air entering the lungs per minute.

Alveolar Ventilation

Alveolar ventilation $\dot{V}_A$ represents the room air delivered to the respiratory zone per breath.

- The first 150 mL of each inspiration comes from the anatomic dead space and does not contribute to alveolar ventilation.
- However, every additional mL beyond 150 does contribute to alveolar ventilation.

$$\dot{V}_A = (V_T - V_D)\ f$$
$$= (500\ mL - 150\ mL)\ 15 = 5250\ mL/min$$

$\dot{V}_A$: alveolar ventilation

V_T: tidal volume

V_D: dead space

f: respiratory rate

The alveolar ventilation per inspiration is 350 mL. This equation implies that the volume of fresh air that enters the respiratory zone per minute depends on the pattern of breathing (how large a V_T and the rate of breathing).

Increases in the Depth of Breathing

There are equal increases in total and alveolar ventilation per breath, since dead space volume is constant.

If the depth of breathing increases from a depth of 500 mL to a depth of 700 mL, the increase in total and alveolar ventilation is 200 mL per breath.

Increases in the Rate of Breathing

There is a greater increase in total ventilation per minute than in alveolar ventilation per minute, because the increased rate causes increased ventilation of dead space and alveoli.

For every additional inspiration with a tidal volume of 500 mL, total ventilation increases 500 mL, but alveolar ventilation only increases by 350 mL (assuming dead space is 150 mL).

For example, given the following, which person has the greater alveolar ventilation?

	Tidal Volume	Rate	Total Ventilation
Person A	600 mL	10/min	6,000 mL/min
Person B	300 mL	20/min	6,000 mL/min

Answer: Person A. Person B has rapid, shallow breathing. This person has a large component of dead-space ventilation (first 150 mL of each inspiration). Even though total ventilation may be normal, alveolar ventilation is decreased. Therefore, the individual is hypoventilating.

In rapid, shallow breathing, total ventilation may be above normal, but alveolar ventilation may be below normal.

LUNG MECHANICS

Muscles of Respiration

Inspiration

The major muscle of inspiration is the diaphragm. Contraction of the diaphragm enlarges the vertical dimensions of the chest. Also utilized are the external intercostal muscles of the chest wall. Contraction of these muscles causes the ribs to rise and thus increases the anterior-posterior dimensions of the chest.

Expiration

Under resting conditions, expiration is normally a passive process, i.e., it is due to the relaxation of the muscles of inspiration and the elastic recoil of the lungs. For a forced expiration, the muscles of the abdominal wall and the internal intercostals contract. This compresses the chest wall down and forces the diaphragm up into the chest.

Included would be external oblique, rectus abdominal, internal oblique, and transverse abdominal muscles.

- Increased compliance means more air will flow for a given change in pressure.
- Reduced compliance means less air will flow for a given change in pressure.
- In the preceding curve, although the slope is changing during inflation, its value at any point is the lung's compliance. It is the relationship between the change in lung volume (tidal volume) and the change in intrapleural or surrounding pressure.
- The steeper the line, the more compliant the lungs. Restful breathing works on the steepest, most compliant part of the curve.
- With a deep inspiration, the lung moves toward the flatter part of the curve, and thus it has reduced compliance. Lung compliance is less at TLC compared to FRC.

Figure VII-1-10 shows pathologic states in which lung compliance changes.

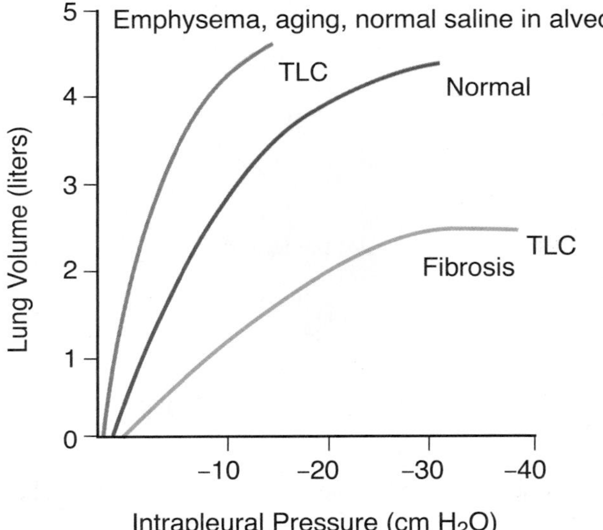

Figure VII-1-10. Lung Compliance

Increased lung compliance also occurs with aging and with a saline-filled lung.

In summary:

- Compliance is an index of the effort required to expand the lungs (to overcome recoil). It does not relate to airway resistance.
- Compliance decreases as the lungs are inflated because the curve is not a straight line.
- For any given fall in intrapleural pressure, large alveoli expand less than small alveoli.
- Very compliant lungs (easy to inflate) have low recoil. Stiff lungs (difficult to inflate) have a large recoil force.

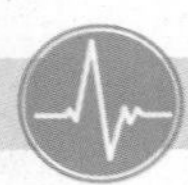

Components of Lung Recoil

Lung recoil has the following components:

- **The tissue itself;** more specifically, the collagen and elastin fibers of the lung.

  The larger the lung, the greater the stretch of the tissue and the greater the recoil force.

- **The surface tension forces in the fluid lining the alveoli.** Surface tension forces are created whenever there is a liquid–air interface (Figure VII-1-11).

  Surface tension forces tend to reduce the area of the surface and generate a pressure. In the alveoli, they act to collapse the alveoli; therefore, these forces contribute to lung recoil.

- **Surface tension forces are the greatest component of lung recoil.**

  The relationship between the surface tension and the pressure inside a bubble is given by the law of LaPlace.

$$P \propto \frac{T}{r}$$

P: pressure

T: tension

r: radius

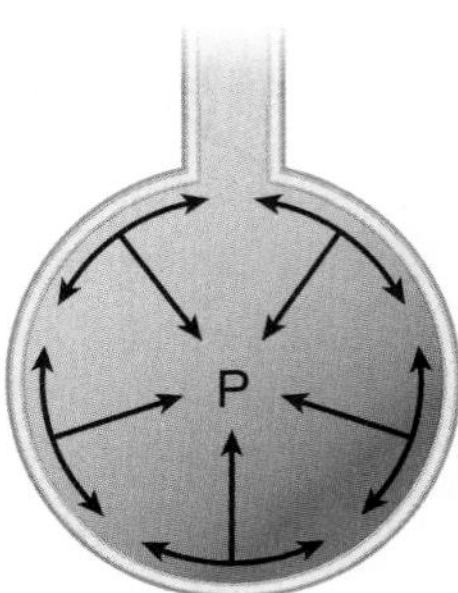

Figure VII-1-11. Surface Tension

If wall tension is the same in two bubbles, the smaller bubble will have the greater pressure.

Although the situation is more complex in the lung, it follows that small alveoli tend to be unstable. They have a great tendency to empty into larger alveoli and collapse (creating regions of atelectasis). This is illustrated in Figure VII-1-12. Collapsed alveoli are difficult to reinflate.

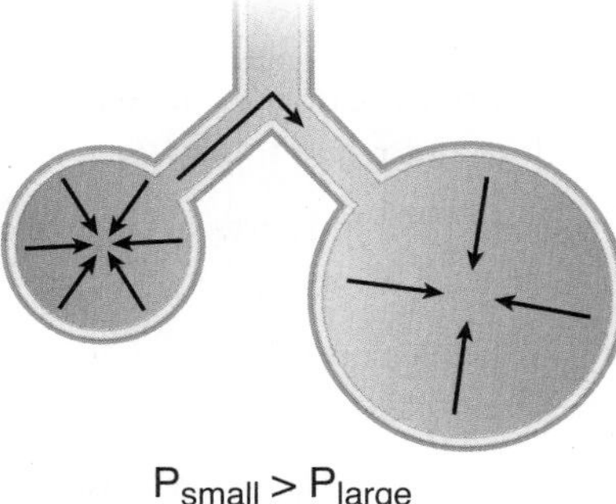

$P_{small} > P_{large}$

Figure VII-1-12. Atelectasis

If the alveoli were lined with a simple electrolyte solution, lung recoil would be so great that lungs theoretically should not be able to inflate. This is prevented by a chemical (produced by alveolar type II cells), surfactant, in the fluid lining a normal lung.

Surfactant has 2 main functions:

- It lowers surface tension forces in the alveoli. In other words, surfactant lowers lung recoil and increases compliance.
- It lowers surface tension forces more in small alveoli than in large alveoli. This promotes stability among alveoli of different sizes by decreasing the tendency of small alveoli to collapse (decreases the tendency to develop atelectasis).

Respiratory Distress Syndrome (RDS)

Infant respiratory distress syndrome (hyaline membrane disease) is a deficiency of surfactant.

Adult respiratory distress syndrome (ARDS) is an acute lung injury via the following:

- Bloodstream—Sepsis—develops from injury to the pulmonary capillary endothelium, leading to interstitial edema and increased lymph flow. This leads to injury and increased permeability of the alveolar epithelium and alveolar edema. The protein seepage into the alveoli reduces the effectiveness of surfactant. Neutrophils have been implicated in the progressive lung injury from sepsis.
- Airway—Gastric aspirations—direct acute injury to the lung epithelium increases permeability of the epithelium followed by edema.

Curve A in Figure VII-1-13 represents respiratory distress syndrome. The curve is shifted to the right, and it is a flatter curve (lung stiffer).

- A greater change in intrapleural pressure is required to inflate the lungs.
- The tendency for collapse is increased, thus PEEP is sometimes provided.

Curve B represents atelectasis.

- Once alveoli collapse, it is difficult to reinflate them.
- Note the high TPP required to open atelectic alveoli (green line, B in Figure VII-1-13).

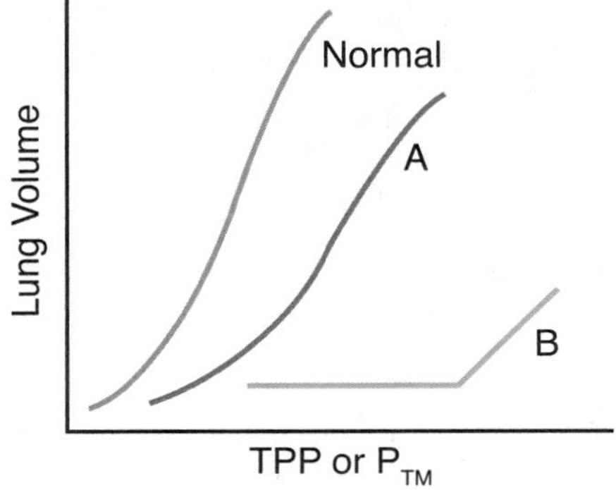

Figure VII-1-13. Deficiency of Surfactant

AIRWAY RESISTANCE

Radius of an Airway

$$\text{Resistance} = \frac{1}{\text{radius}^4}$$

In the branching airway system of the lungs, it is the first and second bronchi that represent most of the airway resistance.

- Parasympathetic nerve stimulation produces bronchoconstriction. This is mediated by M3 receptors. In addition, M3 activation increases airway secretions.
- Circulating catecholamines produce bronchodilation. Epinephrine is the endogenous agent and it bronchodilates via β2 receptors.

Mechanical Effect of Lung Volume

Figure VII-1-14 demonstrates the mechanical effect of lung volume.

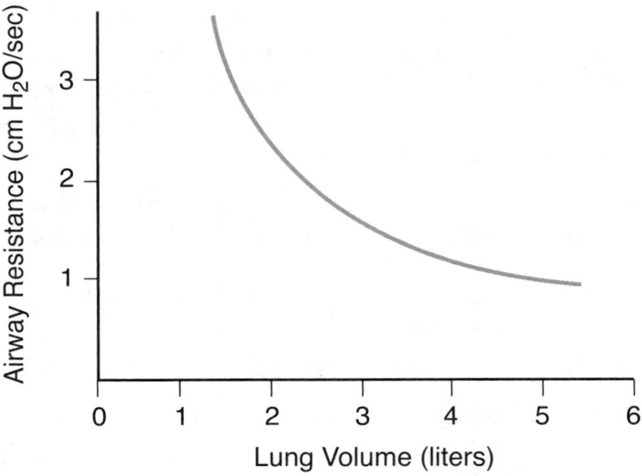

Figure VII-1-14. Airway Resistance

The figure illustrates that, as lung volume increases, airway resistance decreases. The mechanisms for this are:

- **P_{TM}:** To get to high lung volumes, IPP becomes more and more negative. This increases the P_{TM} across small airways, causing them to expand. The result is decreased resistance.
- **Radial traction:** The walls of alveoli are physically connected to small airways. Thus, as alveoli expand, they pull open small airways. The result is decreased resistance.

PULMONARY FUNCTION TESTING

Vital Capacity (VC)

The VC is the maximum volume of air that an individual can move in a single breath. The most useful assessment of the VC is to expire as quickly and forcefully as possible, i.e., a "timed" or forced vital capacity (FVC). During the FVC maneuver, the volume of air exhaled in the first second is called the forced expiratory volume in 1 sec (FEV_1). This is illustrated in Figure VII-1-15.

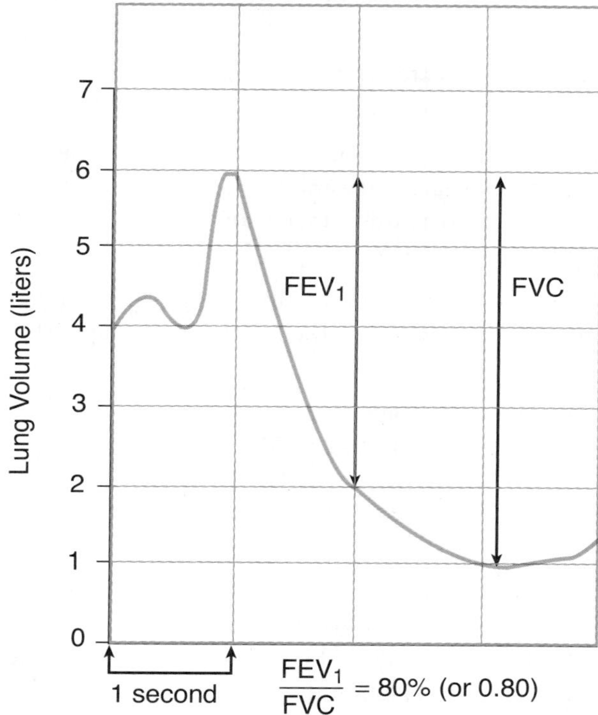

Figure VII-1-15. Pulmonary Function Test of Forced Vital Capacity (FVC)

Note

Figure VII-1-15 and the following figures differ from the output of a spirometer, because they show actual lung volumes (including residual volume) instead of showing only changes in volume.

There are 2 key pieces of data from a pulmonary function test (PFT) involving the measurement of FVC:

- **FVC:** This is total volume exhaled.
  - Because age, gender, body size, etc., can influence the absolute amount of FVC, it is expressed as a percent of predicted (100% of predicted being the "ideal").
- **FEV1 (forced expiratory volume in 1 second):** Although this volume can provide information on its own, it is commonly compared to the FVC such that one determines the FEV1/FVC ratio.
  - This ratio creates a flow parameter; 0.8 (80%) or greater is considered normal.
- Thus, this PFT provides a volume and a flow.
- Restrictive pulmonary disease is characterized by reduced volume (low FVC, but normal flow).
- Obstructive disease is characterized by reduced flow (low FEV1/FVC)

Physiology of a PFT

The picture on the left of Figure VII-1-16 shows that at the end of an inspiratory effort to TLC, IPP is very negative. This negative IPP exists throughout the lungs during a passive expiration and thus the P_{TM} is positive for both alveoli and airways.

The picture on the right of Figure VII-1-16 shows the situation during a maximal forced expiration.

- A forced expiration compresses the chest wall down and in, creating a positive IPP. The level of positive IPP generated is dependent upon effort.
- This forced expiration creates a very positive alveolar pressure, in turn creating a large pressure gradient to force air out of the lungs.
- However, this positive IPP creates a negative P_{TM} in the airways. It is more negative in the large airways, e.g., trachea and main-stem bronchi. These regions have structural support and thus do not collapse even though P_{TM} is very negative.
- Moving down the airways toward alveoli, the negative P_{TM} ultimately compresses airways that lack sufficient structural support. This is dynamic compression of airways.
- This compression of airways creates a tremendous resistance to airflow. In fact, the airway may collapse, producing infinite resistance. Regardless, this compression creates a level of resistance that overwhelms any and all other resistors that exist in the circuit and is thus the dominant resistor for airflow.
- Once this occurs, elastic recoil of the lung becomes the effective driving force for airflow and airflow becomes independent of the effort. This means airflow is a property of the patient's respiratory system, hence the reason this test is very diagnostic.
- Because this resistance is created in small airways, the entire volume of the lungs cannot be expired, creating residual volume (RV).

Because PFTs measure flow (FEV1/FVC) and volume, they accurately diagnose obstructive (low flow) and restrictive disease (low volume, normal flow).

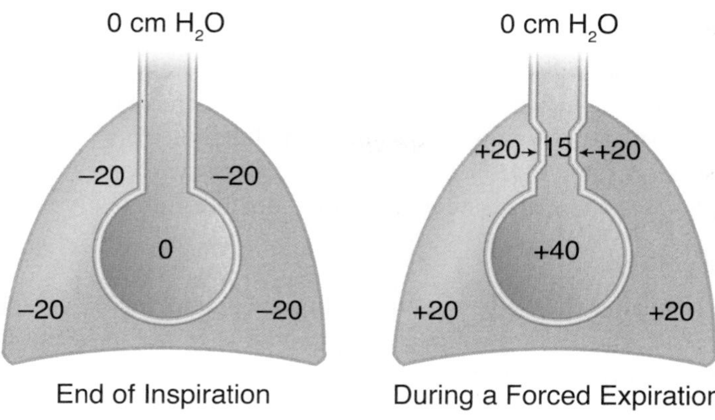

Figure VII-1-16. Dynamic Airway Compression

Obstructive versus Restrictive Patterns

The following figures (Figures VII-1-17 and VII-1-18) demonstrate a standard pulmonary function test, the measurement of FVC, FEV_1, and FEV_1/FVC.

Obstructive pulmonary disease

Obstructive disease is characterized by an increase in airway resistance that is measured as a decrease in expiratory flow. Examples are chronic bronchitis, asthma, and emphysema.

Obstructive pattern

- Total lung capacity (TLC) is normal or larger than normal, but during a maximal forced expiration from TLC, a smaller than normal volume is slowly expired.
- Depending upon the severity of the disease, FVC may or may not be reduced. If severe enough, then FVC is diminished.

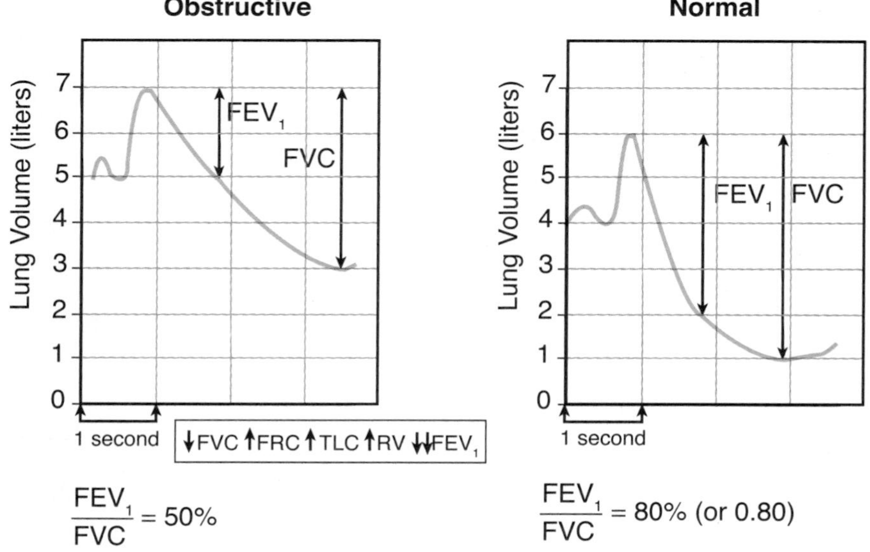

Figure VII-1-17. Obstructive Pattern

Bridge to Pathology

There are 4 basic pathologic alterations that can occur in obstructive disease:

- Bronchoconstriction
- Hypersecretion
- Inflammation
- Destruction of lung parenchyma (emphysema)

Bridge to Pharmacology

Treatment of obstructive disease includes β2-agonists (short- and long-acting), M3 blockers such as ipratropium, PDE inhibitors, mast cell stabilizers, leukotriene-receptor blockers, and steroids.

Restrictive pulmonary disease

Restrictive pulmonary disease is characterized by an increase in elastic recoil—a decrease in lung compliance—which is measured as a decrease in all lung volumes. Reduced vital capacity with low lung volumes are the indicators of restrictive pulmonary diseases. Examples are acute respiratory distress syndrome (ARDS) and interstitial lung diseases such as sarcoidosis and idiopathic pulmonary fibrosis (IPF).

Restrictive pattern

- TLC is smaller than normal, but during a maximal forced expiration from TLC, the smaller volume is expired quickly and more completely than in a normal pattern.
- Therefore, even though FEV_1 is also reduced, the FEV_1/FVC is often increased.
- However, the critical distinction is low FVC with low FRC and RV.

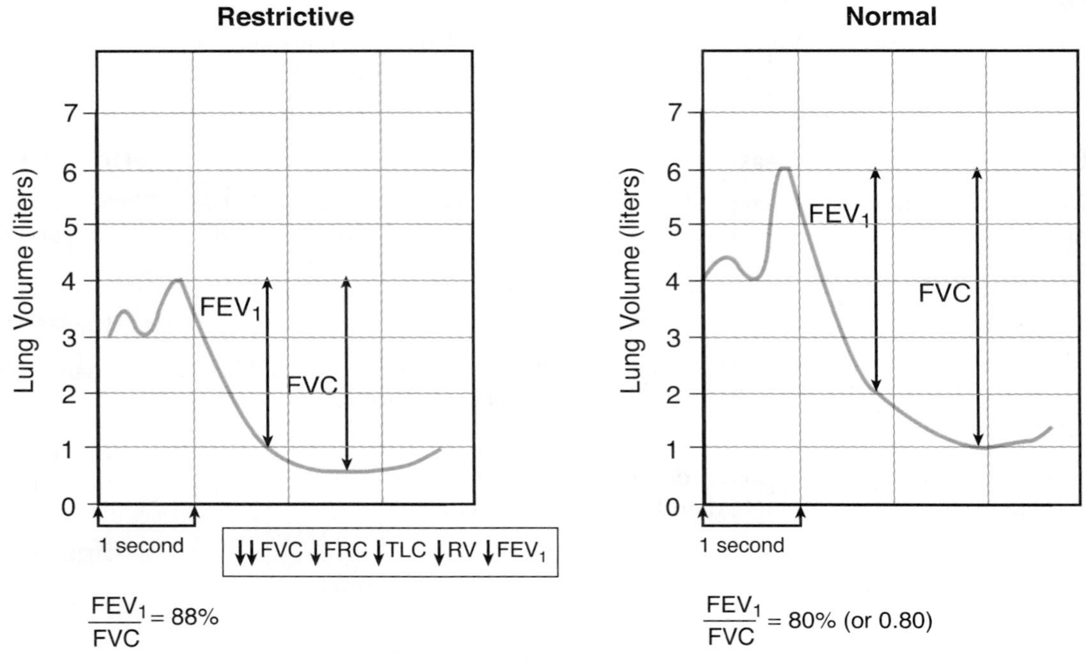

Figure VII-1-18. Restrictive Pattern

Table VII-1-1. Summary of Obstructive Versus Restrictive Pattern

Variable	Obstructive Pattern (e.g., Emphysema)	Restrictive Pattern (e.g., Fibrosis)
TLC	↑	↓↓
FEV_1	↓↓	↓
FVC	↓	↓↓
FEV_1/FVC	↓	↑ or normal
Peak flow	↓	↓
FRC	↑	↓
RV	↑	↓

FVC is always decreased when pulmonary function is significantly compromised.

A decrease in FEV_1/FVC ratio is evidence of an obstructive pattern. A normal or increased FEV_1/FVC ratio is evidence of a restrictive pattern, but a low TLC is diagnostic of restrictive lung disease.

Flow–Volume Loops

The instantaneous relationship between flow (liters/sec) and lung volume is useful in determining whether obstructive or restrictive lung disease is present. In the loop shown in Figure VII-1-19, expiration starts at total lung capacity and continues to residual volume. The width of the loop is the FVC.

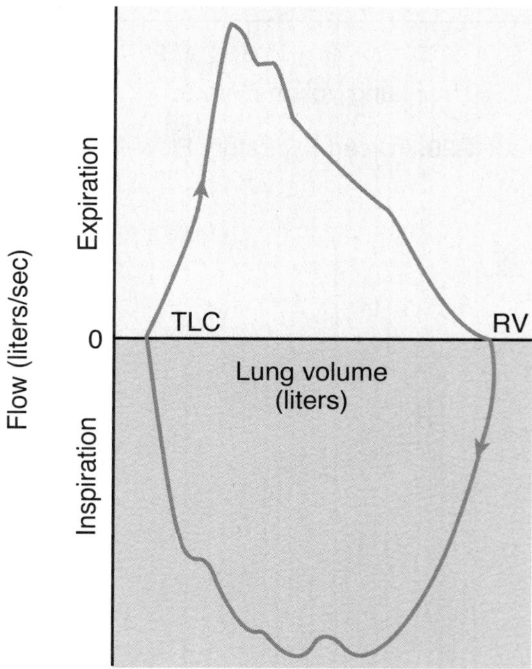

Figure VII-1-19. Flow–Volume Loop

Loops found in obstructive and restrictive disease are shown in Figure VII-1-20.

Obstructive disease

In obstructive disease, the flow–volume loop begins and ends at abnormally high lung volumes, and the expiratory flow is lower than normal. In addition, the downslope of expiration "scallops" or "bows" inward. This scalloping indicates that at any given lung volume, flow is less. Thus, airway resistance is elevated (obstructive).

Restrictive disease

In restrictive disease, the flow–volume loop begins and ends at unusually low lung volumes. Peak flow is less, because overall volume is less. However, when expiratory flow is compared at specific lung volumes, the flow in restrictive disease is somewhat greater than normal.

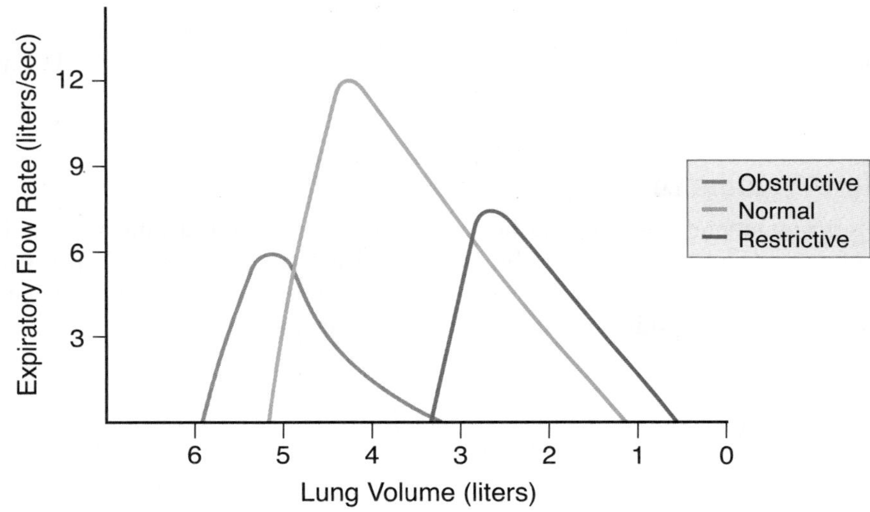

Figure VII-1-20. Forced Expiratory Flow–Volume Loop

Chapter Summary

- Functional residual capacity is the equilibrium point of the respiratory system. Residual volume is the air remaining in the respiratory system after a maximal expiration. Vital capacity is the difference between total lung capacity and residual volume.
- Dead space is air in the respiratory system that is not exchanging gas with capillary blood.
- The first 150 mL of an inspiration fills the anatomical dead space with room air. This volume contributes to total but not alveolar ventilation. Alveolar ventilation represents the inspired volume beyond 150 mL. It is the inspired air that actually reaches the respiratory zone.
- Inspiration decreases IPP, which in turn causes P_{TM} to increase. This increases alveolar volume, which decreases alveolar pressure.
- During restful breathing, intrapleural pressure is always negative. It becomes more negative during inspiration and more positive (less negative) during expiration. Alveolar pressure is slightly negative during inspiration and slightly positive during expiration.
- Compliant lungs are easy to inflate and possess low recoil. Noncompliant or stiff lungs are difficult to inflate and have a large recoil force.
- The main component of lung recoil is the surface tension forces of the fluid lining the alveoli. Surfactant reduces surface tension forces.
- A deficiency of surfactant reduces lung compliance and promotes atelectasis and the development of pulmonary edema.
- A maximal expiration is associated with a partial collapse of the small airways, which increases resistance and limits the maximum flow rate.
- An obstructive pattern is often associated with a diminished FEV_1/FVC, elevated TLC, FRC, and RV.
- A restrictive pattern is associated with a normal FEV_1/FVC, but a reduced FVC, TLC, FRC, and RV.

Alveolar–Blood Gas Exchange 2

Learning Objectives

- ❑ Answer questions about the normal lung
- ❑ Solve problems concerning factors affecting alveolar PCO_2
- ❑ Use knowledge of factors affecting alveolar PO_2
- ❑ Interpret scenarios on alveolar-blood gas transfer: Fick law of diffusion
- ❑ Use knowledge of diffusing capacity of the lung

THE NORMAL LUNG

Partial Pressure of a Gas in Ambient Air

$$Pgas = Fgas \times Patm$$

By convention, the partial pressure of the gas is expressed in terms of its dry gas concentration. For example, the PO_2 in ambient air is:

$$PO_2 = 0.21 \times 760 = 160 \text{ mm Hg}$$

Patm: atmospheric pressure

Pgas: partial pressure of a gas

Fgas: concentration of a gas

Partial Pressure of a Gas in Inspired Air

Inspired air is defined as air that has been inhaled, warmed to 37°C, and completely humidified, but has not yet engaged in gas exchange. It is the fresh air in the anatV_D that is about to enter the respiratory zone.

The partial pressure of H_2O is dependent only on temperature and at 37°C is 47 mm Hg. Humidifying the air reduces the partial pressure of the other gases present.

$$PIgas = Fgas\,(Patm - PH_2O)$$

PIgas: partial pressure of inspired gas

PH_2O: partial pressure of H_2O vapor

For example, the PO_2 of inspired air is:

$$PIO_2 = 0.21(760 - 47) = 150 \text{ mm Hg}$$

Figure VII-2-1 shows the pressures of oxygen and carbon dioxide in the alveolar, pulmonary end capillary, and systemic arterial blood.

In a Nutshell

Dalton's law of partial pressures states that the total pressure exerted by a mixture of gases is the sum of the pressures exerted independently by each gas in the mixture. Also, the pressure exerted by each gas (its partial pressure) is directly proportional to its percentage in the total gas mixture.

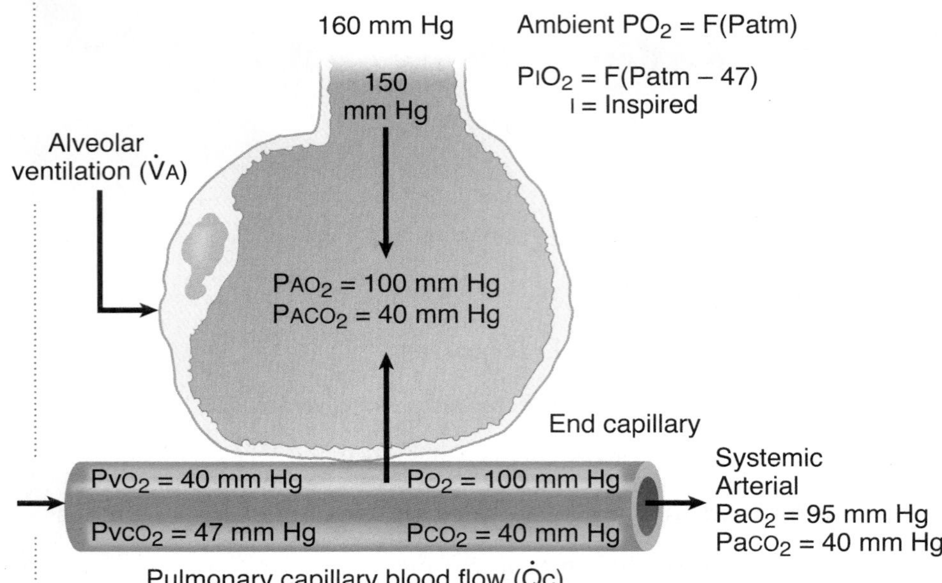

Figure VII-2-1. Pulmonary Capillary Gases

A = alveolar
a = systemic arterial

- Under normal conditions, the PO_2 and PCO_2 in the alveolar compartment and pulmonary end capillary blood are the same (perfusion-limited).
- There is a slight change (PO_2 ↓) between the end capillary compartment and systemic arterial blood because of a small but normal shunt through the lungs.
- Alveolar–systemic arterial PO_2 differences = A – a O_2 gradient.
- This difference (5–10 mm Hg) often provides information about the cause of a hypoxemia.

FACTORS AFFECTING ALVEOLAR PCO_2

Only two factors affect alveolar PCO_2: metabolic rate and alveolar ventilation.

$$P_ACO_2 \propto \frac{\text{metabolic } CO_2 \text{ production}}{\text{alveolar ventilation}}$$

At rest, unless there is fever or hypothermia, CO_2 production is relatively constant; so you can use changes of P_ACO_2 to evaluate alveolar ventilation.

Alveolar Ventilation

There is an inverse relationship between P_ACO_2 and alveolar ventilation. This is the main factor affecting alveolar PCO_2. Therefore, if ventilation increases, P_ACO_2 decreases; if ventilation decreases, P_ACO_2 increases.

Hyperventilation

During hyperventilation, there is an inappropriately elevated level of alveolar ventilation, and P_ACO_2 is depressed.

If $\dot{V}_A$ is doubled, then P_ACO_2 is decreased by half.

e.g., $P_ACO_2 = 40$ mm Hg

$2 \times \dot{V}_A$; $P_ACO_2 = 20$ mm Hg

Hypoventilation

During hypoventilation, there is an inappropriately depressed level of alveolar ventilation, and P_ACO_2 is elevated.

If $\dot{V}_A$ is halved, then P_ACO_2 is doubled.

e.g., $P_ACO_2 = 40$ mm Hg

$1/2\ \dot{V}_A$; $P_ACO_2 = 80$ mm Hg

Metabolic Rate

There is a direct relationship between alveolar PCO_2 and body metabolism. For P_ACO_2 to remain constant, changes in body metabolism must be matched with equivalent changes in alveolar ventilation.

- If $\dot{V}_A$ matches metabolism, then P_ACO_2 remains constant.
- For example, during exercise, if body metabolism doubles, then $\dot{V}_A$ must double if P_ACO_2 is to remain constant.
- If body temperature decreases and there is no change in ventilation, P_ACO_2 decreases, and the individual can be considered to be hyperventilating.

FACTORS AFFECTING ALVEOLAR PO_2

Alveolar Air Equation

The alveolar air equation includes all the factors that can affect alveolar PO_2.

$$P_AO_2 = (P_{atm} - 47)F_IO_2 - \frac{P_ACO_2}{RQ}$$

Practical application of the equation includes differential diagnosis of hypoxemia by evaluating the alveolar arterial (A–a) gradient of oxygen.

Three important factors can affect P_AO_2:

Patm = atmospheric pressure, at sea level 760 mm Hg

An increase in atmospheric pressure (hyperbaric chamber) increases alveolar PO_2, and a decrease (high altitude) decreases alveolar PO_2.

F_IO_2 = fractional concentration of oxygen, room air 0.21

In a Nutshell

What is the difference between respiratory quotient (RQ) and respiratory exchange ratio (RER)?

Answer: RQ is the ratio between CO_2 production and O_2 consumption at the cellular level. RER is the ratio of CO_2 output and oxygen uptake occurring in the lung. In a steady state, RQ and RER are equal.

An increase in inspired oxygen concentration increases alveolar PO_2.

$$\mathbf{P_ACO_2} = \text{alveolar pressure of carbon dioxide, normally 40 mm Hg}$$

An increase in alveolar PCO_2 decreases alveolar PO_2, and a decrease in alveolar PCO_2 increases alveolar PO_2. For most purposes, you can use arterial carbon dioxide ($PaCO_2$) in the calculation.

The fourth variable is RQ.

$$RQ = \text{respiratory exchange ratio} = \frac{CO_2 \text{ produced mL/min}}{O_2 \text{ consumed mL/min}} \text{; normally 0.8}$$

For example, a person breathing room air at sea level would have:

$$PAO_2 = (760 - 47)\ 0.21 - 40/0.8 = 100 \text{ mm Hg}$$

Effect of $PACO_2$ on PAO_2

PIO_2 = P inspired O_2, i.e., the PO_2 in the conducting airways during inspiration

Because P_ACO_2 affects alveolar PO_2, hyperventilation and hypoventilation also affect P_AO_2.

Hyperventilation (e.g., P_ACO_2 = 20 mm Hg)

$$P_AO_2 = P_IO_2 - P_ACO_2 \text{ (assume R = 1)}$$

normal = 150 – 40 = 110 mm Hg

hyperventilation = 150 – 20 = 130 mm Hg

Hypoventilation (e.g., P_ACO_2 = 80 mm Hg)

normal = 150 – 40 = 110 mm Hg

hypoventilation = 150 – 80 = 70 mm Hg

ALVEOLAR–BLOOD GAS TRANSFER: FICK LAW OF DIFFUSION

Simple diffusion is the process of gas exchange between the alveolar compartment and pulmonary capillary blood. Thus, those factors that affect the rate of diffusion also affect the rate of exchange of O_2 and CO_2 across alveolar membranes. (An additional point to remember is that each gas diffuses independently.)

$\dot{V}$gas = rate of gas diffusion

$$\dot{V}\mathbf{gas} = \frac{\mathbf{A}}{\mathbf{T}} \times \mathbf{D} \times (\mathbf{P_1} - \mathbf{P_2})$$

Two structural factors and two gas factors affect the rate of diffusion.

Structural Features That Affect the Rate of Diffusion

A = surface area for exchange, ↓ in emphysema, ↑ in exercise

T = thickness of the membranes between alveolar gas and capillary blood, ↑ in fibrosis and many other restrictive diseases

A structural problem in the lungs is any situation in which there is a loss of surface area and/or an increase in the thickness of the membrane system between the alveolar air and the pulmonary capillary blood. In all cases, the rate of oxygen and carbon dioxide diffusion decreases. The greater the structural problem, the greater the effect on diffusion rate.

Factors Specific to Each Gas Present

D (diffusion constant) = main factor is solubility

The only clinically significant feature of D is solubility. The more soluble the gas, the faster it diffuses across the membranes. CO_2 is the most soluble gas with which we will be dealing. The great solubility of CO_2 is the main reason why it diffuses faster across the alveolar membranes than O_2.

Gradient across the membrane

($P_1 - P_2$): This is the gas partial pressure difference across the alveolar membrane. The greater the partial pressure difference, the greater the rate of diffusion.

Under resting conditions, when blood first enters the pulmonary capillary, the gradient for O_2 is:

$$100 - 40 = 60 \text{ mm Hg}$$

An increase in the PO_2 gradient across the lung membranes helps compensate for a structural problem. If supplemental O_2 is administered, alveolar PO_2 increases, because of the elevated gradient. However, supplemental O_2 does not improve the ability of the lungs to remove CO_2 from blood. This increased gradient helps return the rate of O_2 diffusion toward normal. The greater the structural problem, the greater the gradient necessary for a normal rate of O_2 diffusion.

The gradient for CO_2 is $47 - 40 = 7$ mm Hg.

Even though the gradient for CO_2 is less than for O_2, CO_2 still diffuses faster because of its greater solubility.

DIFFUSING CAPACITY OF THE LUNG (DLCO)

There are 2 terms that describe the dynamics of the transfer of individual substances between the interstitium and the capillary:

- If the substance equilibrates between the capillary and interstitium, it is said to be in a **perfusion-limited situation**.
- If the substance does not equilibrate between the capillary and interstitium, it is said to be in a **diffusion-limited situation**.

Carbon monoxide is a unique gas in that it typically doesn't equilibrate between the alveolar air and the capillary blood. Thus, it is a diffusion-limited gas. This is taken advantage of clinically, and the measurement of the uptake of CO in mL/min/mm Hg is referred to as the diffusing capacity of the lung. It is an index of the lung's structural features.

Carbon Monoxide: A Gas That Is Always Diffusion Limited

Carbon monoxide has an extremely high affinity for hemoglobin. When it is present in the blood, it rapidly combines with hemoglobin, and the amount dissolved in the plasma is close to zero (therefore, partial pressure in the plasma is considered zero). Thus, the alveolar partial pressure gradient ($P_1 - P_2$) is simply P_1 (alveolar partial pressure), since P_2 is considered to be zero. At a constant and known alveolar partial pressure, the uptake of carbon monoxide depends only on the structural features of the lung, as illustrated in Figure VII-2-2.

$$\dot{V}gas = \frac{A}{T} \times D \times (P_1 - P_2)$$

$$\dot{V}CO = \frac{A}{T} \times D \times P_ACO$$

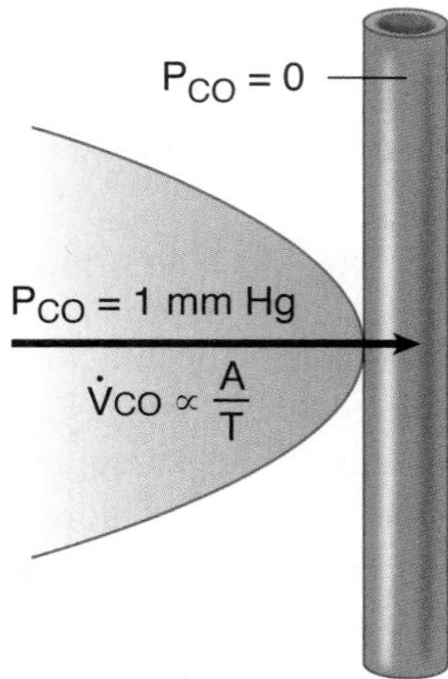

Figure VII-2-2. Carbon Monoxide

- This measured uptake of carbon monoxide is called the diffusing capacity of the lung (DL; mL/min/mm Hg).
- It is an index of overall surface area and membrane thickness.
- With a structural problem, it correlates with the extent of lung damage and is particularly useful when measured serially over time.
- DL (rate of CO diffusion) decreases in emphysema and fibrosis but increases during exercise.

Chapter Summary

- In a normal resting individual at sea level, the partial pressures of oxygen and carbon dioxide are not different between the alveolar and pulmonary end capillary compartments (PO_2 = 100 mm Hg and PCO_2 = 40 mm Hg).
- P_ACO_2 is the same as alveolar, but P_AO_2 is less than alveolar (A–a gradient), which is primarily the result of shunt blood flow.
- Only two factors affect alveolar PCO_2: body metabolism and alveolar ventilation. If body metabolism is constant, there is an inverse relationship between alveolar ventilation and alveolar PCO_2.
- Three important factors affect alveolar PO_2: atmospheric pressure, oxygen concentration in the inspired air, and alveolar PCO_2.
- A change in alveolar PCO_2 causes a change in alveolar PO_2. They change in opposite directions by approximately the same amount in mm Hg.
- Two structural factors and two gas factors affect the rate of gas diffusion across lung membranes.
- Diffusing capacity is directly proportional to membrane surface area and inversely proportional to membrane thickness.
- The partial pressure gradient is the driving force for diffusion.
- Because CO_2 is an extremely soluble gas, it diffuses across the lung membranes faster than oxygen even though it has a small gradient.
- Supplemental oxygen raises the oxygen gradient and can compensate for a diffusion problem.
- Diffusing capacity of the lung is an index of the overall surface area and membrane thickness. It is measured as the uptake of CO from the alveolar air to the blood in mL/min/mm Hg.

Transport of O_2 and CO_2 and the Regulation of Ventilation

3

Learning Objectives

- ❑ Interpret scenarios on transport of oxygen
- ❑ Answer questions about transport of carbon dioxide
- ❑ Interpret scenarios on neural regulation of alveolar ventilation
- ❑ Answer questions about respiratory stress: unusual environments

TRANSPORT OF OXYGEN

Units of Oxygen Content

Oxygen content = concentration of oxygen in the blood, e.g., arterial blood
= 20 volumes %
= 20 volumes of oxygen per 100 volumes of blood
= 20 mL of oxygen per 100 mL of blood
= 0.2 mL of oxygen per mL of blood

Dissolved Oxygen

Oxygen dissolves in blood and this dissolved oxygen exerts a pressure. Thus, PO_2 of the blood represents the pressure exerted by the dissolved gas, and this PO_2 is directly related to the amount dissolved (Figure VII-3-1).

The amount dissolved (PO_2) is the primary determinant for the amount of oxygen bound to hemoglobin (Hb).

There is a direct linear relationship between PO_2 and dissolved oxygen (Figure VII-3-1). When PO_2 is 100 mm Hg, 0.3 mL O_2 is dissolved in each 100 mL of blood (0.3 vol%). Maximal hyperventilation can increase the PO_2 in blood to 130 mm Hg (0.4 vol%).

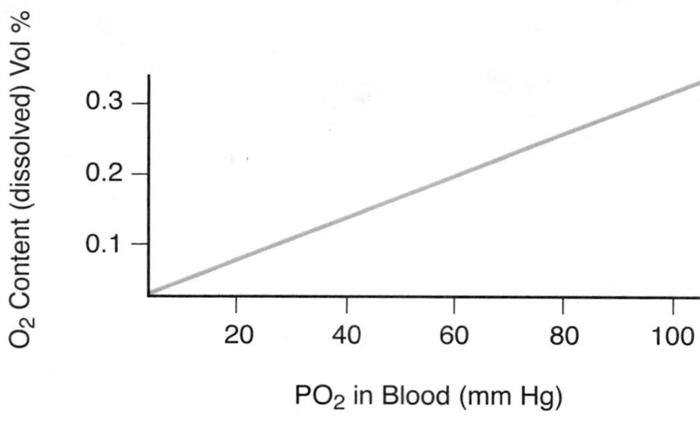

Figure VII-3-1. Dissolved Oxygen in Plasma

Oxyhemoglobin

Each Hb molecule can attach and carry up to four oxygen molecules. Binding sites on Hb have different affinities for oxygen. Also, the affinity of a site can and does change as oxygen is loaded or unloaded from the Hb molecule and as the chemical composition of the plasma changes.

Site 4 – O_2 attached when the minimal $PO_2 \cong 100$ mm Hg	systemic arterial blood = 97% saturated
Site 3 – O_2 attached when the minimal $PO_2 \cong 40$ mm Hg	systemic venous blood = 75% saturated (resting state)
Site 2 – O_2 attached when the minimal $PO_2 \cong 26$ mm Hg	P_{50} for arterial blood. P_{50} is the PO_2 required for 50% saturation

Site 1 – O_2 usually remains attached under physiologic conditions. Under physiologic conditions, only sites 2, 3, and 4 need to be considered.

Most of the oxygen in systemic arterial blood is oxygen attached to Hb. The only significant form in which oxygen is delivered to systemic capillaries is oxygen bound to Hb.

Hemoglobin O_2 Content

The number of mL of oxygen carried in each 100 mL of blood in combination with Hb depends on the Hb concentration [Hb]. Each gram of Hb can combine with 1.34 mL of O_2.

If the [Hb] is 15 g/100 mL (15 g%), then the maximal amount of O_2 per 100 mL (100% saturation) in combination with Hb is:

$$1.34([Hb]) = 1.34(15) = 20 \text{ mL } O_2/100 \text{ mL blood} = 20 \text{ vol\%}$$

This volume represents the "carrying capacity" of the blood.

The Hb in systemic arterial blood is about 97% saturated with oxygen, which means slightly less than 20 vol% is carried by Hb.

When blood passes through a systemic capillary, it is the dissolved oxygen that diffuses to the tissues. However, if dissolved oxygen decreases, PO_2 also decreases, and there is less force to keep oxygen attached to Hb. Oxygen comes off Hb and dissolves in the plasma to maintain the flow of oxygen to the tissues.

Hyperventilation or supplementing the inspired air with additional oxygen in a normal individual can significantly increase the PaO2 but has effect on total oxygen content. For example:

	Dissolved O_2	HbO_2	Total O_2 Content
If PaO_2 = 100 mm Hg	0.3	≅ 19.4	≅ 19.7 vol%
If PaO_2 = 130 mm Hg (hyperventilation)	0.4	≅ 19.4	≅ 19.8 vol%

Oxygen–Hb Dissociation Curves

Figure VII-3-2 represents 3 major points on the oxygen–hemoglobin dissociation curve. The numbered sites refer to the hemoglobin site numbers discussed just previously.

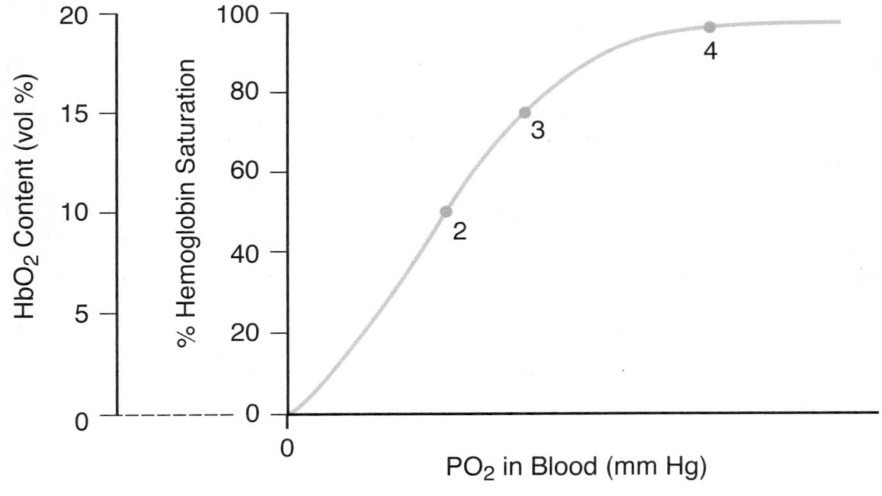

Figure VII-3-2. Oxygen–Hb Dissociation Curves

Shifting the curve

The following factors shift the curve to the right: increased CO_2 (Bohr effect), increased hydrogen ion (decrease pH), increased temperature, increased 2,3-bisphosphoglycerate (2,3-BPG).

In each case, the result can be explained as a reduced affinity of the Hb molecule for oxygen. However, carrying capacity is not changed, and systemic arterial blood at a PO_2 of 100 mm Hg is still close to 100% saturation.

The opposite chemical changes shift the curve to the left.

Figure VII-3-3 shows the result of a shift in the O2–Hb dissociation curve. Note that only points on the steep part of the curve are affected.

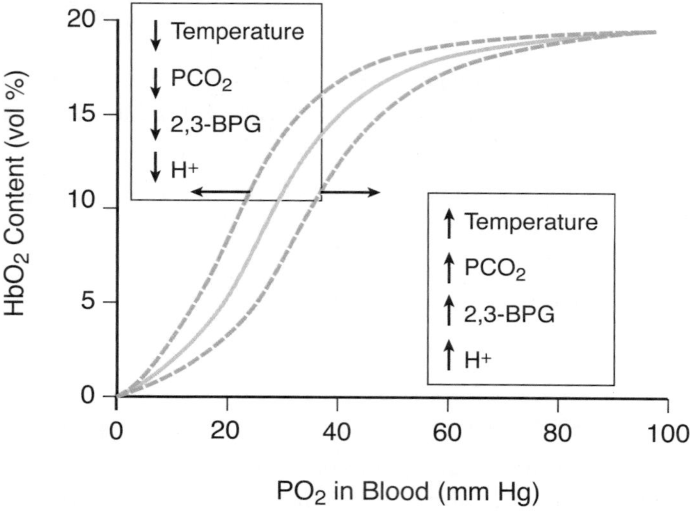

Figure VII-3-3. Shifts in Hb-O_2 Dissociation Curve

Shift to the Right	Shift to the Left
Easier for tissues to extract oxygen	More difficult for tissues to extract oxygen
Steep part of curve, O_2 content decreased	Steep part of curve, O_2 content increased
P_{50} increased	P_{50} decreased

Stored blood loses 2,3-bisphosphoglycerate, causing a left shift in the curve, while hypoxia stimulates the production of 2,3-bisphosphoglycerate, thereby causing a right shift.

Hb Concentration Effects

Anemia

Characterized by a reduced concentration of Hb in the blood.

Polycythemia

Characterized by a higher than normal concentration of Hb in the blood.

P_{50}

In simple anemia and polycythemia, the P_{50} does not change without tissue hypoxia; e.g., a PO_2 of 26 mm Hg produces 50% saturation of arterial hemoglobin.

Figure VII-3-4 illustrates the effects of an increase and a decrease in hemoglobin concentration. The main change is the plateau or carrying capacity of the blood. Note that the point halfway up each curve, the P_{50}, is still close to 26 mm Hg.

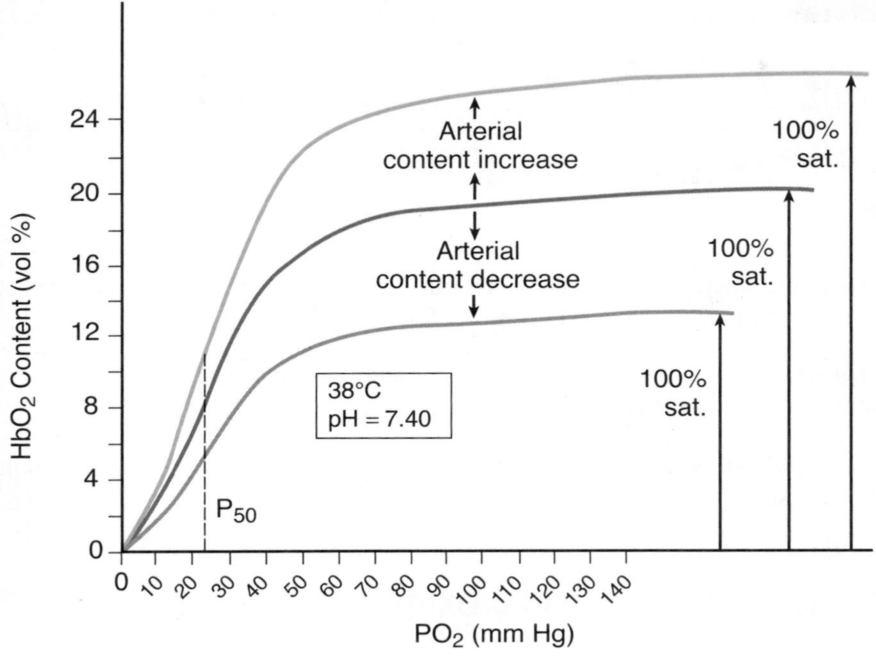

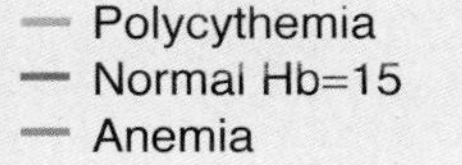

Figure VII-3-4. Effect of Hemoglobin Content on O_2 Content

Effects of Carbon Monoxide

Carbon monoxide (CO) has a greater affinity for Hb than does oxygen (240 times greater). Figure VII-3-5 shows that with CO the O_2–Hb dissociation curve is shifted to the left (CO increases the affinity of Hb for O_2) and HbO_2 content is reduced.

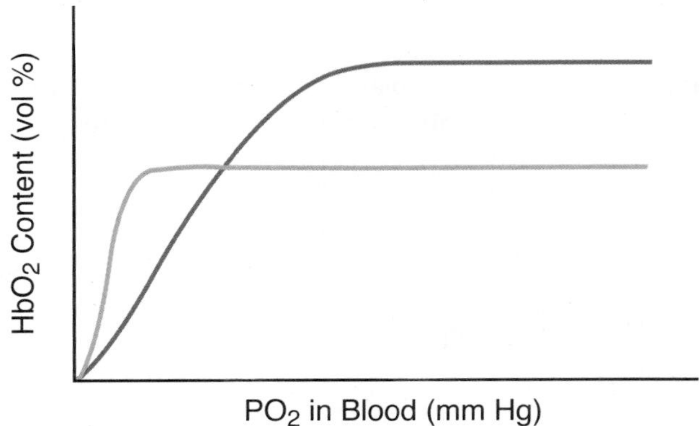

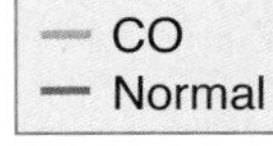

Figure VII-3-5. Carbon Monoxide Poisoning

Table VII-3-1 is a summary of the effects of anemia, polycythemia, and carbon monoxide poisoning.

Table VII-3-1. Systemic Arterial Blood

	PO_2	Hb Concentration	O_2 per g Hb	O_2 Content
Anemia	N	↓	N	↓
Polycythemia	N	↑	N	↑
CO poisoning (acute)	N	N	↓	↓

N = normal; O_2 per g Hb = % saturation.

In **anemia**, hemoglobin is saturated but arterial oxygen content is depressed because of the reduced concentration of hemoglobin.

In **polycythemia**, arterial oxygen content is above normal because of an increased hemoglobin concentration.

In **CO poisoning**, arterial PO_2 is normal, but oxygen saturation of hemoglobin is depressed.

TRANSPORT OF CARBON DIOXIDE

Dissolved Carbon Dioxide

Carbon dioxide is 24 times more soluble in blood than oxygen is. Even though the blood has a PCO_2 of only between 40 and 47 mm Hg, about 5% of the total CO_2 is carried in the dissolved form.

Carbamino Compounds

Carbon dioxide reacts with terminal amine groups of proteins to form carbamino compounds. The protein involved appears to be almost exclusively hemoglobin. About 5% of the total CO_2 is carried as carbamino compounds. The attachment sites that bind CO_2 are different from the sites that bind O_2.

Bicarbonate

About 90% of the CO_2 is carried as plasma bicarbonate. In order to convert CO_2 into bicarbonate or the reverse, carbonic anhydrase (CA) must be present.

$$CO_2 + H_2O \overset{CA}{\leftrightarrow} H_2CO_3 \leftrightarrow H^+ + HCO_3^-$$

Figure VII-3-6 illustrates the steps in the conversion of CO_2 into bicarbonate in a systemic capillary.

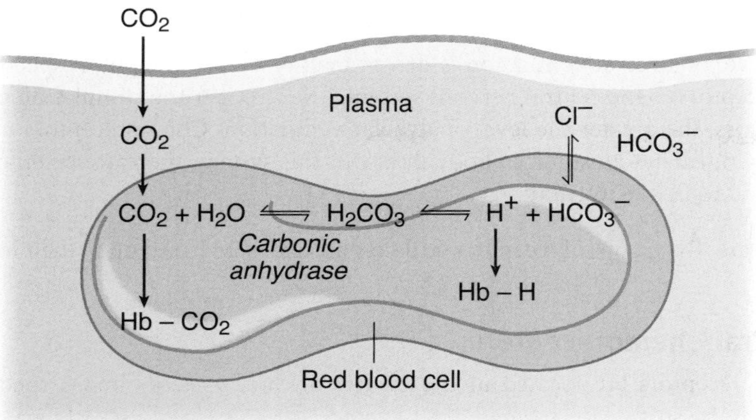

Figure VII-3-6. Formation of Bicarbonate Ion

Plasma contains no carbonic anhydrase; therefore, there can be no significant conversion of CO_2 to HCO_3^- in this compartment.

Because deoxygenated Hb is a better buffer, removing oxygen from hemoglobin shifts the reaction to the right and thus facilitates the formation of bicarbonate in the red blood cells (Haldane effect).

To maintain electrical neutrality as HCO_3^- moves into the plasma, Cl^- moves into the red blood cell (chloride shift).

In summary:

- Bicarbonate is formed in the red blood cell but it is carried in the plasma compartment.
- The PCO_2 determines the volume of CO_2 carried in each of the forms listed above. The relationship between the PCO_2 and the total CO_2 content is direct and nearly linear, as shown in Figure VII-3-7.
- Thus, hyperventilation not only lowers the PCO_2 (mm Hg), it also lowers the CO_2 content (vol%).

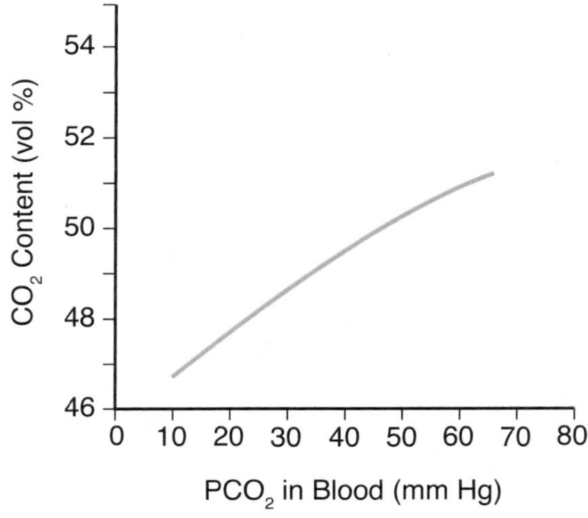

Figure VII-3-7. CO_2 Content in Blood

NEURAL REGULATION OF ALVEOLAR VENTILATION

The level of alveolar ventilation is driven mainly from the input of specific chemoreceptors to the central nervous system. The stronger the stimulation of these receptors, the greater the level of alveolar ventilation. Chemoreceptors monitor the chemical composition of body fluids. In this system, there are receptors that respond to pH, PCO_2, and PO_2.

There are two groups of receptors, and they are classified based upon their location.

Central Chemoreceptors

These receptors are located in the central nervous system—more specifically, close to the surface of the medulla.

- Stimulation of central chemoreceptors increases ventilation.
- The receptors directly monitor and are stimulated by cerebrospinal fluid $[H^+]$ and CO_2. The stimulatory effect of increased CO_2 may be due to the local production of H^+ from CO_2.
- Because the blood–brain barrier is freely permeable to CO_2, the activity of these receptors changes with increased or decreased systemic arterial PCO_2.
- H^+ does not easily penetrate the blood-brain barrier. Thus, an acute rise in arterial H^+, not of CO_2 origin, does not stimulate central chemoreceptors.
- These receptors are very sensitive and represent the main drive for ventilation under normal resting conditions at sea level.
- Therefore, the main drive for ventilation is CO_2 (H^+) on the central chemoreceptors.

Figure VII-3-8 illustrates the relationship between the central chemoreceptors and the systemic arterial blood.

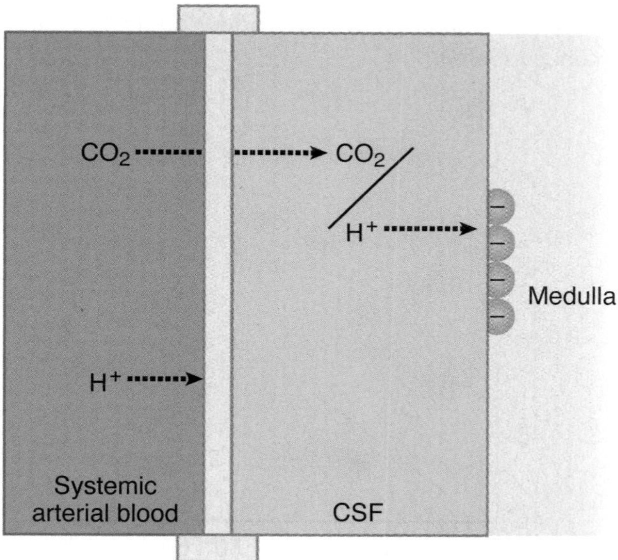

Figure VII-3-8. Central Chemoreceptors

The system does adapt, usually within 12 to 24 hours. The mechanism of adaptation may be the normalization of CSF H^+ by the pumping of HCO_3^- into or out of the CSF. There are no central PO_2 receptors.

Peripheral Chemoreceptors

These receptors are found within small bodies at 2 locations:

Carotid bodies: near carotid sinus, afferents to CNS in glossopharyngeal nerve IX

Aortic bodies: near aortic arch, afferents to CNS in vagus nerve X

The peripheral chemoreceptors are bathed in arterial blood, which they monitor directly. These bodies have 2 different receptors:

- **H^+/CO_2 receptors**
  - These receptors are less sensitive than the central chemoreceptors, but they still contribute to the normal drive for ventilation.
  - Therefore, under normal resting conditions at sea level, for all practical purposes, the total drive for ventilation is CO_2, mainly via the central chemoreceptors but with a small contribution via the peripheral chemoreceptors.
- **PO_2 receptors**
  - The factor monitored by these receptors is PO_2, not oxygen content.
  - Because they respond to PO_2, they are actually monitoring dissolved oxygen and not oxygen on Hb.
  - When systemic arterial PO_2 is close to normal (≅100 mm Hg) or above normal, there is little if any stimulation of these receptors.
- They are strongly stimulated only by a dramatic decrease in systemic arterial PO_2.
- Sensitivity to hypoxia increases with CO_2 retention.

These receptors do not adapt.

Bridge to Pathology/Pharmacology

The normal CO_2 drive to breath is suppressed in COPD patients, and by narcotics and general anesthetics.

Clinical Correlate

Although oxygen content is reduced in anemia, the PaO_2 is normal; thus, anemia does not directly stimulate ventilation. However, the reduced oxygen delivery can cause excess lactic acid production, which would in turn stimulate peripheral chemoreceptors.

Central Respiratory Centers

Medullary centers

Site of the inherent rhythm for respiration.

Inspiratory center

Expiratory center

For spontaneous breathing, an intact medulla must be connected to the diaphragm (via the phrenic nerve). Thus a complete C1 or C2 lesion will prevent diaphragmatic breathing but not a complete C6 or lower lesion.

Figure VII-3-9 illustrates the main features involved in the central control of ventilation.

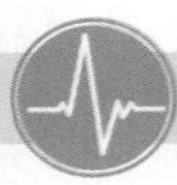

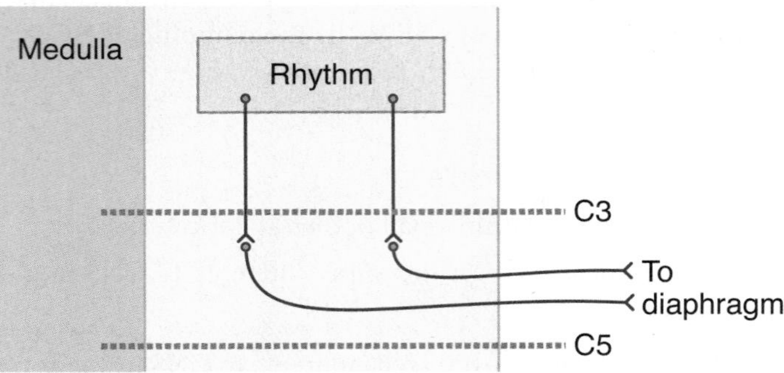

Figure VII-3-9. CNS Respiratory Centers

Abnormal Breathing Patterns

Apneustic breathing: prolonged inspirations alternating with a short period of expiration. This pattern is attributed to the loss of the normal balance between vagal input and the pons-medullary interactions. Lesions in patients with apneustic breathing are usually found in the caudal pons.

Cheyne-Stokes breathing: periodic type of breathing which has cycles of gradually increasing depth and frequency followed by a gradual decrease in depth and frequency between periods of apnea. It may result from midbrain lesions or congestive heart failure.

RESPIRATORY STRESS: UNUSUAL ENVIRONMENTS

High Altitude

At high altitude, atmospheric pressure is reduced from 760 mm Hg of sea level. Because atmospheric pressure is a factor that determines room air and alveolar PO_2, these two values are also reduced. These two values are permanently depressed unless enriched oxygen is inspired.

Therefore, PAO_2 <100 mm Hg, PaO_2 <100 mm Hg, and the low arterial PO_2 stimulates the peripheral chemoreceptors and increases alveolar ventilation. At high altitude, then, the main drive for ventilation changes from CO_2 on the central chemoreceptors at sea level to a low PO_2 drive of the peripheral chemoreceptors, and hyperventilation ensues.

Table VII-3-2. Acute Changes and Long-Term Adaptations (Acclimatization)

	Acute Changes	Acclimatization
PAO_2 and PaO_2	decreased	remains decreased
$PACO_2$ and $PaCO_2$	decreased	remains decreased
Systemic arterial pH	increased	decreases to normal via renal compensation
Hb concentration	no change	increases (polycythemia)
Hb % sat	decreased	remains decreased
Systemic arterial O_2 content	decreased	increases to normal

At high altitude, hypoxia can develop, resulting in increased circulating levels of erythropoietin and red cell concentration of 2,3-bisphosphoglycerate (right shifts the oxygen-hemoglobin dissociation curve). Erythropoietin increases red blood cell production and eventually causes an adaptive polycythemia.

High-Pressure Environment

In a hyperbaric environment breathing room air (21% O_2 and 79% N_2), the partial pressure of O_2 and N_2 increase in the alveoli and systemic arterial blood. The pressure of nitrogen also increases in other body compartments.

Oxygen

- Adverse effect is oxygen toxicity due to the production of oxygen radicals.
- Clinical uses include carbon monoxide poisoning, compromised tissue grafts, and gas gangrene.

Nitrogen

- **Rapture of the deep:** a feeling of euphoria associated with high nitrogen levels
- **The bends** (Caisson's disease, or decompression sickness) too-rapid decompression after exposure to high nitrogen pressures. It can result in nitrogen coming out of solution in joints (bends) or in the blood, resulting in air emboli in the vasculature.

Note

What principle explains the physiology of why nitrogen will be forced into solution?

Answer: Henry's law. The amount of gas that will dissolve in a liquid varies directly with the pressure above that liquid. High pressures force gas into solution. However, solubilities and temperature also come into play when considering Henry's law. Even though a huge N_2 gradient may exist between the air and plasma, nitrogen is barely soluble at all.

Bridge to Microbiology

Gas gangrene is caused by the bacteria *Clostridium perfringens*. This bacteria thrives in an anaerobic environment, explaining why hyperbaric oxygen can be helpful. *Staphylococcus aureus* and *Vibrio vulnificus* can cause similar infections.

Chapter Summary

- The only significant form in which oxygen is delivered to systemic tissues is oxygen attached to hemoglobin. However, PaO_2 created by dissolved oxygen is a force necessary to keep oxygen bound to hemoglobin.
- Normal hemoglobin in the systemic arterial system is almost completely saturated with oxygen when PaO_2 is 100 mm Hg. Mixed venous hemoglobin in a resting individual is about 75% saturated.
- Increased H^+, CO_2, temperature, and 2,3-bisphosphoglycerate shift the Hb–O_2 curve to the right. This assists in the unloading of oxygen to systemic tissues but does not prevent complete loading of oxygen in lung capillaries.
- The normal drive for ventilation is CO_2, mainly on the central chemoreceptors.
- When the systemic arterial PO_2 dramatically decreases, the main drive for ventilation is the low PO_2 on the peripheral chemoreceptors.
- Spontaneous rhythmic breathing requires an intact medulla connected, via the phrenic nerve, to the diaphragm.
- At high altitude, there is a permanent depression in alveolar and systemic arterial PO_2. The low PO_2 stimulates the peripheral chemoreceptors, inducing a hyperventilation and a decrease in alveolar and systemic arterial PCO_2. The loss of CO_2 produces a respiratory alkalosis. To compensate, the kidney loses bicarbonate to return arterial pH close to normal. Acutely, arterial oxygen content is depressed because of reduced hemoglobin saturation. Acclimatization returns oxygen content toward normal because of an increase in hemoglobin concentration.

Causes and Evaluation of Hypoxemia 4

Learning Objectives

- ❑ Demonstrate understanding of ventilation-perfusion differences in the lung
- ❑ Demonstrate understanding of review of the normal lung
- ❑ Answer questions about causes of hypoxemia
- ❑ Use knowledge of left-to-right shunts

VENTILATION–PERFUSION DIFFERENCES IN THE LUNG

Regional Differences in Intrapleural Pressure (IPP)

At FRC, the mean value for intrapleural pressure is –5 cm H_2O. However, there are regional differences, and the reason for these differences is gravity.

- Recall that the pleura is a fluid-filled space.
- Similar to the cardiovascular system, it is subject to gravitational influences
  - (P = height × gravity × density)
- Thus, IPP is higher (less negative) at the base (bottom) of the lung compared to the apex (top).

Clinical Correlate

The regional difference of alveolar and arterial pressure in the lung is referred to as "west zones" of the lung. The take-home message is that ventilation perfusion ratio is higher in the apex of the lung (zone 1) in an upright individual than it is in the base of the lung (zone 3).

Regional Difference in Ventilation

- Because IPP is higher (less negative) at the base, the P_{TM} is less, resulting in less distension of alveoli, i.e., there is less volume.
- In contrast, IPP is more negative at the apex, thus the P_{TM} is higher, resulting in a greater volume in alveoli near the apex.
- As described in chapter 1, alveolar compliance decreases as lung volume increases. Thus, alveoli near the base are more compliant than alveoli near the apex. Stated another way, alveoli near the base are on a much steeper portion of the pressure-volume curve than alveoli near the apex (Figure VII-4-2).
- Because alveoli near the base are more compliant, there is more ventilation in this region compared to the apex.

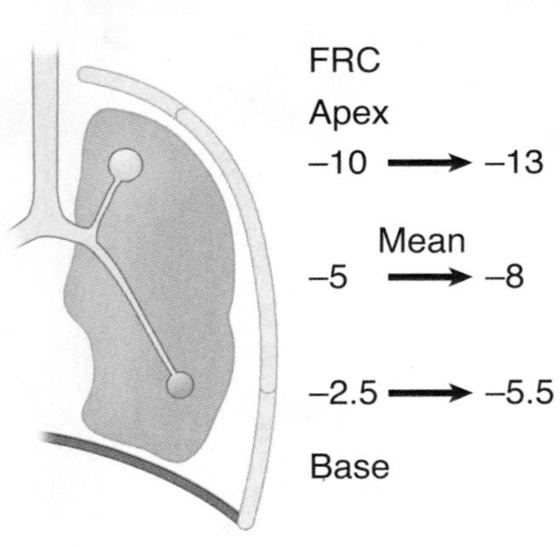

Figure VII-4-1. Upright Posture

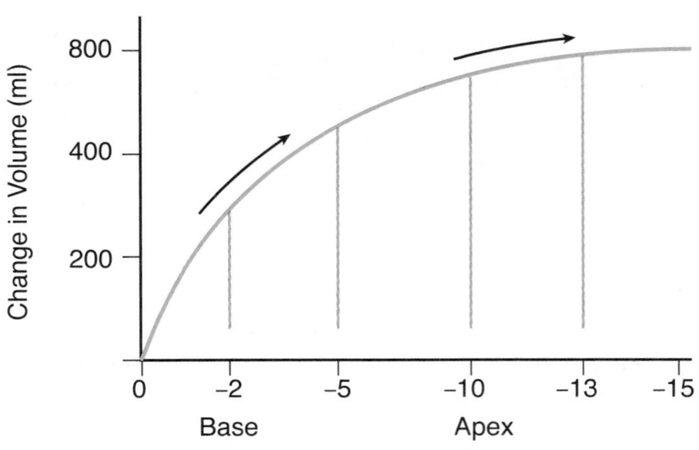

Figure VII-4-2. Regional Ventilation

Regional Differences in Blood Flow

Even in a normal individual, there are regional differences in blood flow through the pulmonary circuit. These differences, for the most part, can be attributed to the effect of gravity.

- Moving toward the base (with gravity), pressure in the pulmonary arteries is higher compared to pressure in the pulmonary arteries of the apex (against gravity).
- Since the intravascular pressure in arteries is higher, there is more blood flow to the base of the lung compared to the apex.

Ventilation–Perfusion Relationships

The partial pressures of O_2 and CO_2 in alveoli are determined by the combination of ventilation (adding O_2, removing CO_2) and perfusion (removing O_2 and adding CO_2). However, it is not the absolute amount of either that determines the composition of alveolar gases. Instead, it is the relative relationship between ventilation and perfusion that ultimately determines the alveolar gases. This is **ventilation-perfusion matching**.

In the normal situation, it would be "ideal" if ventilation and perfusion (blood flow) matched, i.e., the ventilation-perfusion ratio is one (Figure VII-4-3). If this were the case, then:

- P_AO_2 = 100 mm Hg
- P_ACO_2 = 40 mm Hg
- The blood draining the alveolus would have a pH = 7.40 (normal blood pH)

Although the above is "ideal," it is not often encountered. Figure VII-4-3 illustrates ventilation, blood flow (Q) or perfusion, and the relative ventilation-perfusion relationship for an **upright individual**. Toward the base of the lung:

- Alveolar ventilation is high relative to the apex (described above).
- Q is high relative to the apex (described above).
- However, relative to one another, Q is higher than alveolar ventilation, thus the ventilation-perfusion relationship is less than 1.0.
- In short, the alveoli are under-ventilated relative to the perfusion. If alveolar ventilation is inadequate, then it follows that PO_2 falls, PCO_2 rises, and blood pH falls (remember that CO_2 generates H^+).
- Thus, the P_AO_2 at the base is <100 mm Hg and the P_ACO_2 is >40 mm Hg.

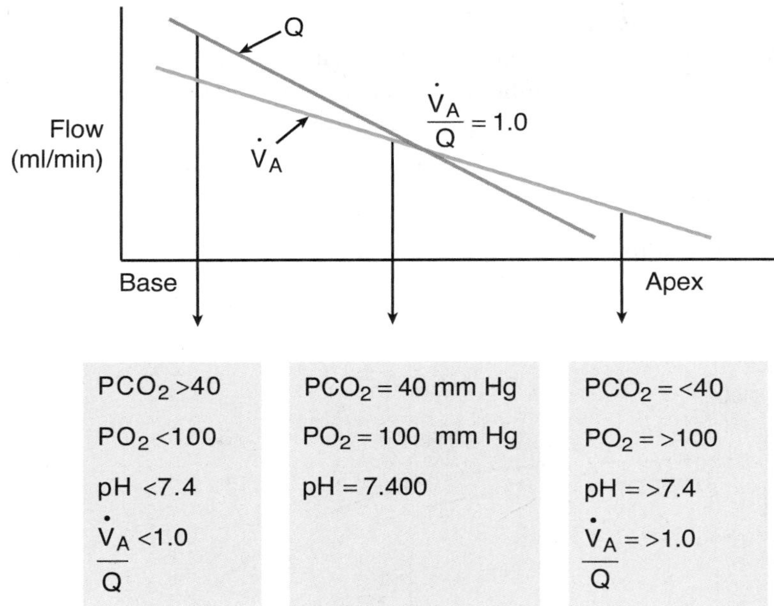

Figure VII-4-3. Ventilation–Perfusion Relationships

Moving toward the apex, the situation reverses (Figure VII-4-3):

- Alveolar ventilation is less relative to the base (described above).
- Q is less relative to the base (described above).
- However, relative to one another, Q is less than alveolar ventilation, thus the ventilation-perfusion relationship is greater than 1.0.
- In short, the alveoli are over-ventilated relative to the perfusion. If alveolar ventilation is excessive, then it follows that PO_2 rises, PCO_2 falls, and blood pH increases (remember that CO_2 generates H^+).
- Thus, the P_AO_2 at the apex is >100 mm Hg and P_ACO_2 is <40 mm Hg.

The effect of the ventilation-perfusion relationship is a continuum and this is illustrated in Figure VII-4-4.

- As **$\dot{V}_A/Q$ falls**, PO_2 falls and PCO_2 rises.
- As **$\dot{V}_A/Q$ rises**, PO_2 rises and PCO_2 falls.

Extremes of $\dot{V}A/Q$ Mismatch

- **Shunt:** If ventilation is zero but there is blood flow, then $\dot{V}A/Q = 0$.
  - This is a right-to-left shunt, and the blood gases leaving the alveoli are the same as venous blood (low PO_2, and high PCO_2; Y-axis intercept in Figure VII-4-4). This causes arterial hypoxemia, which is discussed later in this chapter.
- **Alveolar dead space:** If blood flow is zero but there is ventilation, then $\dot{V}A/Q = \infty$.
  - This is alveolar dead space, and alveolar gases become the same as inspired (high PAO_2 and $PACO_2 = 0$; X-axis intercept in Figure VII-4-4).

To summarize:

- As $\dot{V}A/Q$ falls, PO_2 falls and PCO_2 rises. The extreme is a shunt.
  - Remember, however, that the lower the $\dot{V}A/Q$, the more it "behaves" as a shunt, i.e., the alveolar and blood gases get closer and closer to venous gases. Similar to a shunt, this can lead to arterial hypoxemia, both of which are discussed later in this chapter.
- As $\dot{V}A/Q$ rises, PO_2 rises and PCO_2 falls. The extreme is alveolar dead space.
  - Similar to above, the higher the $\dot{V}A/Q$, the more the situation looks like alveolar dead space.

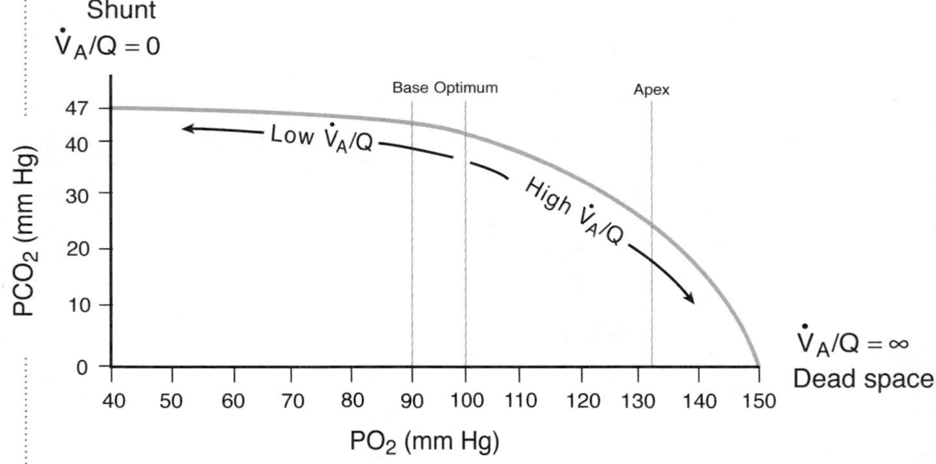

Figure VII-4-4. Shunt and Dead Space

Problem

The following ratios represent two different lung units under resting conditions:

$\dot{V}A/Q$

A = 0.62

B = 0.73

Both lung units A and B are underventilated, but of the two, B is better ventilated.

Which lung unit had the greatest:

$PACO_2$, end capillary PCO_2? (Answer: A)

PAO_2, end capillary PO_2? (Answer: B)

end capillary pH? (Answer: B)

Hypoxic Vasoconstriction

This is a clinically important phenomenon that is unique to the pulmonary circulation. Whenever there is a decrease in alveolar PO_2, a local vasoconstriction of pulmonary blood vessels is produced. The result is a lowering of blood flow through that lung unit and a redistribution of blood to better-ventilated units.

Problem

If a person inhales a peanut that lodges in a peripheral airway, what changes would you expect for the following variables in the peanut-occluded unit?

P_{ACO_2} (increase)

P_{AO_2} (decrease)

pulmonary end capillary pH (decrease)

blood flow in that lung unit (decrease)

All answers here are based on the fact that blocking the airway produces a shunt, as shown in Figure VII-4-4. The blood flow decreases because of hypoxic vasoconstriction. Low $\dot{V}_A/Q$ ratios are associated with hypoxic vasoconstriction. If the pulmonary disease is severe and widespread, the alveolar hypoxia and subsequent arteriolar vasoconstriction increases pulmonary arterial pressure.

Problem

If a small thrombus lodges in a pulmonary artery, what changes would you expect for the following variables in the thrombus-occluded unit?

P_{ACO_2} (decrease)

P_{AO_2} (increase)

pulmonary end capillary pH (increase)

All answers here are based on the fact that the thrombus increases the $\dot{V}_A/Q$ ratio. This produces lung units that act as dead space, as shown in Figure VII-4-4.

Exercise

In exercise, there is increased ventilation and pulmonary blood flow. However, during exercise, ventilation increases more than cardiac output and $\dot{V}_A/Q$ goes well above 1.0 as one approaches maximal oxygen consumption. Also, the base–apex flows are more uniform.

Clinical Correlate

As one ages, the A–a gradient increases because ventilation-perfusion matching becomes less and less "ideal." One formula for taking this into account is:

$$\frac{(\text{age} + 4)}{4}$$

REVIEW OF THE NORMAL LUNG

Before discussing the causes of hypoxemia let's review the normal state using standard values (Figure VII-4-5):

- The blood entering the alveolar-capillary unit is mixed venous blood.
  - $PO_2 = 40$ and $PCO_2 = 45$ mm Hg
- $P_AO_2 = 100$ mm Hg and $P_ACO_2 = 40$ mm Hg
- Both gases are perfusion-limited and thus their partial pressures at the end of the capillary are the same as alveolar.
- Arterial blood gas (ABG) sample shows $PaO_2 = 95$ mm Hg, and $PaCO_2 =$ 40 mm Hg.
  - The A–a gradient is 5 mm Hg (ranges 5-10 mm Hg but is influenced by age; see Clinical Correlate) and is primarily the result of anatomic shunts.

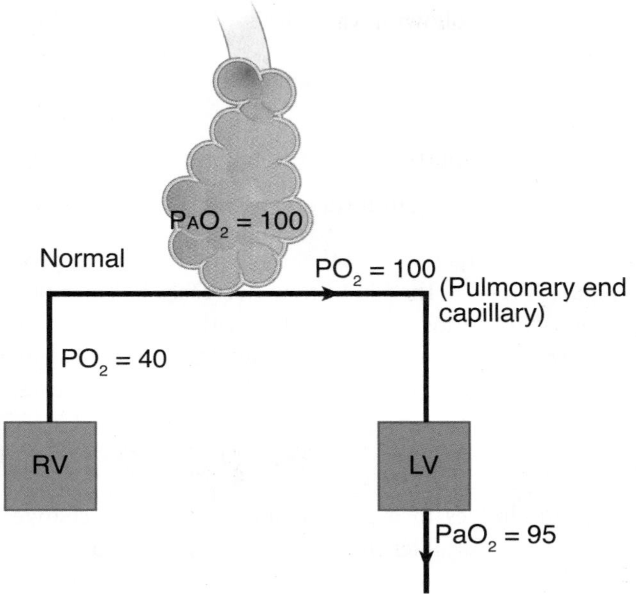

Figure VII-4-5. Normal State

CAUSES OF HYPOXEMIA

Hypoventilation

Hypoventilation of the entire lung elevates alveolar PCO_2, and the increase in PCO_2 decreases PO_2. For example, if alveolar ventilation decreases by 50%, alveolar PCO_2 becomes 80 mm Hg (an increase of 40 mm Hg). Assuming a respiratory ratio close to 1.0, alveolar PO_2 decreases by about 40 mm Hg to 60 mm Hg. If no other problem exists, pulmonary end capillary and systemic arterial PO_2 also decreases by 40 mm Hg. This is illustrated in Figure VII-4-6.

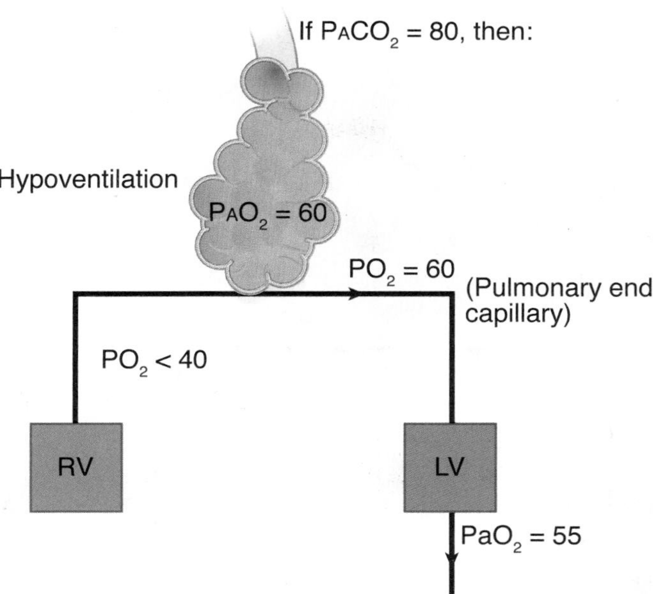

Figure VII-4-6. Hypoventilation

Hypoventilation is characterized as an equal decrease in PO_2 in all 3 compartments. **As a result, A–a is normal and end-tidal PO_2 is still be a good index of systemic arterial PO_2** (provided A–a gradient is taken into consideration).

The hypoxemia can be relieved by increasing the inspired oxygen, however CO_2 remains elevated because ventilation is unchanged.

In summary

- There is no increase in the A–a oxygen gradient.
- Supplemental oxygen can relieve the hypoxemia.
- End-tidal air still reflects the systemic arterial compartment.
- The problem is not within the lung itself.

Diffusion Impairment

Diffusion impairment means a structural problem in the lung. As described in chapter 2, this can be produced by a decreased surface area and/or increased thickness of lung membranes. The consequences of diffusion impairment are illustrated in Figure VII-4-7 and summarized in the following figure.

Clinical Correlate

High altitude is sometimes categorized as a fifth cause of hypoxemia. High altitude causes low P_AO_2, similar to hypoventilation. All the observations described here apply, except for PCO_2. At high altitude, a subject hyperventilates, and thus P_ACO_2 and $PaCO_2$ are reduced.

Bridge to Pathology

Acutely, hypoventilation can be caused by narcotics and general anesthetics. More chronic conditions include COPD, kyphoscoliosis, and neuromuscular disorders such as Guillain-Barré, Lambert-Eaton, and myasthenia gravis.

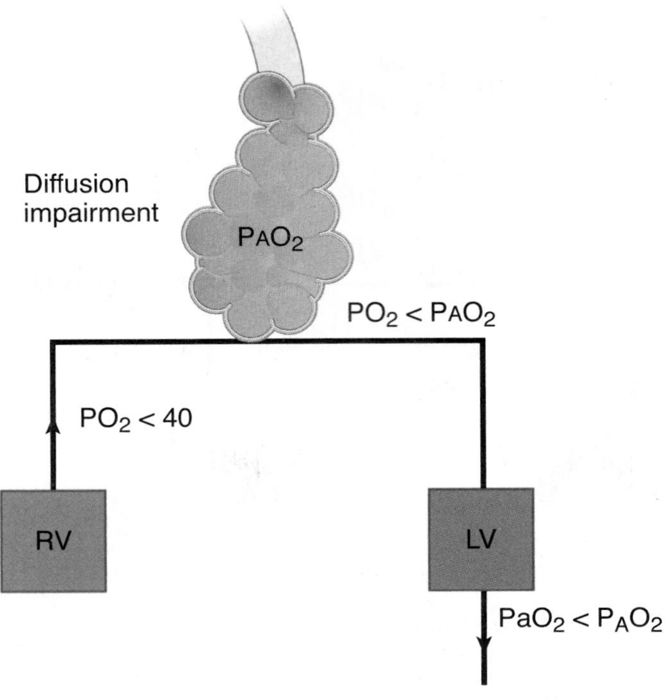

Figure VII-4-7. Diffusion Impairment

In marked diffusion impairment, pulmonary end capillary PO_2 is less than alveolar PO_2. End-tidal PO_2 is not a good index of systemic arterial PO_2.

In diffusion impairment, supplemental oxygen corrects the hypoxemia. Note that although the arterial PO_2 may be restored to normal, or even be above normal by supplemental oxygen, there is still an abnormally large A–a gradient.

Bridge to Pathology

Diffusion problems often occur in restrictive pulmonary diseases, such as pulmonary fibrosis, asbestosis, and sarcoidosis. In addition, pulmonary edema can cause a diffusion impairment.

In summary

- There is an increase in A–a oxygen gradient.
- Supplemental oxygen can relieve the hypoxemia.
- End-tidal air does not reflect the arterial values.
- It is characterized by a decrease in DLCO.

Bridge to Pathology

Some conditions that often result in significant $\dot{V}A/Q$ mismatch include: severe obstruction (status asthmaticus, cystic fibrosis, anaphylaxis), infection (pneumonia), and partial occlusion of an airway (mucus plug, foreign object).

Ventilation-Perfusion Mismatch: Low $\dot{V}_A/Q$ Units

If ventilation to a significant portion of the lungs is markedly compromised, then $\dot{V}_A/Q$ is << 1.0. As described earlier, low $\dot{V}_A/Q$ creates alveolar and end-pulmonary capillary blood gases that are approaching venous gases (low PO_2, and high CO2). The blood from these low $\dot{V}_A/Q$ units mixes in with blood draining normal alveolar-capillary units, resulting in systemic hypoxemia.

Because P_AO_2 is normal in areas that don't have low $\dot{V}_A/Q$, the A–a gradient is elevated. Supplemental oxygen corrects the hypoxemia because the problem regions still have some ventilation—it is just much lower than normal. Similar to diffusion impairment described above, the increased A–a gradient means end-tidal PO_2 is not reflective of PaO_2.

In summary:

- There is an increased A–a oxygen gradient.
- Supplemental oxygen corrects the hypoxemia.
- End-tidal air does not reflect the arterial values.

Intrapulmonary Shunt

By definition, systemic venous blood is delivered to the left side of the heart without exchanging oxygen and carbon dioxide with the alveoli. A right-to-left shunt leads to hypoxemia.

Figure VII-4-8 illustrates the consequences of an intrapulmonary shunt. The solid-line regions represent the normal areas of the lung. The dashed line represents the shunted blood, which is passing from the right heart to the left heart without a change in chemical composition.

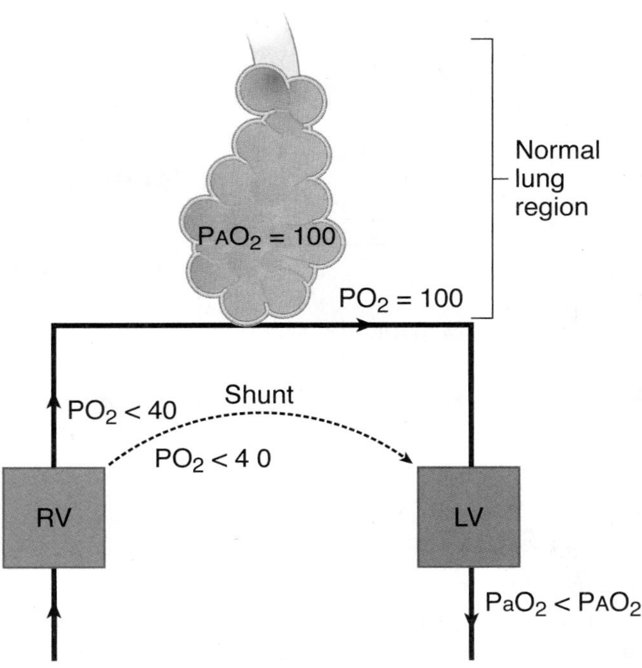

Figure VII-4-8. Pulmonary Shunt

With an intrapulmonary shunt, systemic arterial PO_2 is less than alveolar, resulting in an elevated A–a gradient. End-tidal PO_2 does not reflect systemic arterial PO_2.

When a significant intrapulmonary shunt exists, breathing pure O_2 elevates systemic arterial PO_2 a small amount, but it often doesn't correct the hypoxemia. See Figure VII-4-9 for response of PaO_2 with shunt.

The failure to obtain a significant increase in arterial PO_2 following the administration of supplemental oxygen in hypoxemia is strong evidence of the presence of a shunt.

Bridge to Pathology

Intrapulmonary shunts are caused by atelectatic lung regions (pneumothorax, ARDS), complete occlusion of an airway (mucus plug, foreign body), and the right-to-left shunts created by heart defects, tetralogy of Fallot, for example.

In summary

- Increase in A–a oxygen gradient
- Supplemental oxygen ineffective at returning arterial PO_2 to normal
- End-tidal air does not reflect the arterial values

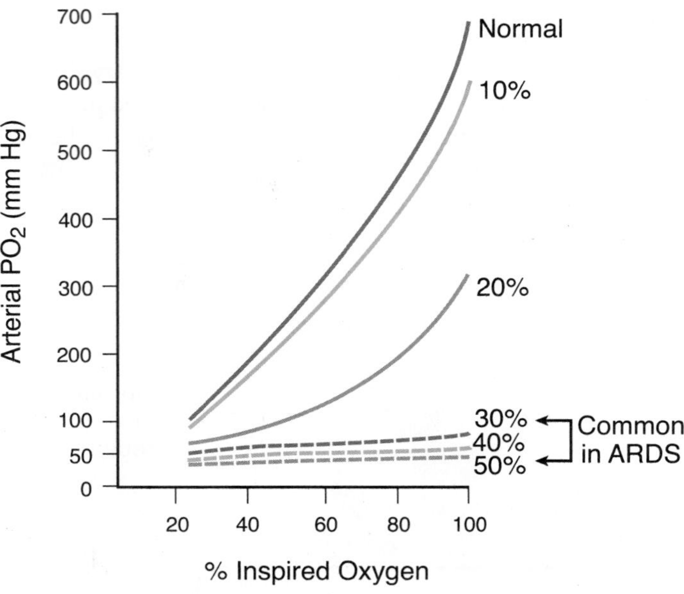

Figure VII-4-9. Response to Supplemental Oxygen

LEFT-TO-RIGHT SHUNTS

Pressures are usually higher on the left side of the heart (atria and ventricles), and thus flow is normally left to right. A major characteristic is that hypoxemia never develops in a left-to-right shunt. The principal example is an atrial or ventricular septal defect.

Figure VII-4-10 illustrates the normal PO_2 values in the left and right compartments. Note from the descriptions that follow where the first increase in PO_2 develops on the right side.

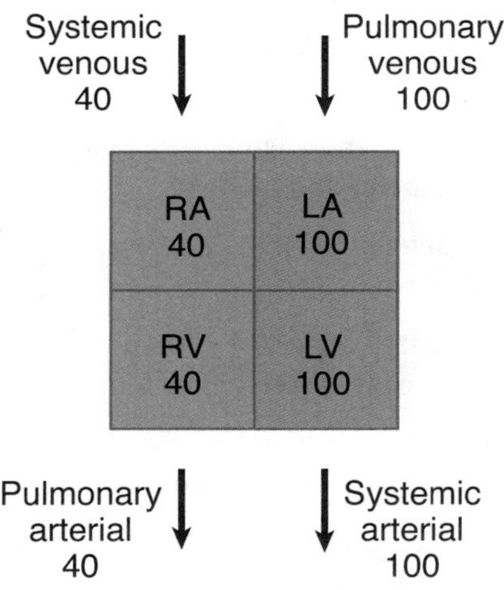

Figure VII-4-10. Left-to-Right Cardiac Shunts

Numbers refer to normal PO_2 in mm Hg

- Diagnosed clinically with echocardiogram with bubble study
- Most intracardiac shunts are left-to-right shunts. However, longstanding uncorrected shunts result in a reversal of the shunt.

Table VII-4-1. Consequences of 3 Different Left-to-Right Shunts

	Atrial Septal Defect	Ventricular Septal Defect	Patent Ductus (newborn)
Systemic arterial PO_2	no change	no change	no change
Right atrial PO_2	↑	no change	no change
Right ventricular PO_2	↑	↑	no change
Pulmonary arterial PO_2	↑	↑	↑
Pulmonary blood flow	↑	↑	↑
Pulmonary arterial pressure	↑	↑	↑

Atrial septal defect: PO_2 increase first appears in right atrium
Ventricular septal defect: PO_2 increase first appears in right ventricle
Patent ductus: PO_2 increase appears in pulmonary artery

Chapter Summary

- As a consequence of gravity, there is more ventilation and blood flow near the base of the lung compared to the apex.
- The $\dot{V}A/Q$ relationship determines the alveolar gases and thus the gases of the blood draining the alveolus.
- The ideal $\dot{V}A/Q$ ratio at rest is close to 1.0. A ratio >1.0 is an overventilated lung unit and a ratio <1.0 is an underventilated lung unit.
- A low $\dot{V}A/Q$ ratio or any other decrease in alveolar PO_2 initiates a vasoconstriction of the pulmonary vasculature.
- Hypoventilation is associated with equal decreases in the PO_2 of the alveolar, pulmonary end capillary, and systemic arterial compartments. There is no widening of the A–a gradient, and an increase in alveolar ventilation returns arterial PO_2 to normal. This can also be achieved with supplemental oxygen.
- Diffusion impairment is a structural problem of the lung. When it is severe, blood leaving a pulmonary capillary does not equilibrate with alveolar air. There is a widening of the A–a gradient, and supplemental oxygen returns arterial PO_2 toward normal.
- The development of regions of the lung with very low $\dot{V}A/Q$ causes hypoxemia with an elevated A–a gradient. The hypoxemia is corrected by providing supplemental oxygen.
- A pulmonary (right-to-left) shunt produces a widening of the A–a gradient and is the only cause of hypoxemia that typically does not respond significantly to supplemental oxygen.
- A left-to-right shunt can lead to pulmonary hypertension but does not produce hypoxemia.

SECTION VIII

Renal Physiology

Renal Structure and Glomerular Filtration

1

Learning Objectives

- ❑ Use knowledge of overview of the renal system
- ❑ Demonstrate understanding of nephron hemodynamics
- ❑ Demonstrate understanding of glomerular filtration

OVERVIEW OF THE RENAL SYSTEM

Functions of the Kidney

- Excretes waste products: urea, uric acid, creatinine
- Water and electrolyte balance
- Acid/base balance
- Secretes the hormone erythropoietin and the enzyme, renin into the circulation
- Hydroxylates 25-hydroxy-Vit D to form the active form of Vitamin D (1,25 dihydroxy-Vit D)

Functional Organization of the Kidney

Figure VI-1-1 illustrates the cortical versus the medullary organization of the kidney. Nephrons (the funcionting unit of the kidney) with glomeruli in the outer cortex have short loops of Henle (cortical nephrons). Those with glomeruli in the inner cortex have long loops of Henle that penetrate the medullary region (juxtamedullary nephrons).

- 7/8 of all nephrons are cortical nephrons
- 1/8 of all nephrons are juxtamedullary nephrons

Nephron structures in the medulla consist of the long loops of Henle and the terminal regions of the collecting ducts. All other structures, including the first section of the collecting ducts, are in the cortex.

- In the cortex, the proximal and distal tubules, as well as the initial segment of the collecting duct, are surrounded by a capillary network, and the interstitium is close to an isotonic environment (300 mOsm/kg).
- The medullary region has capillary loops organized similar to the loops of Henle, known as the vasa recta.
- The slow flow through these capillary loops preserves the osmolar gradient of the interstitium.

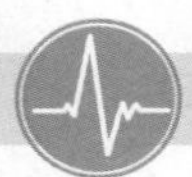

- However, this slow flow also keeps the PO_2 of the medulla lower than that in the cortex and even though the metabolic rate of the medulla is lower than in the cortex, it is more susceptible to ischemic damage.

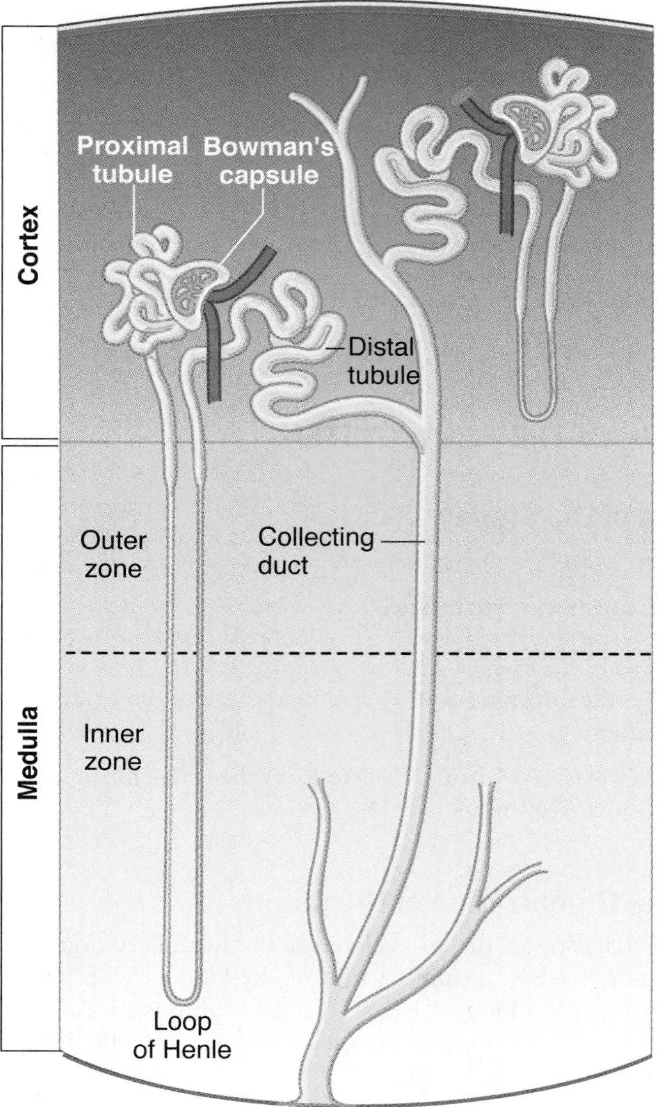

Figure VIII-1-1. Nephron Structures

Function of the Nephron

There are 4 basic renal processes (figure VIII-1-2): filtration, reabsorption, secretion, and excretion.

Filtration

- Blood is filtered by nephrons, the functional units of the kidney.
- Each nephron begins in a renal corpuscle (site of filtration), which is composed of a glomerulus enclosed in a Bowman's capsule.
- An ultrafiltrate resembling plasma enters Bowman's space.
- Filtration is driven by Starling forces.
- The ultrafiltrate is passed through, in turn, the proximal convoluted tubule, the loop of Henle, the distal convoluted tubule, and a series of collecting ducts to form urine.
- Filtration rate or filtered load is the amount of a substance (in mg) that is filtered at the glomeruli in a min (mg/min; see chapter 2 for more details).

Reabsorption

- Tubular reabsorption is the process by which solutes and water are removed from the tubular fluid that was formed in Bowman's space and transported into the blood.
- Reabsorption rate is the amount (in mg) that is reabsorbed from the ultrafiltrate in a min (mg/min; see chapter 2 for more details).

Secretion

- Tubular secretion is the transfer of materials from peritubular capillaries to the renal tubular lumen.
- Tubular secretion is primarily the result of active transport.
- Usually only a few substances are secreted.
- Many drugs are eliminated by tubular secretion.
- Secretion rate is the amount (in mg) that is secreted into the ultrafiltrate in a min (mg/min; see chapter 2 for more details).

Excretion

- Substances that are in the urine are excreted.
- A substance that is filtered and not completely reabsorbed is excreted in the urine.
- A substance that is filtered and then secreted is excreted in large amounts in the urine because it comes from 2 places in the nephron.
- Excretion rate is the amount (in mg) that is excreted in the urine in a min (mg/min; see chapter 2 for more details).

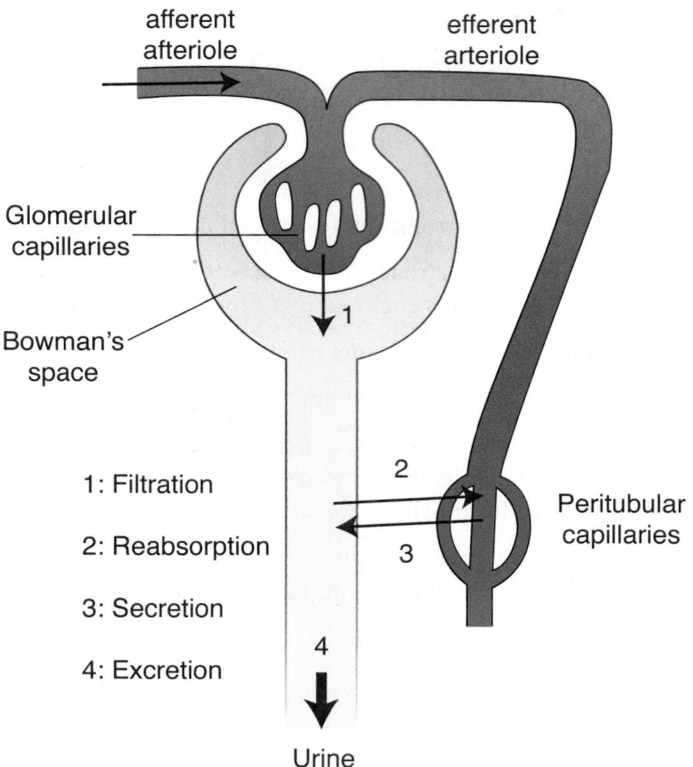

Figure VIII-1-2. Renal Processes

Clinical Correlate

Spinal cord injury can markedly alter the micturition reflex. A lumbar lesion can eliminate voluntary control (motor nerves exit L1–L3) and the sympathetic component (T10–T12). Over time, the PNS component can return (S1–S3) and voiding can be initiated when the bladder is sufficiently filled.

The following equation is central to understanding renal physiology and will be addressed in detail in a later chapter.

Excretion rate (ER) = (filtration rate – reabsorption rate) + secretion rate

Micturition Reflex

Micturition is a reflex regulated by the peripheral nervous system. The autonomic component exists at birth, continuing throughout life, but the motor component requires sufficient maturation of the nervous system (occurs around the age of two). This section discusses the physiologic regulation that occurs in sufficiently mature individuals. In this case, nuclei in the medulla ultimately regulate the phase, switching between the filling and voiding phases.

Filling phase

- This phase is typically the longest and is dominated by the sympathetic nervous system (SNS).
- Sympathetic input relaxes the detrusor muscle via the β-3 receptor (Gs-cAMP). In addition, sympathetic input contracts the internal sphincter via α-1 receptors.
- As a result, the bladder can fill with urine.

Voiding phase

- As the bladder fills, the pressure of the fluid causes distension of the bladder.
- This distension activates sensory afferent neurons (not depicted in figure) resulting in activation of the parasympathetic nervous system (PNS) and inhibition of the SNS (spinal reflex). In addition, in the sufficiently mature individual, it sends input to the medulla and cortex signaling that voiding is needed.
- PNS activation causes contraction of the detrusor muscle (M3). This initiates voiding.
- However, the external sphincter is controlled voluntarily (nicotinic receptor). If voiding is inappropriate at that moment, voluntary contraction of this sphincter stops the voiding process.
- If the voiding reflex is thwarted voluntarily, the bladder initially relaxes (stretch-induced relaxation of smooth muscle), reducing the pressure and the sensory drive to void.
- However, continued filling of the bladder increases pressure and re-initiates the sensory input attempting to start the voiding process.
- Typically, one voluntarily relaxes the external sphincter by inhibiting motor output (Ach via nicotinic receptor) and the bladder is emptied.

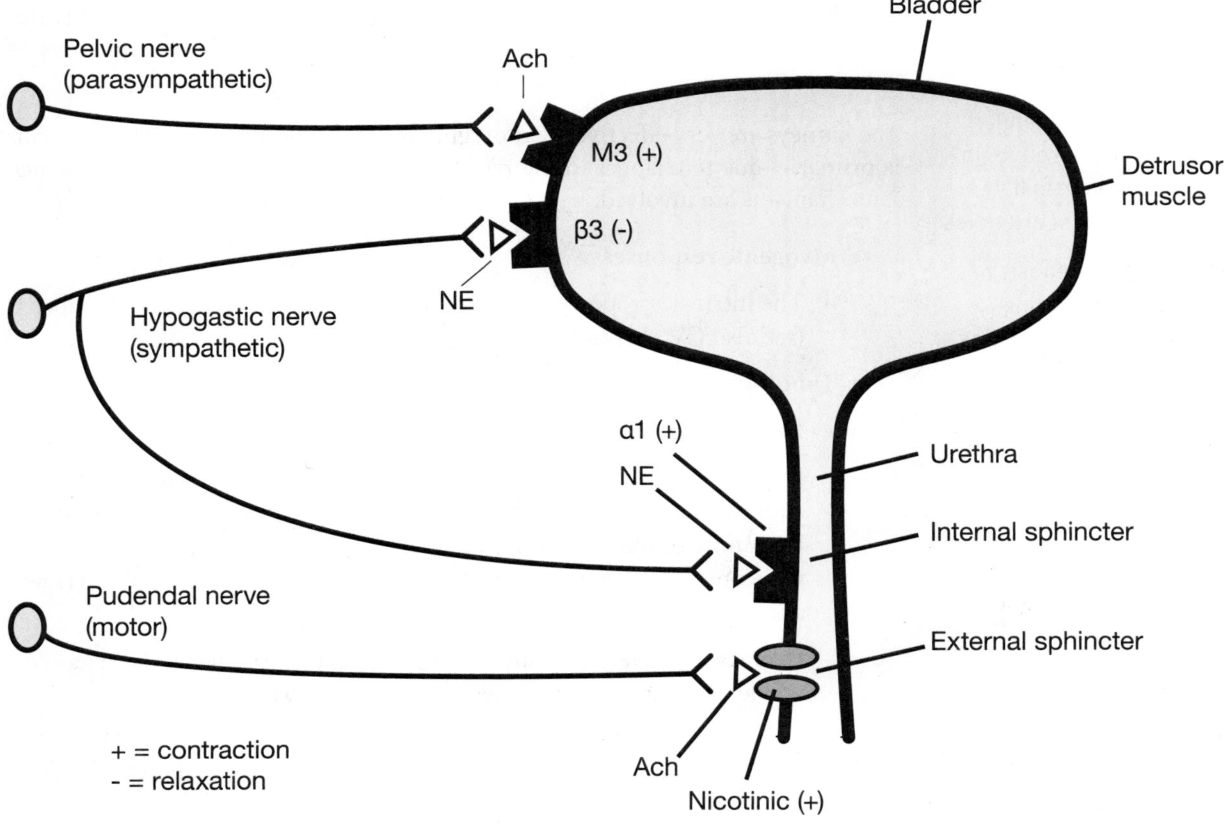

Figure VIII-1-3. Control of Micturition

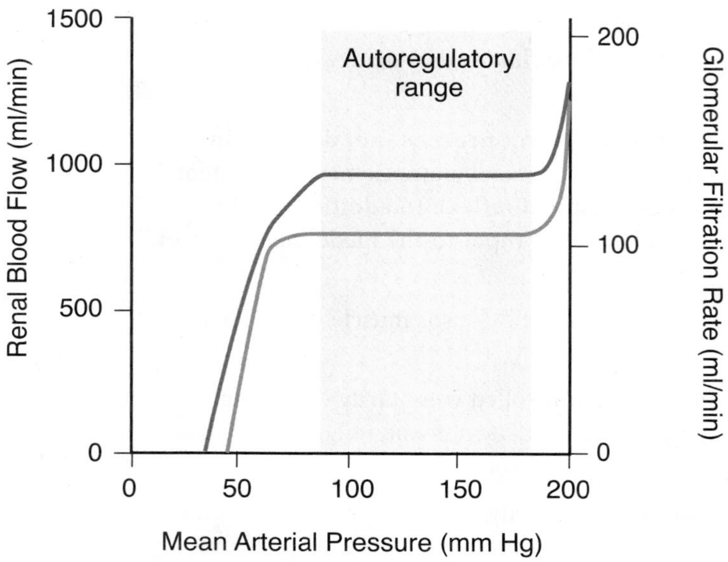

Figure VIII-1-4. Autoregulation and the Renal Function Curve

NEPHRON HEMODYNAMICS

Autoregulation

Blood flow throughout the kidney: renal artery → arcuate artery → afferent arteriole → glomerular capillaries → efferent arterioles → peritubular capillaries → vasa recta → arcuate vein → renal vein

The kidneys are very effective in autoregulating blood flow (figure VIII-1-4). This is primarily due to changes in the resistance of the afferent arterioles, for which 2 mechanisms are involved:

- **Myogenic responses**
  - The intrinsic property of smooth muscle is to contract when stretched (see also CV chapter)
- **Tubuloglomerular feedback (TGF)**
  - Increased MAP leads to an increase in RBF and GFR
  - High delivery of sodium ions to the macula densa (the part of the nephron where the thick ascending loop of Henle connects with the beginning of the distal tubule) → adenosine and ATP secretion → vasoconstriction of the afferent arteriole → decreases renal blood flow and GFR.
  - Decreased delivery of sodium to the macula densa dilates the arteriole and leads to an increase in renal blood flow and GFR.

Clinical Correlate

A patient with essential hypertension has increased renal artery pressure leading to vasoconstriction of the afferent arterioles and vasodilation of the efferent arterioles.

- High pressure the juxtaglomerular apparatus leads to decreased renin secretion → low angiotensin II → vasodilation of the efferent arterioles

A patient with renal artery stenosis has low renal artery pressures, leading to low pressures at the afferent arterioles.

- Vasodilation of the afferent arterioles and vasoconstriction of the efferent arterioles (increased renin secretion leads to increased angiotensin II)

Series Hemodynamics

The individual nephrons that make up both kidneys are connected in parallel. However, the flow through a single nephron represents 2 arterioles and 2 capillary beds connected in series.

Flow must be equal at all points in any series system. If flow changes, it changes equally at all points in the system.

For a brief review of CV hemodynamics, refer back to section V, chapter 1.

Flow (Q) = pressure gradient / resistance (R) = (upstream pressure-downstream pressure)

Blood flows from high pressure to low pressure. Two factors decrease flow:

- Decreasing the pressure gradient (decreasing the upstream pressure or increasing the downstream pressure)
- Increasing resistance at any point throughout the circuit

Therefore, when considering blood flow through the nephron as a series circuit, if resistance increases (vasoconstriction) at the afferent arteriole or efferent arteriole, renal plasma flow decreases.

When an arteriole vasoconstricts, this increases the resistance at that arteriole and there are 2 changes to consider:

- Flow across the entire circuit **decreases**
- Pressure builds up or **increases** before (upstream) the point of resistance **and** pressure **decreases** after (downstream) the point of resistance

When an arteriole vasodilates, this decreases the resistance at that arteriole, and there are 2 changes to consider:

- Flow across the entire circuit **increases**
- Pressure **decreases** before (upstream) the point of resistance **and** pressure **rises** after (downstream) the point of resistance

Hemodynamics of a single nephron

Figure VI-1-5 represents the hemodynamics of a single nephron. Connected in series are the high-pressure filtering capillaries of the glomerulus and the low-pressure reabsorbing peritubular capillaries.

The glomerular capillaries have a very high hydrostatic pressure because the efferent arterioles are very narrow and thus have a very high resistance. Likewise, there is a large pressure drop as blood flows past this high resistant arteriole and the peritubular capillaries have very low hydrostatic pressure.

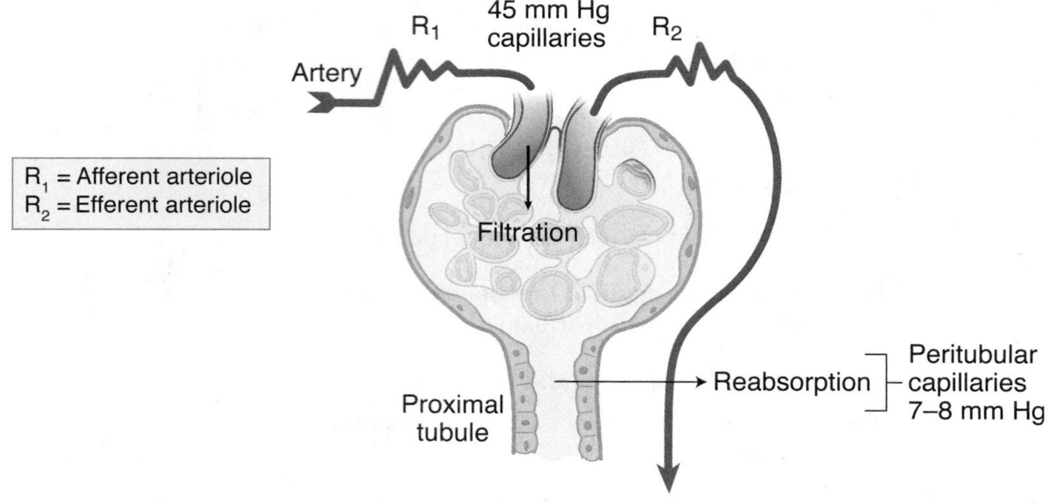

Figure VIII-1-5. Glomerular Hemodynamics

Independent response of the afferent and efferent arterioles

Table VIII-1-1 illustrates the expected consequences of independent isolated constrictions or dilations of the afferent and efferent arterioles.

Table VIII-1-1. Consequences of Independent Isolated Constrictions or Dilations of the Afferent and Efferent Arterioles

	Glomerular Cap Pressure	Peritubular Cap Pressure	Nephron Plasma Flow
Constrict efferent	↑	↓	↓
Dilate efferent	↓	↑	↑
Constrict afferent	↓	↓	↓
Dilate afferent	↑	↑	↑

GLOMERULAR FILTRATION

Glomerular filtration rate (GFR) is the rate at which fluid is filtered into Bowman's capsule. The units of filtration are volume filtered per unit time, e.g., mL/min or liters/day; in a young healthy adult it is about 120 mL/min or 180 L/day.

If one kidney is removed (half of the functioning nephrons lost), GFR decreases only about 25% because the other nephrons compensate.

The 4 Factors Determining Net Filtration Pressure

Figure VIII-1-6 illustrates the role of the 4 factors that determine net filtration pressure.

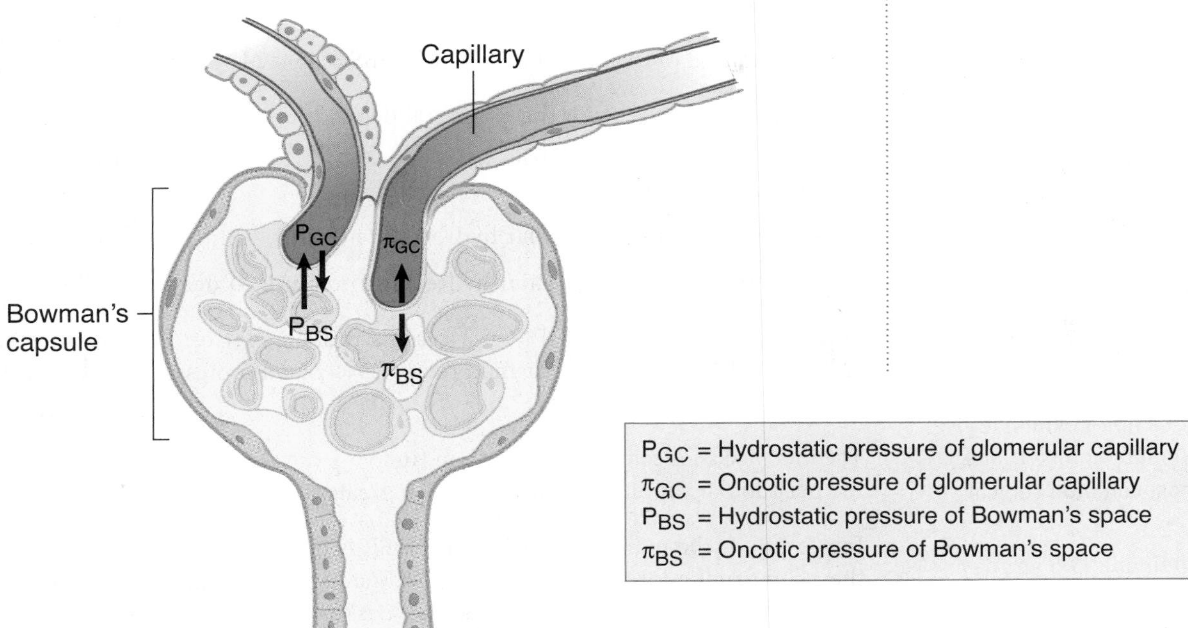

P_{GC}	= Hydrostatic pressure of glomerular capillary
π_{GC}	= Oncotic pressure of glomerular capillary
P_{BS}	= Hydrostatic pressure of Bowman's space
π_{BS}	= Oncotic pressure of Bowman's space

Figure VIII-1-6. Determinants of Filtration

Hydrostatic pressure of the glomerular capillaries

PGC: The hydrostatic pressure of the glomerular capillaries is the only force that promotes filtration. Under normal conditions, this is the main factor that determines GFR.

Oncotic pressure of the plasma

πGC: The oncotic pressure of the plasma varies with the concentration of plasma proteins. Because fluid is filtered but not protein, oncotic pressure, which opposes filtration, increases from the beginning to the end of the glomerular capillaries

Hydrostatic pressure in Bowman's space

PBS: The hydrostatic pressure in Bowman's capsule opposes filtration. Normally, it is low and fairly constant and does not affect the rate of filtration. However, it increases and reduces filtration whenever there is an obstruction downstream, such as a blocked ureter or urethra (postrenal failure).

Protein or oncotic pressure in Bowman's space

πBS: This represents the protein or oncotic pressure in Bowman's space. Very little if any protein is present, and for all practical purposes this factor can be considered zero.

Normal Values

PBS = 8 mm Hg

PGC = 45 mm Hg

πBS = 0 mm Hg

πGC = 24 mm Hg

Net filtration pressure = PGC – πGC – PBS = 45 – 24 – 8 = 13 mm Hg

To summarize, filtration at the glomeruli depends on starling forces:

- The glomerular capillaries have very high hydrostatic pressures → this is why filtration occurs here
- Increasing the glomerular hydrostatic pressure → increases GFR
- Decreasing the glomerular hydrostatic pressure → decreases GFR

Oncotic pressure opposes GFR → ↑ plasma protein → ↑ oncotic pressure → ↓ GFR (no effect on RPF) ↓ plasma protein → ↓ oncotic pressure → ↑ GFR (no effect on RPF)

The increased concentration of protein (increase oncotic pressure) is carried into the peritubular capillaries and promotes a greater net force of reabsorption.

Important: If the main driving force for GFR is the hydrostatic pressure, what is the main driving force the reabsorption at the proximal tubule? The force that is driving reabsorption at the proximal tubule is the oncotic pressure in the peritubular capillaries.

Bridge to Pathology

In nephrotic syndrome, there is marked disruption of the filtering membrane. As a result, plasma proteins now pass through the membrane and are eliminated in the urine. This is typically associated with a non-inflammatory injury to the glomerular membrane system. The most common clinical signs are:

- Marked proteinuria ›3.5 gm/day (because of disrupted glomerular membrane system)
- Edema (loss of plasma oncotic pressure)
- Hypoalbuminemia (albumin lost in urine)
- Lipiduria (disrupted membrane system and proteins in urine)
- Hyperlipidemia (increased lipid synthesis in liver)

In nephritic syndrome, there is an inflammatory disruption of the glomerular membrane system. This disruption allows proteins and cells to cross the filtering membrane. The most common clinical signs are:

- Proteinuria ‹3.5 gm/day (evidence of disrupted membrane)
- Hematuria (disrupted membrane)
- Oliguria (inflammatory infiltrates reduce fluid movement across the membrane)
- Hypertension (inability of kidney to regulate the extracellular volume)
- Azotemia (inability to filter and excrete urea)

Filtering Membrane

The membrane of the glomerulus consists of 3 main structures:

- Capillary endothelial wall with fenestrations that have a magnitude greater than proteins; in addition, the wall is covered with negatively charged compounds
- Glomerular basement membrane made up of a matrix of extracellular negatively charged proteins and other compounds
- Epithelial cell layer of podocytes next to Bowman's space; the podocytes have foot processes bridged by filtration slit diaphragms

Around the capillaries is the mesangium, containing mesangial cells similar to monocytes.

The capillary wall with its fenestrated endothelium, the basement membrane with hydrated spaces, and the interdigitating foot processes of the podocytes combined with an overall large surface area, create a high hydraulic conductivity (permeable to water and dissolved solutes). Passage of large proteins is restricted because of negative charge of the membrane system.

In addition to the net hydraulic force, GFR depends on both the permeability and the surface area of the filtering membrane. The decrease in GFR in most diseased states is due to a reduction in the membrane surface area. This also includes a decrease in the number of functioning nephrons.

Materials Filtered

The following are easily or freely filtered:

- Major electrolytes: sodium, chloride, potassium, bicarbonate
- Metabolic waste products: urea, creatinine
- Metabolites: glucose, amino acids, organic acids (ketone bodies)
- Nonnatural substances: inulin, PAH (p-aminohippuric acid)
- Lower-weight proteins and peptides: insulin, myoglobin

The following are not freely filtered:

- Albumin and other plasma proteins
- Lipid-soluble substances transported in the plasma attached to proteins, such as lipid-soluble bilirubin, T4 (thyroxine), other lipid-soluble hormones; unbound lipid-soluble substances such as free-cortisol are filtered and can appear in the urine

As blood flows though the glomerular capillary, plasma is filtered, but albumin is not, so the plasma albumin concentration and oncotic pressure increase.

Fluid Entering Bowman's Capsule

The fluid entering Bowman's space is an ultrafiltrate of plasma; that is, the filtrate has the same concentration of dissolved substances as plasma, except proteins. The osmolality of the filtrate is 300 mOsm/kg. The criteria for effective osmolality are the same as those previously stated for extracellular fluid (section I).

If a substance is freely filtered by the kidney, the ratio of the filtrate concentration to plasma concentration TF/P = 1.0. This means the concentrations in Bowman's space and the plasma is the same.

Filtration Fraction

The following formula for filtration fraction (FF) and the normal values given should be memorized.

FF = fraction of the material entering the kidney that is filtered normally 0.20 or 20% for a freely filtered substance

$$FF = \frac{GFR}{RPF} \qquad GFR = 120\ mL/min \qquad RPF\ (\text{renal plasma flow}) = 600\ mL/min$$

$$= \frac{120\ mL/min}{600\ mL/min} = 0.20 \text{ or } 20\%$$

- FF affects oncotic pressure in the peritubular capillary (πPC). The greater the FF, the higher the oncotic pressure in the peritubular capillaries; that is because FF represents loss of protein-free fluid into Bowman's space, thereby increasing the concentration of protein in the plasma.
- If FF decreases, then πPC decreases
- Only 20% of the renal plasma flow is filtered. Every minute 600 ml of plasma enters the kidneys. That is the renal plasma flow.
- 20% or 120 mL of plasma is filtered hence a GFR of 120 mL.

Factors Affecting FF

Based on the preceding discussion, the following should be expected for afferent versus efferent constriction:

	Afferent Constriction	Efferent Constriction
Glomerular filtration pressure	↓	↑
GFR	↓	↑
RPF	↓	↓
FF	↔	↑

Effects of Sympathetic Nervous System

Stimulation of the sympathetic neurons to the kidney causes vasoconstriction of the arterioles, but has a greater effect on the afferent arteriole. As a consequence:

- RPF decreases
- PGC decreases
- GFR decreases
- FF increases
- PPC decreases
- πPC increases
- ↑ forces promoting reabsorption in the peritubular capillaries because of a lower peritubular capillary hydrostatic pressure and an increase in plasma oncotic pressure (FF increases)

Effects of Angiotensin II

Angiotensin II (Ang II) is a vasoconstrictor. It constricts both the afferent and efferent arterioles, but is has a bigger effect on the efferent arteriole. As a consequence:

- RPF decreases
- PGC increases
- GFR increases
- FF increases
- PPC decreases
- πPC increases
- ↑ forces promoting reabsorption in the peritubular capillaries because of a lower peritubular capillary hydrostatic pressure and an increase in plasma oncotic pressure (FF increases)

During a stress response, there is an increase in sympathetic input and very high levels of circulating angiotensin II. As a consequence:

- Increased sympathetic tone to the kidneys and very high levels of angiotensin II vasoconstrict both the afferent and the efferent arterioles. Because both arterioles constrict, there is a large drop in the RPF and only a small drop in the GFR.
- The net effect is an increase in FF.
- The increase in FF → increase in oncotic pressure → increase in the reabsorption in proximal tubules

- Overall, less fluid is filtered and a greater percentage of that fluid is reabsorbed in the proximal tubule, leading to preservation of volume in a volume depleted state
- There is also an increase in ADH due to the low volume state
- Activation of the sympathetic nervous system also directly increases renin release

The net effect of angiotensin II is to preserve GFR in volume-depleted state. In a volume-depleted state, a decrease in GFR is beneficial because less fluid filtered results in less fluid excretion (however, a very large decrease in GFR prevents removal of waste products like creatinine and urea). Angiotensin II prevents a large decrease in GFR.

Clinical Correlate

Administration of ACE inhibitors and ARBs

ACE inhibitors and ARBs are used for diabetic nephropathy because they lead to a reduction in glomerular capillary pressure and reduce damage and fibrosis of the glomuli (which will delay the need for hemodialysis). They treat hyperfiltration. In most cases, there is a small and transient drop in GFR.

Inhibition of angiotensin II leads to vasodilation of the efferent arteriole, which leads to decreased glomerular capillary pressure and decreased GFR. It also leads to increased RPF because of the decrease in resistance to flow. The pressure downstream from the efferent arteriole (peritubular capillary pressure) increases because there is a decreased resistance at the EA.

Use the following guidelines for using ACE inhibitors and ARBs:

- Give ACE inhibitors to patients with nephrotic syndrome and stable chronic renal failure.
- Avoid ACE inhibitors and ARBs in patients with severely compromised GFR (risk of hyperkalemia) and with acute renal failure.
- ACE inhibitors and ARBs may cause a type IV RTA because they block aldosterone (leading to hyperkalemia); in this case they must both be held. If ACE inhibitors cause hyperkalemia, so will ARBs.
- Switch from ACE inhibitor to ARB in cases with ACE-inhibitor cough, not for hyperkalemia.
- ACE inhibitors and ARBs are contraindicated in bilateral renal artery stenosis, where both kidneys have such low perfusion that GFR is highly dependent on constriction of EA. When the effect of angiotensin II is removed, the result is a significant drop in GFR and acute renal failure.

There is no parasympathetic innervation of the kidney.

Although prostaglandins seem to play little role in the normal regulation of renal blood flow, they do become important in times of stress. For example, the vasoconstriction produced by sympathetic activation is partially countered by the local release of vasodilating prostaglandins (PGI_2 and PGE_2). This is thought to help prevent ischemic damage during times of stress.

Clinical Correlate

A 25-year-old man spends a week in the desert. Due to severe dehydration, his volume status is depleted → high angiotensin II → vasocontriciton of the efferent arterioles → an increase in GFR and decrease in RPF → an increase in FF → more plasma filtered in the glomeruli → higher albumin concentration (hence higher oncotic pressure) in the glomerular capillaries → higher oncotic pressure in the peritubular capillaries → an increase in peritubular reabsorption. Therefore, an increase in the FF → an increase is reabsorption at the proximal tubules.

A dehydrated patient needs to increase reabsorption of fluid at the proximal tubules to preserve volume. Angiotension II helps preserve GRF and volume in a volume-depleted state.

Clinical Correlate

What would happen if you gave NSAIDs to the 75-year-old man who is hemorrhaging?

During a stress state the increase in sympathetic tone causes vasoconstriction of the afferent arterioles. The same stimuli activate a local production of prostaglandins. Prostaglandins lead to vasodilation of the afferent arterioles, thus modulating the vasoconstriction. Unopposed, the vasoconstriction from the sympathetic nervous system and angiotensin II can lead to a profound reduction in RPF and GFR, which in turn, could cause renal failure. NSAIDs inhibit synthesis of prostaglandins and interfere with these protective effects.

Chapter Summary

- Autoregulatory mechanisms maintain a fairly constant renal blood flow and GFR despite changes in arterial blood pressure.
- Individual nephrons are organized in parallel, but the vascular system of each nephron structure (afferent arteriole, glomerular capillaries, efferent arteriole, and peritubular capillaries) is connected in series.
- The major factor determining GFR is glomerular capillary hydrostatic pressure. The only other important factor in a normal kidney system is the oncotic pressure of the plasma proteins. The glomerular membrane system is permeable to all substances dissolved in plasma except proteins and provides a large surface area for filtration. A loss of surface area can be compensated for by an increase in glomerular capillary pressure.
- FF is the fraction of plasma that is filtered at the glomerular capillary. A decrease in flow tends to increase FF.
- Filtered load is the rate at which a substance is filtered into Bowman's space. For a freely filtered substance it is determined by its plasma concentration and GFR.
- Nephrotic and nephritic syndromes are 2 classic patterns of glomerular disease.
  - **Nephrotic syndrome** characteristically is a noninflammatory injury to the glomerular epithelium or basement membrane, resulting in a large proteinuria but only minimal changes in GFR.
  - **Nephritic syndrome** is an inflammatory response to the glomerular injury, resulting in significantly decreased GFR and red blood cells appearing in the urine.

Solute Transport: Reabsorption and Secretion

2

Learning Objectives

- ❑ Interpret scenarios on solute transport
- ❑ Interpret scenarios on quantifying renal processes (mass balance)
- ❑ Demonstrate understanding of clearance
- ❑ Answer questions about TM tubular reabsorption
- ❑ Solve problems concerning TM tubular secretion
- ❑ Use knowledge of the renal handling of some important solutes

SOLUTE TRANSPORT

Transport proteins in the cell membranes of the nephron mediate the reabsorption and secretion of solutes and water transport in the kidneys. Acquired defects in transport proteins are the cause of many kidney diseases.

In addition the transport proteins are important drug targets.

Transport Mechanisms

Simple diffusion

- Net movement represents molecules or ions moving down their electrochemical gradient.
- This doesn't require energy.

Facilitated diffusion (facilitated transport)

- A molecule or ion moving across a membrane down its concentration gradient attached to a specific membrane-bound protein.
- This doesn't require energy.

Active transport

- A protein-mediated transport that uses ATP as a source of energy to move a molecule or ion against its electrochemical gradient.

Dynamics of Protein-Mediated Transport

Uniport

- Transporter moves a single molecule or ion as in the uptake of glucose into skeletal muscle or adipose tissue. This is an example of facilitated diffusion.

Symport (cotransport)

- A coupled protein transport of 2 or more solutes in the same direction as in Na-glucose, Na-amino acid transporters.

Antiport (countertransport)

- A coupled protein transport of 2 or more solutes in the opposite direction.

Generally, protein carriers transport substances that cannot readily diffuse across a membrane. There are no transporters for gases and most lipid-soluble substances because those substances readily move across membranes by simple diffusion.

Characteristics common to all protein-mediated transport

Rate of transport

A substance is transported more rapidly than it would be by diffusion, because the membrane is not usually permeable to any substance for which there is a transport protein.

Saturation kinetics

- As the concentration of the substance initially increases on one side of the membrane, the transport rate increases.
- Once the transporters become saturated, transport rate is maximal (TM = transport maximum). Rate of transport is dependent upon:
  - Concentration of solute
  - Number of functioning transporters; the only way to increase TM is to add more protein carriers to the membrane
- Once all the protein carriers are saturated, the solutes are transported across the membrane at a constant rate. This constant rate is TM.
- There is no TM is simple diffusion.

Chemical specificity

To be transported, the substance must have a certain chemical structure. Generally, only the natural isomer is transported (e.g., D-glucose but not L-glucose).

Competition for carrier

Substances of similar chemical structure may compete for the same transporter. For example, glucose and galactose generally compete for the same transport protein.

Primary and secondary transport

- In primary active transport, ATP is consumed directly by the transporting protein, (e.g., the Na/K-ATPase pump, or the calcium-dependent ATPase of the sarcoplasmic reticulum).
- Secondary active transport depends indirectly on ATP as a source of energy, as in the cotransport of Na-glucose in the proximal tubule. This process depends on ATP utilized by the Na/K-ATPase pump.
- Glucose moves up a concentration gradient via secondary active transport.

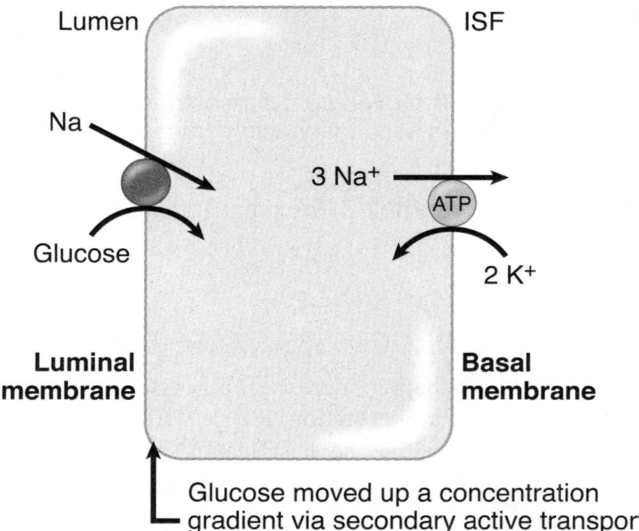

Figure VIII-2-1. Renal Tubule or Small Intestine

Figure VIII-2-1 represents a renal proximal tubular cell. The Na/K-ATPase pump maintains a low intracellular sodium concentration, which creates a large gradient across the cell membrane. It is this sodium gradient across the luminal membrane that drives secondary active transport of glucose.

In summary, the secondary active transport of glucose:

- Depends upon luminal sodium
- Is stimulated by luminal sodium (via increased sodium gradient)
- Is linked to the uptake of sodium
- Depends upon rate of metabolic ATP production

Another example (Figure VIII-2-2) of secondary active transport is the counter transport of Na–H^+ also in the proximal tubule. This process depends on the Na/K-ATPase pump.

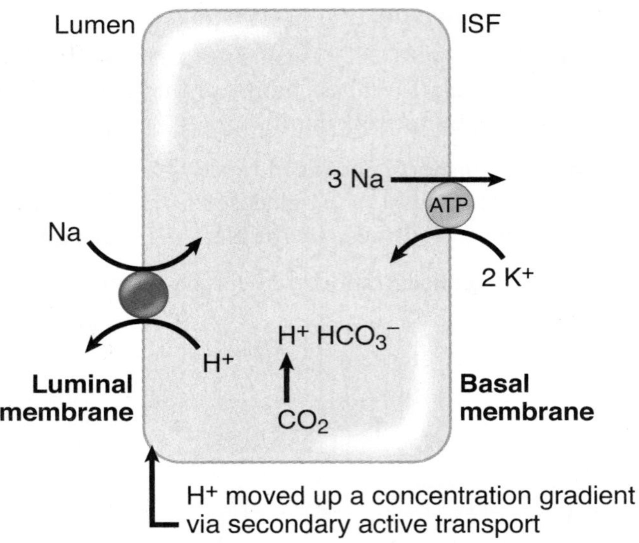

Figure VIII-2-2. Proximal Tubule

QUANTIFYING RENAL PROCESSES (MASS BALANCE)

As indicated in the previous chapter, there are 4 processes in the nephron: filtration, reabsorption, secretion, and excretion. Figure VIII-2-3 illustrates that how the nephron handles any solute, on a net basis, can be derived because the rate at which it enters (filtered load) and its rate of excretion can be measured.

Both variables are expressed as an amount of substance per unit time, and the units are the same, e.g., mg/min.

U_x = Urine concentration of substance
V = Urine flow rate

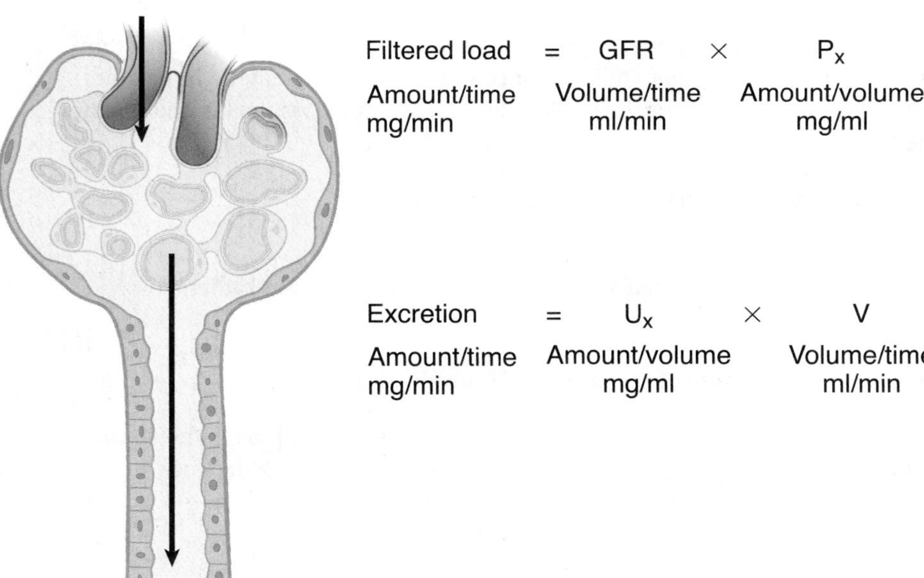

Filtered load = GFR × Px
Amount/time mg/min
Volume/time ml/min
Amount/volume mg/ml
Excretion = Ux × V
Amount/time mg/min
Amount/volume mg/ml
Volume/time ml/min

Figure VIII-2-3. Relationship of Filtered Load and Excretion

No Net Tubular Modification

- Filtered load = excretion rate
- The amount filtered and amount excreted per unit time are always the same, e.g., inulin, mannitol.

Net Reabsorption

- Filtered load > excretion
- Excretion is always less than filtered load, e.g., glucose, sodium, urea.
- If the substance is completely reabsorbed, the rate of filtration and the rate of reabsorption are equal.
- Excretion rate is 0
- If the substance is partially reabsorbed, excretion is less than filtration.

Net Secretion

- Filtered load < excretion
- Excretion is always greater than filtered load, e.g., PAH, creatinine.
- Creatinine is freely filtered, and a very small amount is secreted.

The following formula is sometimes used to calculate net transport. The sign of the calculated number will indicate the 3 basic categories:

0 = no net transport

+ = net reabsorption

– = net secretion

net transport rate = filtered load – excretion rate

= (GFR × Px) – (Ux × V)

GFR: glomerular filtration rate
units: volume/time, e.g., mL/min

P_x: free (not bound to protein) concentration of substance in the plasma

units: amount/volume, e.g., mg/mL

Question: Given the following information, calculate the reabsorption rate for glucose.

GFR = 120 mL/min

Plasma glucose = 300 mg/100 mL

Urine flow = 2 mL/min

Urine glucose = 10 mg/mL

Answer: 340 mg/min

CLEARANCE

Clearance refers to a theoretical volume of plasma from which a substance is removed over a period of time. Applying the principles of mass balance above, if a solute has an ER, then it is cleared by the kidney. In other words, if it is filtered and not fully reabsorbed or is secreted, then it appears in the urine and is thus cleared from the body.

If, on the other hand, it is filtered and then all is reabsorbed, the ER and clearance is zero, and it is not cleared by the kidney.

For example, if the concentration of substance x is 4 molecules per liter and the excretion of x is 4 molecules per minute, the volume of plasma cleared of x is 1 L per minute. If the excretion of x decreases to 2 molecules per minute, the volume cleared of x is only 0.5 L per minute. If the concentration of x decreases to 2 molecules per liter of plasma and excretion is maintained at 2 molecules per minute, the cleared volume is back to 1 L per minute. These numbers are summarized in Table VIII-2-1.

Table VIII-2-1. Example Calculations of Clearance Values

Plasma Concentration (molecules/L)	Excretion Rate (molecules/minute)	Volume Cleared (L/minute)
4	4	1.0
4	2	0.5
2	2	1.0

Ux: urine concentration of x
V: urine flow rate
Px: plasma concentration of x

Thus, the 2 factors that determine clearance are the plasma concentration of the substance and its excretion rate.

$$\text{Clearance of x} = \frac{\text{Excretion rate of x}}{\text{Px}} = \frac{\text{Ux} \times \text{V}}{\text{Px}}$$

The plasma concentration of the substance and its urine concentration must be in the same units, which then cancel.

Urine flow (V) is a volume per unit time, and the units of V become the units of clearance.

Clearance is a volume of plasma cleared of a substance per unit time, mL/min or L/day.

Question: Using the following information, calculate the clearance of x, y, and z.

V = 2 mL/min
Ux = 2 mg/mPx =2 mg/mL
Uy = 0 mg/mPy =13.6 mg/mL
Uz = 0.5 mg/mPz =1 mg/mL

Answer: *x* = 2 mL/min, y = 0, and z = 1 mL/min

TM TUBULAR REABSORPTION

Glucose

Figure VIII-2-4 graphically represents the dynamics of glucose filtration, reabsorption, and excretion. It is the application of the principle of mass balance and clearance discussed above. Many substances are reabsorbed via a TM system, and glucose serves as our prototypical example.

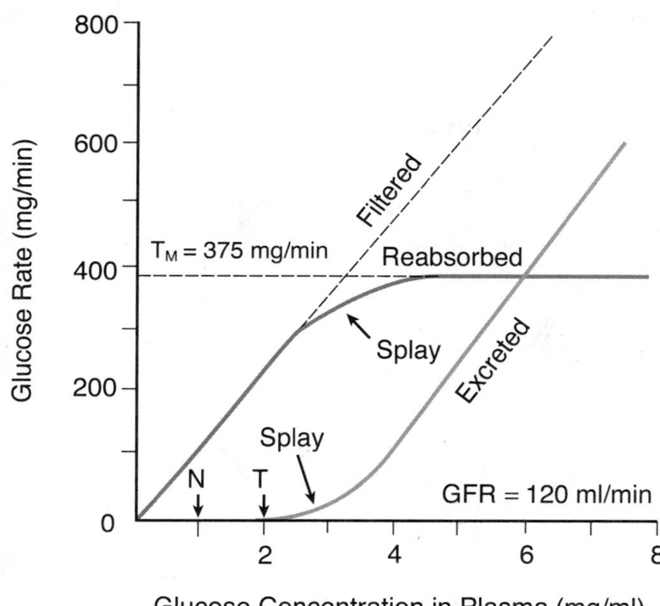

Figure VIII-2-4. Transport Maximum Reabsorption of Glucose

N: normal plasma glucose concentration
T: plasma (renal) threshold

Note the x-axis is glucose rate (mg/min). As was just discussed, there are 3 rates: filtration (dashed line), excretion (blue line); and reabsorption (purple line), which is filtered load (filtration rate) – excretion rate (ER).

- At low plasma levels, the filtration and reabsorption rates of glucose are equal, thus glucose does not appear in the urine and the clearance is zero.
- TM is the maximal reabsorption rate of glucose, i.e., the rate when all the carriers (SGLT-2/1; see chapter 4) are saturated. TM can be used as an index of the number of functioning nephrons.
- The rounding of the reabsorption curve into the plateau is called **splay**. Splay occurs because some nephrons reach TM before others. Thus, TM for the entire kidney is not reached until after the region of splay.
- Plasma (or renal) threshold is the plasma glucose concentration at which glucose first appears in the urine. This occurs at the beginning of splay. Before splay, all of the glucose that is filtered is reabsorbed and the ER is 0.

TM TUBULAR SECRETION

p-aminohippuric acid (PAH) secretion

- PAH secretion from the peritubular capillaries into the proximal tubule is an example of a transport maximum system.
- As a TM system, it has the general characteristics discussed for the reabsorption of glucose except for the direction of transport.

Figure VIII-2-5 illustrates the renal handling of PAH at low plasma concentrations.

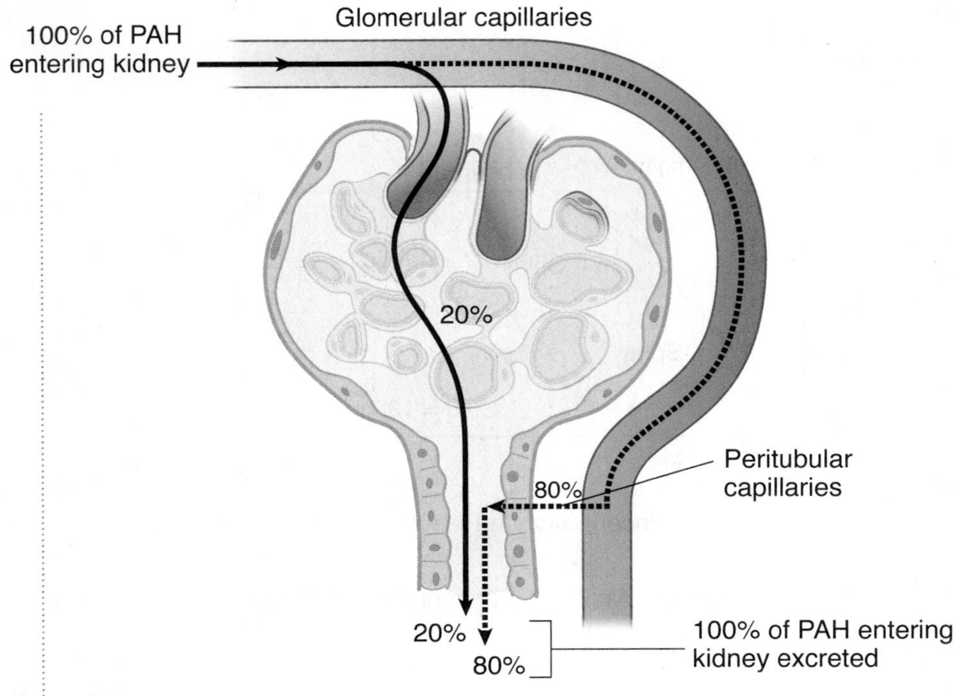

Figure VIII-2-5. Secretion of PAH

<u>Normal values:</u>
Renal plasma flow = 600 mL/min
GFR = 120 mL/min
FF = 0.20

- The renal plasma flow (RPF) is the volume of plasma that enters the kidney in a minute (600 mL/min).
- The RPF contains the total concentration of PAH dissolved in plasma in mg/ml entering the PAH.
- Of the RPF, 20% (120 mL) is typically filtered, regardless of the total amount of PAH entering the kidney (in the RPF).
- Whatever is filtered is excreted, it is NOT reabsorbed; therefore, that 20% is **always** cleared (removed from the plasma) and excreted (placed in the urine)!!

What happens to the rest of the PAH (the 480 mL [80%] of plasma that was not filtered)? That depends on the concentration of PAH in the RPF:

- If the RPF has a low concentration of PAH, 20% of the PAH in the RPF is filtered and the rest of PAH (the remaining 80% of the RPF) is secreted; 100% of PAH in the RPF is excreted in the urine right arrow; therefore, 100% is cleared.
- **All** of the PAH that enters the kidney is removed and is excreted in the urine; it is all cleared from the plasma. If you looked at the renal vein, it would have no PAH.

- When the PAH concentration is below the transport maximum, we can use the clearance of PAH to calculate the estimated RPF.

For example, a concentration of 0.08 mg/ml means that out of the entire 480 mL of plasma (80% of the RPF) that was not filtered, there is only 38.4 mg (0.08 x 480 mL) of PAH because that is well below the transport maximum for PAH (80 mg/min), it is all secreted.

If the concentration of PAH entering the kidneys in the RPF was high and it was past the TM for PAH, you would not be able to secrete it all because the carriers are all saturated. Some would remain in the plasma of the renal vein; the clearance of PAH would decrease but you will always excrete the 20% of the RPF that was filtered (because it is not reabsorbed). Therefore, as the plasma concentration of PAH increases, the clearance of PAH decreases. Figure VIII-2-6 illustrates this mechanism.

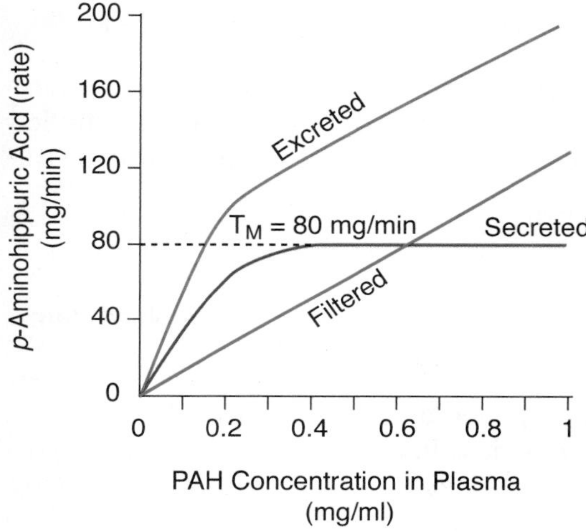

Filtration: linear relationship with plasma concentration and represents 20% of PAH delivered to kidney

Secretion: initially 4× filtration rate and represents 80% of PAH delivered to kidney. Therefore, initially all the PAH delivered to kidney is removed—20% by filtration and 80% by secretion—and the concentration of PAH in the renal venous plasma should be zero. As plasma level rises, secretion increases, reaching maximum rate (T_M) when the carriers are saturated. PAH appears in renal venous plasma at the beginning of splay region in the secretion curve

Excretion: sum of the filtration rate and secretion rate. Once T_M is reached, increases in excretion parallel increases in filtration

Figure VIII-2-6. Excretion of PAH

For example, if the PAH concentration were 80 mg/mL, 20% of the RPF would be filtered (always) and excreted. That 20% is cleared (removed from the plasma). Of the remaining 80% of the RPF, there will be 80 mg/mL of PAH, which means that in 1 mL there will be 80 mg of PAH and you will only be able to secrete the 80 mg (because that is the TM), you will only clear 1 mL of plasma of the remaining RPF. So 479 mL of plasma out of the 600 ml that entered the kidney (the RPF) is not cleared and will be present in the renal vein.

Therefore, you see a dramatic decrease in clearance (because there is more PAH in the renal vein, meaning it was not cleared).

Remember:

- If it is in the renal vein, it was not cleared.
- If it is in the urine, it was cleared.

Most of what was cleared in this case was cleared by filtration, not secretion. Thus, calculating the clearance here is very similar to calculating the GRF, not the RPF.

Regardless of the plasma concentration of PAH, the kidney will always clear the volume filtered (GFR), i.e., the volume of PAH that is filtered (GFR) is cleared from the plasma and excreted in the urine. At low PAH concentrations, as the plasma PAH concentration is increasing, both the secretion rate (SR) and filtered load (FL) are increasing. Thus, there is a very rapid increase in the excretion rate (ER) of PAH and the slope of the line is very steep.

After transport maximum, the SR is constant because all the PAH protein carriers are saturated. The slope of the ER decreases and parallels the FL because now, only the FL is increasing and the SR is constant. The ER still increases, just not as quickly.

The reason why the slope of the line decreases is because the PAH carriers are saturated and the SR has reached transport maximum.

$$\mathbf{ER = FL + SR}$$

After transport maximum, the SR is constant, but as the plasma concentration increases, the FL increases, therefore, the ER increases and parallels the FL.

PAH clearance at low plasma concentrations is referred to as effective renal plasma flow (ERPF) because some plasma perfused the renal capsule. This flow (about 10%) is not cleared of PAH. Thus, PAH clearance is only 90% of the true renal plasma flow.

$$\text{Renal blood flow} = \text{renal plasma flow}/1 - \text{HCT}$$

If renal plasma flow is 600 mL/min and Hct is 50%, then renal blood flow is 1200 mL/min.

PAH is transported by a fairly nonspecific organic anion transporter (OAT). Many compounds compete for the carriers. In addition to PAH, some of those compounds include:

- Penicillin
- Furosemide
- Acetazolamide
- Salicylate

Because the organic anions all compete for the same carriers, elevation of the plasma level of one ion inhibits the secretion and clearance of the others.

There is a similar transport secretory system for many organic cations. A slightly different transport mechanism is involved but, again, the system is fairly nonspecific. Drugs using this pathway include:

- Atropine
- Morphine
- Procainamide
- Cimetidine
- Amiloride

Note that, because of competition for the carrier proteins, the concurrent administration of organic cations can increase the plasma concentration of both drugs to much higher levels than when the drugs are given alone.

THE RENAL HANDLING OF SOME IMPORTANT SOLUTES

The illustrations in Figure VIII-2-7 represent the net transport of specific types of substances for a normal individual on a typical Western diet (contains red meat). The dashed lines represent the route followed by the particular substance. Quantitative aspects are not shown. For example, in B, 20% of the substance entering the kidney is filtered and excreted, and the remaining 80% passes through the kidneys and back into the general circulation without processing.

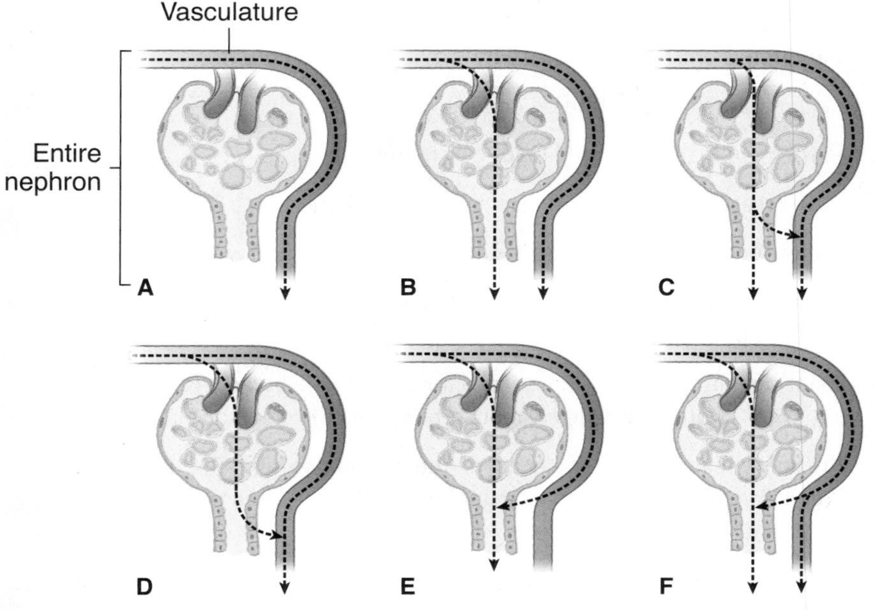

Figure VIII-2-7. Graphical Representation of Transport

Note

These illustrations are meant to show overall net transport only.

A = protein
B = inulin
C = potassium, sodium, urea
D = glucose, bicarbonate
E = PAH
F = creatinine

Chapter Summary

- Simple diffusion and facilitated transport are both passive processes (not energy-dependent) driven by concentration gradients.
- The rate of protein-mediated transport increases with increased substrate delivery until the carriers are saturated. The maximum rate of transport (carrier saturation) is called TM, and this rate is directly proportional to the number of functioning carriers present in the system.
- Secondary active transport is driven by the sodium gradient across the cell membrane, which is maintained by the Na/K–ATPase pump.
- If a substance is freely filtered and exhibits:
  - No net transport, filtered load = excretion rate
  - Net reabsorption, filtered load is $>$ excretion rate
  - Net secretion, filtered load is $<$ excretion rate
- Clearance is the theoretical volume of plasma from which a substance is removed per unit time.
- Renal clearance means a solute is removed from the body because it is in the urine. If a solute is completely reabsorbed, then the clearance is zero.
- The active reabsorption of glucose in the proximal exhibits TM dynamics. Everything filtered is reabsorbed until the carriers in some nephrons are saturated.
  - The plasma level at this point is called plasma (or renal) threshold, and glucose begins to appear in the urine.
  - This is also at the beginning of the region of splay. All transporters in all nephrons become saturated once the plateau is reached, which is after the region of splay. At this point, the glucose reabsorption rate is maximal (TM). TM is an index of the number of functioning nephrons.
- The active secretion of PAH in the proximal tubule exhibits TM dynamics. At plasma levels below carrier saturation, 20% of the PAH entering the kidney is filtered, and 80% is secreted. All the PAH is excreted, and no PAH appears in the renal venous plasma (excluding plasma flow through the capsule). PAH appears in the renal venous plasma once the carriers in a few nephrons become saturated (beginning of splay).

Clinical Estimation of GFR and Patterns of Clearance

3

Learning Objectives

- ❑ Use knowledge of clearance as an estimator of GFR
- ❑ Demonstrate understanding of clearance curves for some characteristic substances
- ❑ Solve problems concerning free water clearance
- ❑ Use knowledge of sodium and urea clearance

CLEARANCE AS AN ESTIMATOR OF GFR

Estimates of GFR are used clinically as an index of renal function and to assess the severity and the course of renal disease. A fall in GFR means the disease is progressing, whereas an increase in GFR suggests a recovery. In many cases a fall in GFR may be the first and only clinical sign of renal dysfunction. Estimations of GFR rely on the concept of clearance.

Substances having the following characteristics can be used to estimate GFR.

- Stable plasma concentration that is easily measured
- Freely filtered into Bowman's space
- Not reabsorbed, secreted, synthesized, or metabolized by the kidney

Ideal substances include inulin, sucrose, and mannitol. Even though the clearance of inulin is considered the gold standard for the measurement of GFR, it is not used clinically. Instead clinical estimates of GFR rely on creatinine.

Creatinine is released from skeletal muscle at a constant rate proportional to muscle mass. Muscle mass decreases with age but GFR also normally decreases with age. Creatinine is freely filtered and not reabsorbed by the kidney, though a very small amount is secreted into the proximal tubule.

Creatinine production = creatinine excretion =
filtered load of creatinine = Pcr × GFR

Thus, if creatinine production remains constant, a decrease in GFR increases plasma creatinine concentration, while an increase in GFR decreases plasma creatinine concentration.

Plasma creatinine, however, is not a very sensitive measure of reduced GFR. It only reveals large changes in GFR. As shown in Figure VIII-3-1, a significant reduction of GFR only produces a modest elevation of plasma or serum creatinine concentration.

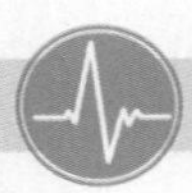

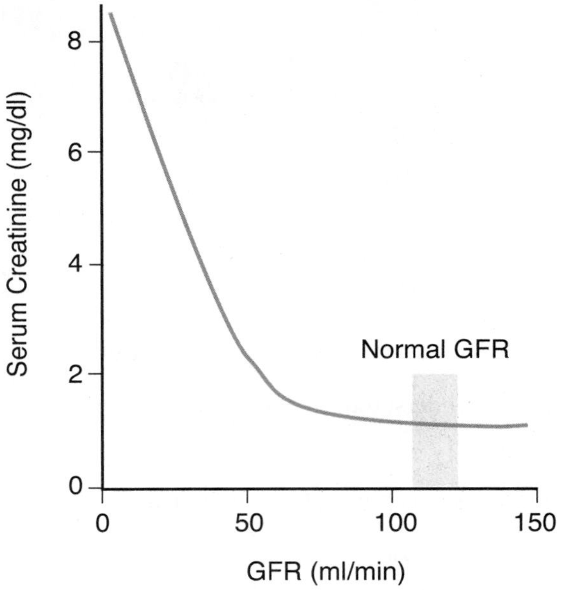

Figure VIII-3-1. Serum Creatinine as Index of GFR

The only practical numerical estimate is the calculated clearance of creatinine. The following is all that is needed:

- Plasma creatinine concentration
- Timed collection of urine and the urine concentration of creatinine

CLEARANCE CURVES FOR SOME CHARACTERISTIC SUBSTANCES

Figure VIII-3-2 plots clearance versus increasing plasma concentration for 4 substances. A description of each curve follows the figure.

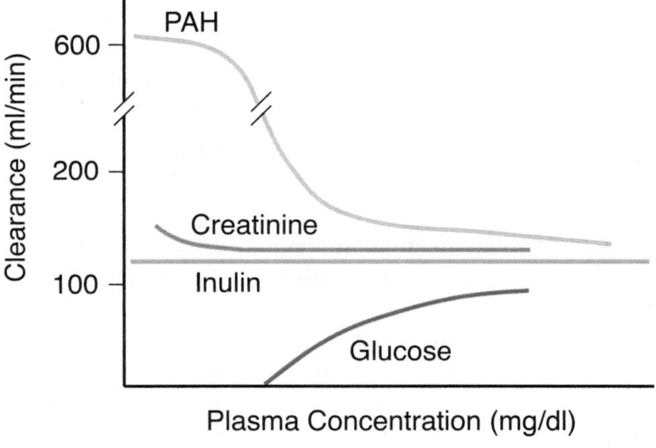

Figure VIII-3-2. Clearance Curves

Inulin

- The clearance of inulin is independent of the plasma concentration, thus plotting it on the graph produces a line parallel to the X-axis. This is because a rise in the plasma concentration produces a corresponding rise in filtered load and thus a corresponding rise in ER (recall that inulin is neither secreted nor reabsorbed). In other words, the numerator and denominator of the clearance equation for inulin change in proportion, leaving the quotient (clearance) unchanged.
- It is always parallel to the x axis, and the point of intersection with the y axis is always GFR.
- If GFR increases, the line shifts upward; likewise, if GFR decreases, the line shifts down.

Glucose

- At low plasma levels, the clearance of glucose is zero because all of the FL is reabsorbed.
- As the plasma levels rise, the FL exceeds the TM in some nephrons and as a result, glucose appears in the urine and thus has a clearance.
- The plasma level at which glucose first appears in the urine is called the plasma (or renal) threshold.
- As the plasma level rises further, the clearance increases and approaches that of inulin. The clearance never equals inulin because some glucose is always reabsorbed.

Creatinine

- Because there is some secretion of creatinine, the clearance is always greater than the clearance of inulin.
- However, because only a small amount is secreted, creatinine clearance parallels inulin clearance and is independent of production rate (excretion rises as plasma concentration increases).
- Because it is endogenously produced, it is not necessary to infuse it to get a clearance measurement, as has to be done to measure inulin clearance. Therefore, the clearance of creatinine is the preferred clinical method for determining GFR (see above).

PAH

- At low plasma concentrations, the clearance equals renal plasma flow.
- As the plasma concentration rises, the carriers in some nephrons hit TM, resulting in some PAH appearing in the renal venous plasma.
- Plasma concentrations above TM reduce the clearance of PAH (described in chapter 2)
- As the plasma level rises further, the clearance approaches but never equals GFR because some PAH is always secreted.

Summary of the highest clearance to the lowest clearance:

PAH > creatinine > inulin > urea > sodium > glucose = albumin

Remember, if it is in the renal vein, it is not cleared. This could be because it was not filtered (like albumin) or it was filtered and all reabsorbed (like glucose).

FREE WATER CLEARANCE

Free water clearance is the best measure of the balance between solute and water excretion. Its use is to determine whether the kidneys are responding appropriately to maintain normal plasma osmolality. Free water clearance is how much solute-free water is being excreted; it is as if urine consisted of plasma (with solutes) plus or minus pure water.

- If urine osmolality is 300 mOsm/kg (isotonic urine), free water clearance is zero.
- If plasma osmolality is too low, urine osmolality should be lower still (positive free water clearance) in order to compensate.
- Positive-free water clearance tends to cause increased plasma osmolality; negative free water clearance causes reduced plasma osmolality.
- C_{H_2O} (+) = hypotonic urine is formed (osmolality <300 mOsm/kg)
- C_{H_2O} (–) = hypertonic urine is formed (osmolality >300 mOsm/kg)

$$C_{H_2O} = V - \frac{U_{osm} V}{P_{osm}}$$

V = urine flow rate

U_{osm} = urine osmolarity

P_{osm} = plasma osmolarity

$$V = C_{H_2O} + C_{osm}$$

Sample Calculation

$\dot{V} = 3.0$ mL/min

$U_{osm} = 800$ mOsm/L

$P_{osm} = 400$ mOsm/L

$C_{H_2O} = -3$ mL/min

Conclusion: The kidneys are conserving water; this is appropriate compensation for the excessive plasma osmolarity in this patient.

SODIUM AND UREA CLEARANCE

Sodium

- Sodium always appears in the urine, thus sodium always has a positive clearance.
- The fractional excretion of Na^+ (F_ENa^+; equation not shown) indicates the fraction (percentage) of the filtered Na^+ that is excreted. It is very useful in differentiating prerenal from intrarenal acute renal failure (see next chapter).

- Since almost the entire filtered load of sodium is reabsorbed its clearance is just above zero. Aldosterone, by increasing the reabsorption of sodium, decreases the $FeNa^+$. Atrial natriuretic increases the $FeNa^+$ by causing a sodium diuresis.

Urea

- Urea is freely filtered but partially reabsorbed.
- Because some urea is always present in the urine, you always clear a portion of the 120 mL/min filtered into Bowman's space.
- Since urea tends to follow the water and excretion is flow dependent, a diuresis increases urea clearance and an antidiuresis decreases urea clearance.
- ADH increases reabsorption of urea in the medullary collecting duct → increase in BUN → decrease in clearance → if the plasma concentration is increasing in the renal venous plasma, less is cleared from the plasma
- With a small volume of concentrated urine, the concentration of urea is relatively high, but the excretion is less than in a diuresis that has a much lower concentration of urea. It is the large volume in the diuresis that increases the urea excretion and clearance.

Chapter Summary

- Substances that do not appear in the urine have a clearance of zero.
- Substances freely filtered and partially reabsorbed have a clearance less than the GFR.
- Substances freely filtered with no net transport like inulin have a clearance equal to GFR.
- Substances freely filtered and with net secretion like creatinine have a clearance greater than the GFR. Because only a very small amount of creatinine is secreted, it always has a clearance slightly greater than GFR. However, because the amount secreted is small, and it is a solute naturally produced in the body, estimating its clearance serves as an indicator of GFR.
- Substances freely filtered with the remainder entering the kidney completely secreted, have a clearance equal to renal plasma flow.
- Free water clearance is a volume excreted without solute. It is used to evaluate if the renal balance of solute and water excretion is appropriate.
- There is an obligatory solute loss from the kidney. The primary solutes lost are sodium and urea.

Regional Transport 4

Learning Objectives

- ❑ Solve problems concerning the proximal tubule
- ❑ Explain information related to loop of Henle
- ❑ Use knowledge of distal tubule
- ❑ Use knowledge of collecting duct
- ❑ Answer questions about renal tubular acidosis
- ❑ Explain information related to disorders of potassium homeostasis
- ❑ Demonstrate understanding of renal failure

THE PROXIMAL TUBULE

The fluid that enters the proximal tubule is an isotonic ultrafiltrate (300 mOsm/kg). The concentration of a freely filtered substance in this fluid equals its plasma concentration. Figure VIII-4-1 illustrates the main cellular transport processes of the proximal tubular cells.

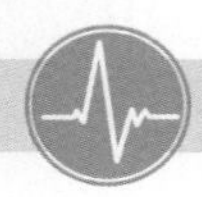

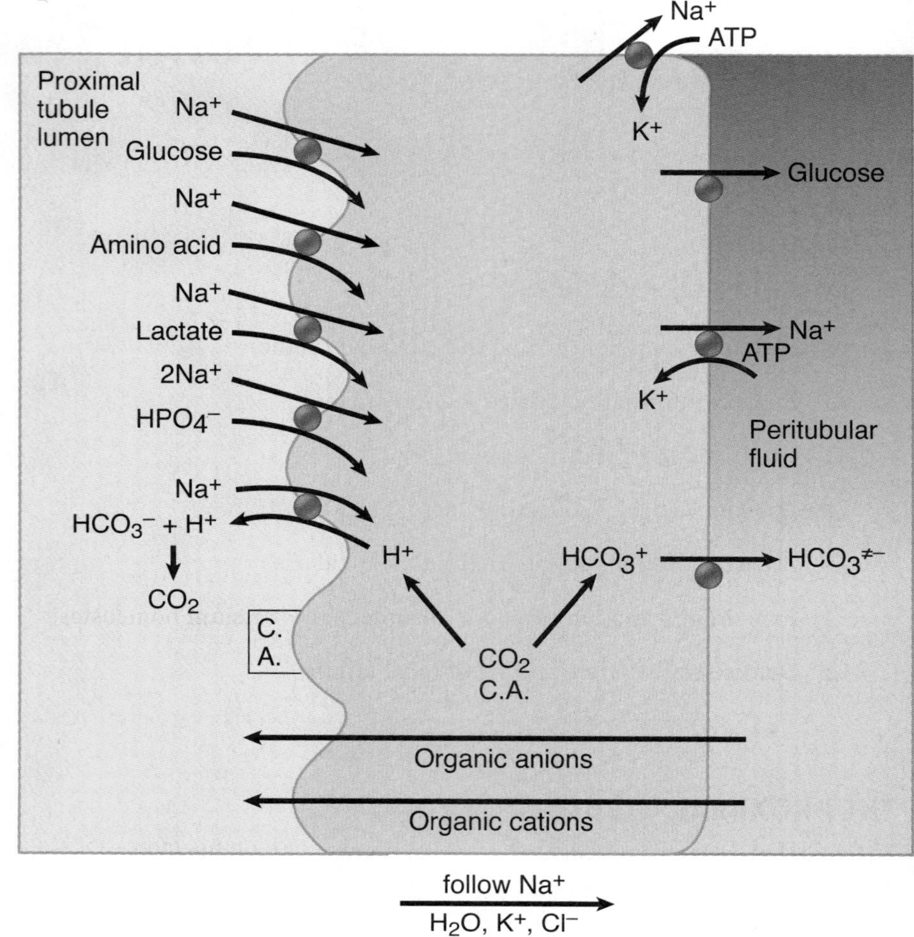

Figure VIII-4-1. Transport in Proximal Tubule

Proximal Tubule (PT) Changes

Sodium

- Approximately two-thirds of the filtered sodium is reabsorbed in the proximal tubule (PT). The basolateral Na^+--K^+ ATPase creates the gradient for Na^+ entry into the cell and its removal from the cell back into the bloodstream.
- Although it can be modified some, the PT captures two-thirds of the filtered sodium (referred to as glomerulotubular balance). Recapturing two-thirds of the sodium helps protect extracellular volume despite any changes that may occur in GFR.
- Catecholamine and angiotensin II stimulate the basolateral ATPase and thus enhance the fraction of sodium reabsorbed in the proximal tubule.

Water and electrolytes

- About two-thirds of the filtered H_2O, K^+ and almost two-thirds of the filtered Cl^- follow the sodium (leaky system to these substances), and the osmolality at the end of the proximal tubule remains close to 300 mOsm/kg (isosmotic reabsorption). The chloride concentration rises slightly through the proximal tubule because of the large percentage of bicarbonate reabsorbed here.
- Therefore, at the end of the proximal tubule, osmolality and the concentrations of Na^+ and K^+ have not changed significantly from plasma, but only one-third of the amount originally filtered remains.

Metabolites

- Normally, all of the filtered glucose is reabsorbed in the PT via secondary active transport linked to sodium. This transporter is termed the sodium glucose-linked transporter (SGLT) and type 2 (SGLT-2) is the predominant form in the kidney.
- In addition, all proteins, peptides, amino acids, and ketone bodies are reabsorbed here via secondary active transport (requires luminal sodium, linked to sodium reabsorption).
- Therefore, the concentration of the above should be zero in the tubular fluid leaving the proximal tubule (clearance is zero).

Bridge to Pharmacology

SGLT-2 blocker canagliflozin inhibits proximal tubule reabsorption of glucose and is used to treat type 2 DM.

Bicarbonate

About 80% of the filtered bicarbonate is reabsorbed here. The mechanism for this reabsorption is:

- Bicarbonate combines with free H^+ in lumen and is converted into CO_2 and H_2O, catalyzed by the luminal carbonic anhydrase enzyme (CA). H^+ is pumped into the lumen in exchange with sodium (antiporter). Although not pictured, there is a H^+--ATPase on the luminal membrane that contributes to pumping H^+ into the lumen.
- CO_2, being very soluble, crosses the luminal membrane where it combines with water to reform H^+ and bicarbonate (note CA in the cell). The H^+ is then pumped back into the lumen, while bicarbonate exits the baslolateral membrane to complete its reabsorption.
- Because of this mechanism, bicarbonate reabsorption is dependent upon H^+ secretion and the activity of CA.
- The most important factor for H^+ secretion is the concentration of H^+ in the cell. Thus, H^+ secretion and bicarbonate reabsorption are increased during an acidosis and they decrease with an alkalosis.
- Angiotensin II stimulates the Na^+--H^+ antiporter. Thus, in volume-depleted states, the amount of bicarbonate reabsorption in the PT increases. This is thought to be the mechanism preventing bicarbonate loss when a patient develops a contraction alkalosis.

The small amount of bicarbonate that leaves the proximal tubule is normally reabsorbed in subsequent segments.

Bridge to Pharmacology

The primary site of action for carbonic anhydrase inhibitors is the PT. Blocking CA reduces bicarbonate reabsorption and the activity of the Na^+--H^+ exchanger.

Clinical Correlate

An 85-year-old woman presents to the emergency room with confusion. She is on hydrochlorothiazide. Her bicarbonate is 34 mEq/L (normal = 24 mEq/L). What is the cause of the metabolic alkalosis?

This is what is called a contraction alkalosis. The thiazide diuretic is causing a decrease in the intravascular volume. You can see the same in sweating in the desert or vomiting (not diarrhea because you lose bicarbonate in the stools and get a metabolic acidosis). The low volume state increases renin secretion leading to high angiotensin II. Angiotensin II activates the sodium/hydrogen exchanger →, increasing the reabsorption of bicarbonate → maintaining the metabolic alkalosis.

Clinical Correlate

Administration of a solute that is freely filtered but not reabsorbed (mannitol) and/or reducing/preventing the normal reabsorption of a solute results in the osmotic pull of water into the lumen and diuresis occurs. From the standpoint of the PT, glucose exceeding the TM is an important example.

Urate (uric acid)

The details of the renal handling of urate are too complex for the scope of this book. In short:

- Urate is formed by the breakdown of nucleotides
- Xanthine oxidase is the enzyme that catalyzes the final reaction to form urate.
- About 90% of the filtered urate is reabsorbed by the proximal tubule.
- If the FL of urate is high enough and the luminal pH is low, then more of the urate exists as uric acid, which can precipitate and form a kidney stone.
  - This is not the most common type of kidney stone, but it can occur in patients with gout.

Secretion

The proximal tubule is where many organic anions and cations are secreted and cleared from the circulation including PAH, penicillin, atropine, and morphine.

Energy requirements

Notice that all of the active processes illustrated in Figure VIII-4-1 are powered by the Na/K- ATPase primary active pump. This pump is located in the proximal tubule basal and basolateral borders and is directly or indirectly responsible for most of the water and electrolyte reabsorption in the nephron. It thus represents the most energy-demanding process of the nephron.

Figure VIII-4-2 depicts the ratio of the concentration of the substance in the proximal tubular fluid (TF) to the concentration in the plasma (P), beginning in Bowman's space through the end of the PT.

A = PAH
B = Inulin
C = Substance reabsorbed somewhat less rapidly than water, e.g., chloride
D = Major electrolytes such as sodium, potassium
E = Substance reabsorbed somewhat more rapidly than water
F = Substance completely reabsorbed in proximal tubule, e.g., glucose

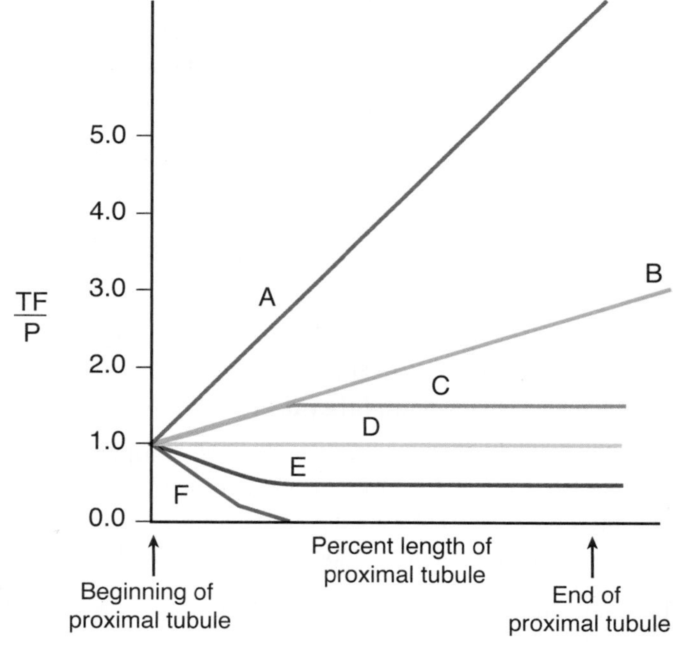

Figure VIII-4-2. Proximal Tubule Transport

Concentration of Inulin in the Nephron Tubule

- The concentration of inulin along the nephron tubule is an index of water reabsorption.
- Inulin is freely filtered; thus, its concentration in Bowman's space is the same as it is in the plasma. Because water is reabsorbed but inulin is not, the concentration of inulin increases throughout the nephron. The greater the water reabsorption, the greater the increase in inulin concentration.
- Since two-thirds of the water is reabsorbed in the proximal tubule, the inulin concentration should triple TF/P = 3.0. Its concentration should further increase in the descending limb of the loop of Henle, distal tubule, and the collecting duct (assuming ADH is present).
- The segment of the nephron with the highest concentration of inulin is the terminal collecting duct. The segment of the nephron with the lowest concentration of inulin is Bowman's space.

LOOP OF HENLE

- Fluid entering the loop of Henle is isotonic (300 mOsm/kg), but the volume is only one-third the volume originally filtered into Bowman's space.
- The loop of Henle has countercurrent flow and it acts as a countercurrent multiplier, the details of which are not imperative to learn. In short, the loop of Henle creates a concentrated medullary interstitium.
- The osmolality of the medulla can reach a maximum of about 1200 mOsm/kg, and the predominant osmoles are NaCl and urea (see Figure VIII-4-3).
- Juxtamedullary nephrons are responsible for this extremely high medullary osmolality. They are surrounded by vasa recta and slow flow in the vasa recta is crucial for maintaining the concentrated medullary interstitium.

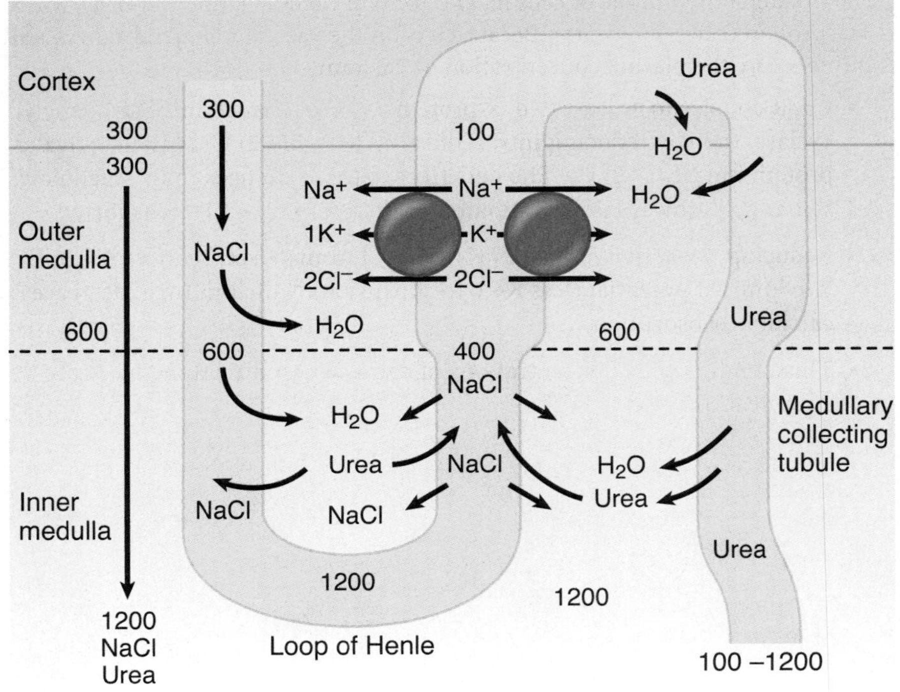

Figure VIII-4-3. Countercurrent and the Loop of Henle

Clinical Correlate

For a patient who has diarrhea, vomiting, or hemorrhaging, it is important to preserve extracellular volume; one way to do so is to increase reabsorption of fluid and electrolytes at the **proximal tubules.**

Clinical Correlate

In nephrogenic diabetes insipidus (DI), ADH receptors are not functioning and it is not possible to increase reabsorption at the collecting duct. The patient loses free water and develops hypernatremia. Treatment is reduction of extracellular volume with a thiazide diuretic. This increases peritubular oncotic pressure, in turn increasing water reabsorption in the proximal tubule. The elevated water reabsorption, along with sodium loss in the urine (action of thiazide diuretics), corrects the hypernatremia.

Clinical Correlate

A 65-year-old man presents with hyponatremia. His serum osmolarity is low and urine osmolarity high. He is diagnosed with SIADH. He is started on fluid restriction but is not able to comply. He is started on a loop diuretic, and plasma sodium increases.

Loop diuretics decrease the reabsorption of sodium and chloride at the loop of Henle. This removes the concentrating effect of the loop of Henle, decreaseing the osmolar gradient. This, in turn, decreases the reabsorption for free water from the collecting duct.

Bridge to Pharmacology

Loop diuretics block the Na^+--K^+--$2Cl^-$ transporter in ATL, thereby reducing their reabsorption. Blocking this transporter also reduces calcium and magnesium reabsorption, all of which results in a marked diuresis.

Bridge to Pathology

Bartter's syndrome is a genetic mutation resulting in diminished function of the Na^+--K^+--$2Cl^-$ transporter in ATL. This leads to a low volume state, which causes an increase in renin and aldosterone (know as a secondary hyperaldosteronism). Patients exhibit hypokalemia, alkalosis, and elevated urine calcium.

Bridge to Pathology

Familial hypocalciuric hypercalcemia (FHH) is an autosomal dominant genetic disorder resulting in hypercalcemia. In this condition, the CaSR is mutated such that it does not respond to plasma calcium. The CaSR is inactive and "fooled" into thinking that the plasma calcium is low, when it is in fact elevated. Thus, calcium reabsorption in the kidney is elevated despite the hypercalcemia. Patients also have high levels of parathyroid hormone (PTH) because CaSR is expressed in cells of the parathyroid gland. The mutation prevents the inhibition of PTH that normally occurs in response to hypercalcemia.

Descending Limb

- Permeable to water (about 15% of filtered is reabsorbed here)
- Relatively impermeable to solute

Ascending Limb

- Impermeable to water
- Solutes transported out

Figure VIII-4-4 shows a typical cell in the ascending thick limb (ATL) of the loop of Henle. Similar to the PT, there is a luminal Na^+--H^+ antiporter and bicarbonate is reabsorbed here.

Na^+--K^+--$2Cl^-$ transporter

This is an electroneutral transport resulting in the reabsorption of about 25% of the filtered sodium, chloride, and potassium.

- The luminal membrane contains a K^+ channel (Figure VIII-4-4), allowing diffusion of this ion back into lumen (recall that the concentration of K^+ inside cells is very high compared to the extracellular concentration).
- This back diffusion of K^+ into the lumen creates a positive luminal potential, which in turn, promotes calcium and magnesium reabsorption (about 25% of FL) via a paracellular pathway (primarily). This positive luminal potential also causes sodium reabsorption via a paracellular pathway.

Calcium-sensing receptor (CaSR)

The basolateral membrane of cells in ATL contain CaSR (Figure VIII-4-4), which is a G-protein coupled receptor. Because it is on the basolateral membrane, CaSR is influence by the plasma concentration of calcium.

- CaSR couples to at least two G-proteins: 1) $G_{I/O}$, which inhibits adenylyl cyclase, thereby reducing intracellular cAMP, and 2) G_q, which activates protein kinase C (PKC). The net effect of these changes in intracellular signaling pathways is an inhibition of the Na^+--K^+--$2Cl^-$ transporter.
- Reducing the activity of the Na^+--K^+--$2Cl^-$ transporter reduces the positive luminal potential (less K+ back diffusion), which in turn, decreases calcium reabsorption.
- Thus, high plasma concentrations of calcium can directly reduce calcium reabsorption in ATL.

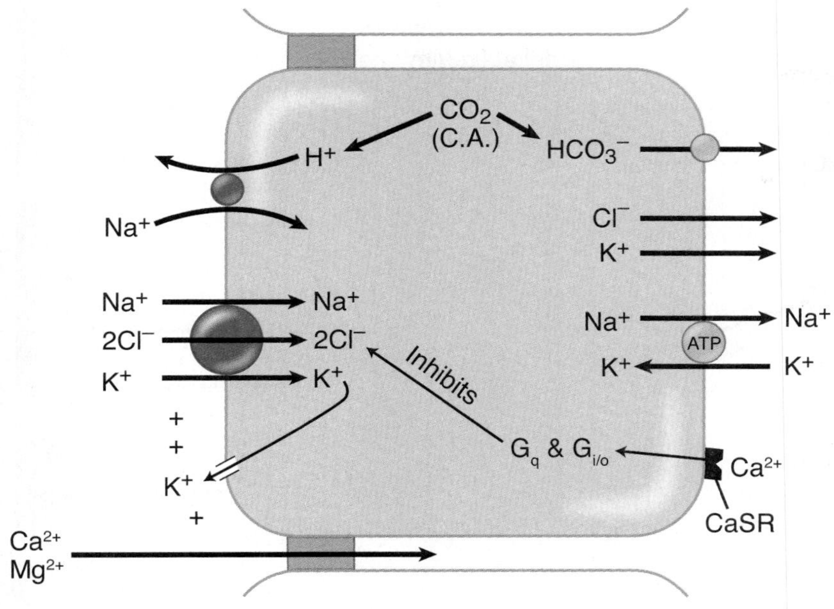

Figure VIII-4-4. Loop of Henle

DISTAL TUBULE

The early distal tubule reabsorbs Na^+, Cl^-, and Ca^{2+}. Transporters in the distal tubule are summarized in Figure VIII-4-5.

NaCl

- NaCl crosses the apical membrane via a Na^+-Cl^{--} symporter.
- The Na^+ is pumped across the basal membrane via the Na/K-ATPase proteins and Cl^- diffuses down its electrochemical gradient through channels.
- This section is impermeable to water. Thus, osmolality decreases further. In fact, the ultrafiltrate in the early distal tubule has the lowest osmolality of the entire nephron.

Calcium

- Calcium enters the cell from the luminal fluid passively through calcium channels.
- The opening of these channels is primarily regulated by parathyroid hormone (PTH).
- Calcium is actively extruded into the peritubular fluid via Ca^{2+}-ATPase or a $3Na^+$-Ca^{2+} antiporter.
- These cells also express the calcium binding protein, calbindin, which facilitates calcium reabsorption. Calbindin synthesis is increased by the active form of vitamin D, and thus vitamin D enhances PTH's action on the distal tubule.

Bridge to Pharmacology

Thiazide diuretics block the NaCl symporter in the distal tubule. Blocking this transporter enhances calcium reabsorption in the distal tubule and can result in hypercalcemia. In addition, thiazide diuretics are sometimes used to increase plasma calcium.

Bridge to Pathology

Gitelman's syndrome is a genetic disorder resulting in a mutated (reduced function) NaCl transporter. These patients are hypokalemic, alkalotic, and have a low urine calcium.

Cal: calbindin

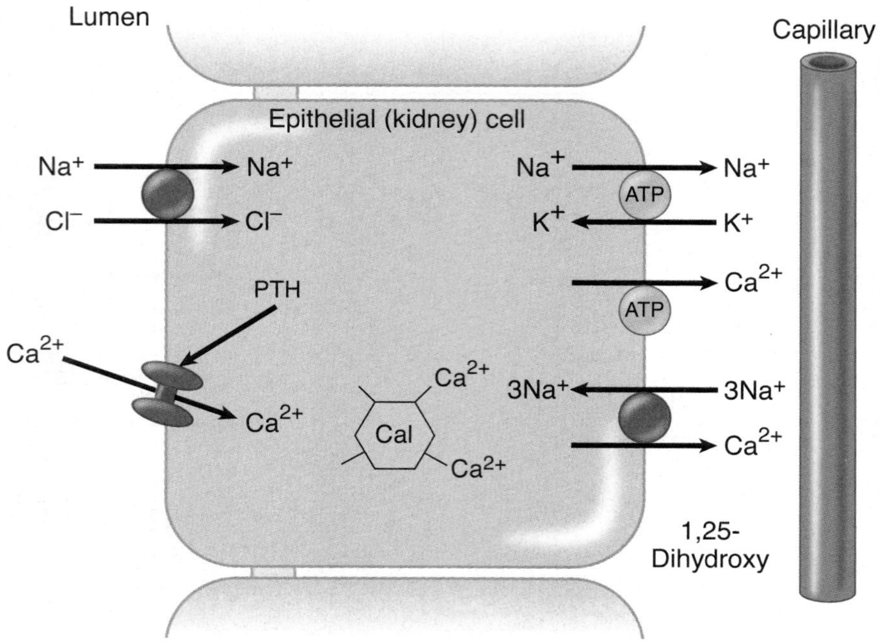

Figure VIII-4-5. Transporters in Distal Tubule

COLLECTING DUCT

The collecting duct (DC) is composed of principal cells and intercalated cells, both of which are illustrated in figure VIII-4-6.

Principal Cells

- The luminal membrane of principal cells contains sodium channels, commonly referred to as epithelial Na^+ channels (ENaC). Because of these channels, sodium follows its electrochemical gradient (created by the basolateral Na^+--K^+ ATPase) into the cell.
- Some chloride does not follow the sodium, thus the reabsorption of sodium produces a negative luminal potential. This negative luminal potential causes potassium secretion.
- Thus, the reabsorption of sodium and secretion of potassium are linked.
- Mineralcorticoids such as aldosterone exert an important effect on these cells. Activation of the mineralcorticoid receptor increases the number of luminal ENaC channels, increases their open time, and induces synthesis and trafficking of the basolateral Na^+--K^+ ATPase. The net effect is increased sodium reabsorption and potassium secretion.
- Although not illustrated on the slide, principal cells express aquaporins, which are regulated by anti-diuretic hormone (ADH), also known as arginine vasopressin (AVP). ADH acts on V2 (Gs—cAMP) receptors to cause insertion of aquaporins, which in turn, causes water (and urea) reabsorption.

Intercalated Cells

- Intercalated cells are intimately involved in acid-base regulation. The amount of fixed acid generated by an individual is mainly determined by diet. A high percentage of animal protein in the diet generates more fixed acid than a vegetarian-based diet.
- The luminal membrane contains a H^+--ATPase, which pumps H^+ into the lumen. Although free H^+ is pumped into the lumen, luminal pH can only go so low before it causes damage to cells, and thus most of the H^+ is eliminated from the body via buffers, phosphate and ammonia being the two most common.
- Monoprotonated phosphate is freely filtered at the glomerulus. About 80% is reabsorbed in the PT and another 10% is reabsorbed in the distal tubule. The remaining phosphate serves as a buffer for the secreted H^+. The H^+ pumped into the lumen binds to phosphate to form diprotonated phosphate, which is poorly reabsorbed, thus eliminating H^+ from the body. Phosphate is the primary titratable acid.
- In addition, the H^+ pumped into the lumen can combine with ammonia to form ammonium, which is not reabsorbed and is thus excreted. Ammonia is produced by the catabolism of glutamine and this occurs in cells of the PT.
- For every H^+ excreted by the above buffers, bicarbonate is added to the body (new bicarbonate).
- Aldosterone stimulates the H^+--ATPase of intercalated cells. Thus, excess aldosterone results in a metabolic alkalosis.

Bridge to Pharmacology

Potassium sparing diuretics work by blocking ENaC, e.g., amiloride, or by blocking aldosterone receptors, e.g., spironolactone, or the production of aldosterone, e.g., blockers of the RAAS system. Because sodium reabsorption is reduced, potassium secretion is diminished.

Bridge to Pathology

Liddle's syndrome is a genetic disorder resulting in a gain of function of ENaC channels in the CD. This results in enhanced sodium reabsorption and potassium secretion. Patients are hypertensive, hypokalemic, and alkalotic.

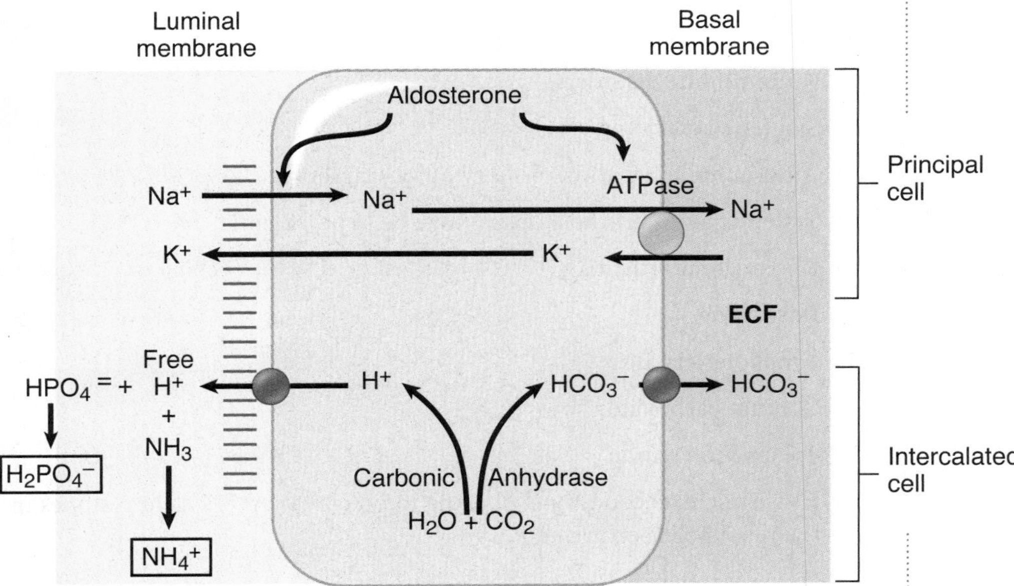

Figure VIII-4-6. Late Distal Tubule and Collecting Duct

RENAL TUBULAR ACIDOSIS

Proximal Renal Tubular Acidosis (Type II)

- Due to a diminished capacity of the proximal tubule to reabsorb bicarbonate.
- Transient appearance of bicarbonate in the urine until the filtered load is reduced to match the reduced capacity of reabsorption.
- Steady-state characterized by a low plasma bicarbonate and acid urine.
- An example would be Fanconi syndrome, which involves a general defect in the proximal tubular transport processes and carbonic anhydrase inhibitors.
- Serum potassium is also low. When bicarbonate is lost in the urine, it is lost as sodium bicarbonate and that pulls water with it creating an osmotic diuresis. The diuresis leads to loss of potassium in the urine.

Distal Renal Tubular Acidosis (Type I)

- Due to an inability of the distal nephron to secrete and excrete fixed acid, thus an inability to form an acid urine. Urine pH >5.5 – 6.0
- Mechanisms would include impairment of the transport systems for hydrogen ions and bicarbonate and an increased permeability of the luminal membrane allowing the back diffusion of the hydrogen ions from the tubular lumen.
- The result is a metabolic acidosis with an inappropriately high urine pH.
- Serum potassium is also low.

Causes:

- Autoimmune disorders
- Sjögren's syndrome
- Autoimmune hepatitis/primary biliary cirrhosis
- Systemic lupus erythematosus (may be hyperkalemic)
- Rheumatoid arthritis
- Ifosfamide
- Amphotericin B
- Lithium carbonate
- Toluene inhalation
- Hypercalciuric conditions (leading to precipitation of calcium stones in the renal pelvis or ureters)
- Hyperparathyroidism
- Vitamin D intoxication
- Sarcoidosis
- Idiopathic hypercalciuria

Renal Tubular Acidosis Type IV: Hypoaldosterone States

- Inability to secrete potassium leading to hyperkalemia
- Decreased secretion of protons leading to metabolic acidosis

Causes:

- Diabetic nephropathy, due to low renin secretion with loss of kidney function
- Any drug that inhibits the RAAS system, such as ACE-inhibitors, ARBs, spironolactone, and aliskiren
- Trimethoprim
- Addison's disease due to loss of aldosterone secretion from the adrenal cortex

DISORDERS OF POTASSIUM HOMEOSTASIS

Potassium Balance

To keep the body amount constant, excretion of potassium must match dietary intake, and the kidneys regulate potassium excretion. A small percentage of ingested potassium is lost in the stool but this is not a major regulatory route under normal conditions.

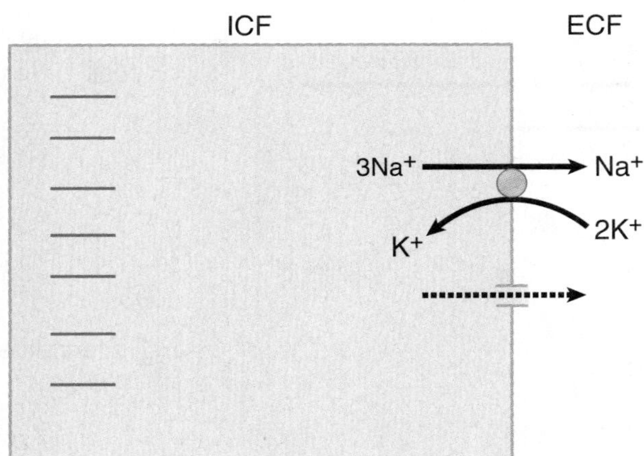

The large concentration gradient is due to membrane potential and cell membrane permeability to potassium.

Figure VIII-4-7. ICF and ECF Potassium Distribution

- 98% of potassium inside cells (150 mEq/L)
- 2% of potassium in ECF (4 mEq/L)
- >5.0 mEq/L = hyperkalemia
- <3.5 mEq/L = hypokalemia
- The large concentration gradient across the cell membrane is mainly due to the negative intracellular potential and the permeability of the cell membrane to potassium.
- The NaK-ATPase maintains the membrane potential as well as a small net diffusion gradient from the ICF to the ECF.

- Insulin and epinephrine stimulate the Na/K ATPase and can thus reduce plasma potassium.
- Long term balance is maintained via aldosterone's effect on potassium secretion in the distal tubule and collecting ducts of the nephrons.
- Acidosis and increased ECF osmolality (cell shrinkage) shifts potassium from the ICF to the ECF. Inorganic fixed acid > organic acids > respiratory acidosis
- Alkalosis and decreased ECF osmolality (cell swelling) shifts potassium from the ECF to the ICF. Metabolic alkalosis > respiratory alkalosis

Potassium secretion and excretion by the kidney

Potassium secretion is determined mainly by 2 factors: filtrate flow and sodium reabsorption (creates negative potential of the lumen).

- Increased flow and/or aldosterone increases potassium secretion and excretion.
- Decreased flow and/or aldosterone decreases potassium secretion and excretion.

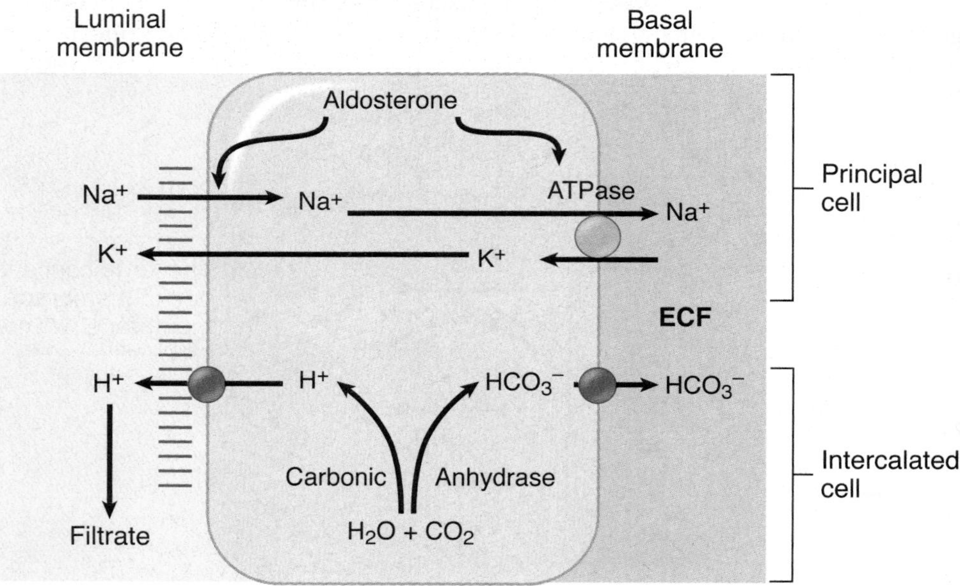

Figure VIII-4-8. Late Distal Tubule and Collecting Duct

Acid–Base Disorders

Acidosis: shifts potassium from the ICF to ECF. Decreased intracellular potassium reduces the potassium gradient, thus potassium secretion falls. (both promote hyperkalemia). However, this negative potassium balance in acidosis is not typically sustained because hyperkalemia stimulates aldosterone.

Alkalosis: shifts potassium from ECF to ICF. Increased intracellular potassium increases potassium secretion (both promote hypokalemia).

Summary of Potassium Balance

Promoters of hyperkalemia

- Transcellular shifts: metabolic acidosis, hyperglycemia, insulin deficiency or resistance, muscle trauma
- GI: excessive intake (on rare occasions)
- Kidney: acute oligouric kidney disease, chronic kidney disease where GFR decreases dramatically from normal, hypoaldosteronism

Consequences of hyperkalemia

- Neuromuscular function: muscle weakness, general fatigue if chronic
- Cardiac: high T wave, eventually in severe hyperkalemia ventricular fibrillation
- Metabolic: metabolic acidosis

Promoters of hypokalemia

- Transcellular shifts: metabolic alkalosis, sudden increases in insulin and catecholamines
- GI: diarrhea, vomiting, low potassium diet (rarely has an effect on its own)
- Kidney: diuretics due to increased flow (thiazides, loop diuretics, osmotic diuresis), hyperaldosteronism (adrenal adenoma, renal arterial stenosis), increased excretion of negative ions (bicarbonate, ketone bodies), renal tubular acidosis types I and II.

Consequences of hypokalemia

- Neuromuscular function: muscle weakness, general fatigue
- Cardiac: hyperpolarization affects excitability and delays repolarization.
- EKG effects: low T wave, high U wave
- Metabolic: decreased insulin response to carbohydrate load, decrease growth rate in children, nephrogenic diabetes insipidus, metabolic alkalosis

RENAL FAILURE

Acute Renal Failure

Acute renal failure is a rapid loss of renal function that is often reversible. Loss of renal function results in the accumulation of waste products that the kidney excretes, e.g., BUN and creatinine. Depending upon the cause, the fractional excretion of Na^+ ($FeNa^+$) is either elevated or reduced. As its name implies, $FeNa^+$ simply means the % of filtered Na^+ that is excreted: The higher the number, the less reabsorption and vice versa. The causes of acute renal failure are:

Prerenal

With prerenal renal failure, there is decreased renal perfusion as would occur with a decreased renal perfusion pressure, e.g., hypovolumia of hemorrhage,

Clinical Correlate

A 55-year-old woman with a history of end-stage renal failure presents with confusion after missing a dialysis session. Her potassium is elevated. While waiting for the nurse to set up the dialysis, the patient is treated with an injection of bicarbonate and insulin with dextrose.

Giving bicarbonate gives the patient an alkalosis. This causes protons to leave the intracellular space down its concentration gradient. To maintain electroneutrality, potassium shifts into cells. This decreases the extracellular potassium concentration. Insulin activates the sodium/potassium ATPase and that increases the shift of potassium into the cell also.

diarrhea, vomiting; congestive heart failure. Initially, there is no renal injury and it is reversible if corrected early. Characteristic signs are:

- Reduced GFR
- Reduced $FeNa^+$: Tubular function is intact and the low GFR (reduced filtered load) allows for significant reabsorption.
- Na^+ reabsorption: In addition, Ang II and catecholamines are often elevated in this condition, both of which increase Na^+ reabsorption.
- Elevated plasma BUN:Cr: Although both are elevated, the high reabsorption of urea (water reabsorption is elevated in prerenal) elevates BUN more than creatinine.

Intrarenal

In this condition, tubular damage occurs resulting in tubular dysfunction. Toxins, interstitial nephritis, ischemia, rhabdomyolysis, and sepsis are factors that could cause acute tubular necrosis and intrarenal failure. Characteristic signs are:

- Increased $FeNa^+$: Tubules are damaged and thus unable to reabsorb Na^+
- Casts/cells in the urine: Damaged cells are sloughed off into the tubule
- Low plasma BUN:Cr: Tubular damage prevents reabsorption of urea

Postrenal

This condition is caused by obstruction of fluid outflow from the kidney, e.g., renal calculi, enlarged prostate.

- Early: Characteristics are similar to prerenal, i.e., reduced $FeNa^+$, elevated plasma BUN:Cr
- Late: Buildup of pressure results in tubular damage, resulting in characteristics of intrarenal failure, i.e., marked increase in $FeNa^+$, low plasma BUN:Cr

Chronic Renal Failure

Although nephrons often recover from the sloughing of the tubular epithelial cells in acute renal failure, in chronic renal failure there is an irreversible loss of nephrons. In order to compensate, the remaining nephrons have an increased glomerular capillary pressure and hyperfiltration. One way of looking at this is a "hypertension" at the level of the nephron; the hyperfiltration combined with the increased work load promotes further injury leading to fibrosis, scarring, and loss of additional nephrons.

Looking back at the function of the kidney and how it regulates a variety of physiologic variables, many of the consequences of chronic renal failure are predictable. These include:

- Inability to excrete waste products leads to a rise in plasma BUN and creatinine.
- Inability to regulate sodium and water: This can lead to hyponatremia, volume overload, and thus edema. In addition, patients are susceptible to rapid development of hypernatremia and volume depletion following vomiting and diarrhea.
- Inability to regulate potassium excretion leads to hyperkalemia.

- Inability to excrete fixed acids leads to metabolic acidosis (elevated anion gap—see next chapter)
- Inability to excrete phosphate leads to hyperphosphatemia. This hyperphosphatemia reduces plasma calcium, causing a rise in parathyroid hormone (PTH—secondary hyperparathyroidism) resulting in increased bone resorption (renal osteodystrophy).
- Inability to hydroxylate (1-alpha hydroxylase enzyme is in the kidney) 25,OH-cholecalciferol decreases circulating levels of active vitamin D, which contributes to the hypocalcemia.
- Inability to secrete erythropoietin results in anemia.

The most common cause of chronic renal failure is the nephropathy produced by diabetes. The second most common cause is hypertension.

Chapter Summary

- In the proximal tubule, two-thirds of the water and electrolytes are reabsorbed, along with almost all the organic molecules filtered. An exception is urea. Because equal amounts of solutes and fluid are reabsorbed, the fluid remains isotonic.
- The loop of Henle, acting as a countercurrent multiplier, creates an osmotic gradient in the medullary interstitium, with the tip reaching a maximum of 1200 mOsm/kg. This value determines the maximum osmolality of the urine.
- In the early distal tubule, additional electrolytes are reabsorbed and the osmolality decreases further. In the collecting duct, aldosterone regulates the final electrolyte modifications and ADH the final osmolality.
- Net acid lost in the urine is via phosphate and ammonium. Renal tubular acidosis is a metabolic acidosis caused by a failure of nephron cellular processes. Proximal failure is type II, distal failure (distal tubule/ collecting duct) is type I, and type IV is hypoaldosterone.
- Hyperkalemia can be caused either by a transcellular shift in potassium (ICF to ECF) or a failure of the kidney to excrete adequate amounts of potassium.
- Hypokalemia can be caused by a transcellular shift in potassium (ECF to ICF) or to excess loss via the GI tract or kidney.
- Hyper- and hypokalemia affect the excitability of nerves and cardiac muscle.
- Acute renal failure (disease) is a sudden loss of renal function (GFR) and is reversible.
- Chronic renal failure (disease) is a loss of functioning nephrons and is generally not reversible. Diabetes is the major cause of chronic renal failure followed by hypertension.

SECTION IX

Acid–Base Disturbances

Acid–Base Disturbances 1

Learning Objectives

- ❑ Interpret scenarios on buffering systems
- ❑ Explain information related to formulating a diagnosis
- ❑ Explain information related to 3-question method
- ❑ Solve problems concerning the 4 primary disturbances
- ❑ Use knowledge of compensation
- ❑ Solve problems concerning plasma anion gap diagnosis
- ❑ Use knowledge of graphical representation (Davenport plot)
- ❑ Solve problems concerning supplemental information

BUFFERING SYSTEMS

Figure IX-1-1 shows the CO_2-bicarbonate buffer system. This is one of the major buffers systems of the blood and the one we focus on in this chapter.

$$H_2O + CO_2 \overset{CA}{\rightleftharpoons} H_2CO_3 \rightleftharpoons H^+ + HCO_3^-$$

Figure IX-1-1. Production of Carbonic Acid

To demonstrate the changes in the major variables during acid–base disturbances, the scheme can be simplified to the following:

$$CO_2 \longleftrightarrow H^+ + HCO_3^-$$

Recall that the respiratory system plays the key role in regulating CO_2, while the kidneys serve as the long-term regulators of H^+ and HCO_3^-. Thus, these 2 organ systems are paramount in our discussion of acid-base regulation.

FORMULATING A DIAGNOSIS

Acid-base disturbances can be diagnosed from arterial blood gases (ABGs) using a 3-step approach. Given that arterial blood is the source for the diagnostic data, one is actually determining an acidemia or alkalemia. However, an acidemia or alkalemia is typically indicative of an underlying acidosis or alkalosis, respectively.

An overview of this approach is provided here to lay the framework for remainder of the chapter.

THREE-QUESTION METHOD

Question 1: What is the osis?

- If pH <7.35, then acidosis
- If pH >7.45, then alkalosis

The normal value of pH is 7.4 (see below), with the normal range 7.35–7.45, thus the basis of the above numbers. However, one can in fact have an underlying acid-base disorder even though pH is in the normal range.

Question 2: What is the cause of the osis?

To answer this, one looks at bicarbonate next. In the section below, we will go into more detail.

Question 3: Was there compensation?

A calculation must be performed to answer this final question, and this will be covered in detail below. However, bear in mind the following:

- For respiratory disturbances, the kidneys alter total bicarbonate; whether or not compensation has occurred is based upon the patient's measured bicarbonate versus a calculated value of bicarbonate.
- The respiratory system responds quickly and it is important to determine if it has responded appropriately; respiratory compensation compares the patient's measured PCO_2 versus a calculated (predicted) value.

THE 4 PRIMARY DISTURBANCES

There are 4 primary acid-base disturbances, each of which results in an altered concentration of H^+. The basic deviations from normal can be an acidosis (excess H^+) or an alkalosis (deficiency of H^+), either of which may be caused by a respiratory or metabolic problem.

- **Respiratory acidosis**: too much CO_2
- **Metabolic acidosis**: addition of H^+ (not of CO_2 origin) and/or loss of bicarbonate from the body
- **Respiratory alkalosis**: not enough CO_2
- **Metabolic alkalosis**: loss of H^+ (not of CO_2 origin) and/or addition of base to the body

Normal systemic arterial values are as follows:

$$pH = 7.4$$
$$HCO_3^- = 24 \text{ mEq/L}$$
$$PCO_2 = 40 \text{ mm Hg}$$

Follow the Bicarbonate Trail

Question 2 asks for the cause of the osis. To answer this, look at the bicarbonate concentration and remember the basic CO_2–bicarbonate reaction, applying mass action. The table below shows the 4 primary disturbances with the resultant bicarbonate changes.

$$CO_2 \leftrightarrow H+ + HCO_3^-$$

Table IX-1-1. Summary of Acute Changes in pH/HCO_3^-

	pH	HCO_3^-
Respiratory acidosis	↓	↑
Metabolic acidosis	↓	↓↓
Respiratory alkalosis	↑	↓
Metabolic alkalosis	↑	↑↑

Respiratory acidosis is characterized by too much CO_2.

- Increasing CO_2 drives the reaction to the right, thereby increasing HCO_3^-.
  - For every 1 mm Hg rise in $PaCO_2$, there is a 0.1 mEq/L increase in HCO_3^-, as a result of the chemical reaction.
  - Thus, there is a 1 : 0.1 ratio of CO2 increase to HCO3- increase for an acute (uncompensated) respiratory acidosis.

Metabolic acidosis causes a marked decrease in $HCO3^-$ because the addition of H^+ consumes bicarbonate (drives reaction to the left).

- Alternatively, the acidosis could be caused by loss of base (HCO_3^-).

Respiratory alkalosis is characterized by a reduced CO_2.

- Decreasing CO_2 drives the reaction to the left, thereby reducing HCO_3^-.
  - For every 1 mm Hg fall in PaCO2, there is a 0.2 mEq/L decrease in HCO3– as a result of the chemical reaction.
  - Thus, there is a 1 : 0.2 ratio of CO2 decrease to HCO3– decrease for an acute (uncompensated) respiratory alkalosis.

Metabolic alkalosis causes a rise in HCO_3^- because the loss of H^+ drives the reaction to the right.

- Alternatively, an alkalosis can be caused by addition of base (bicarbonate) to the body.

COMPENSATION

Respiratory Acidosis

The kidneys compensate by increasing HCO_3^- and eliminating H^+, but the kidneys take days to fully compensate.

- For every 1 mm Hg increase in $PaCO_2$, HCO_3^- increases 0.35 mEq/L as a result of kidney compensation. Thus, there is a **1:0.35 ratio of CO_2 increase to HCO_3^- increase in a chronic (compensated) respiratory acidosis.**

Note

One can use pH instead of bicarbonate to determine if a respiratory disturbance is acute or chronic; this is provided at the end-of-chapter Supplemental Information.

Metabolic Acidosis

Metabolic acidosis is characterized by low pH and HCO_3^-. The drop in pH stimulates ventilation via peripheral chemoreceptors, thus the respiratory system provides the first, rapid compensatory response.

- Winter's equation is used to determine if the respiratory response is adequate.

$$\text{Predicted } PaCO_2 = (1.5 \text{ x } HCO_3^-) + 8$$

- The patient's $PaCO_2$ should be within 2(±) of this predicted value, and if so, then respiratory compensation has occurred.

Respiratory Alkalosis

The kidneys compensate by eliminating HCO_3^- and conserving H^+, but the kidneys take days to fully compensate.

- For every 1 mm Hg drop in $PaCO_2$, HCO_3^- decreases 0.5 mEq/L as a result of kidney compensation. Thus, there is a **1:0.5 ratio** of CO_2 decrease to HCO_3^- decrease **in a chronic (compensated) respiratory alkalosis.**
- The maximum low for HCO_3^- is 15 mEq/L.

Metabolic Alkalosis

Similar to a metabolic acidosis, the respiratory system is the first-line compensatory mechanism. Ventilation decreases to retain CO_2.

- The following equation is used to determine if compensation occurred. It computes the $PaCO_2$, which denotes appropriate compensation.

$$\text{Expected } PaCO_2 = (0.7 \text{ x rise in } HCO_3^-) + 40$$

- The patient's $PaCO_2$ should be within 2(±) of the computed value, but should not exceed 55 mm Hg. The 40 represents the normal $PaCO_2$ (see above).

Additional Important Points

- The body never overcompensates.
  - If it appears that a patient "overcompensated" for a primary disorder, there is likely a second disorder.
- If CO_2 and HCO_3^- go in opposite directions, there is a combined disturbance—either a combined (mixed) respiratory and metabolic acidosis or a combined (mixed) respiratory and metabolic alkalosis.
- Although the opposite direction rule is true, do not presume that it is **required** for someone to have a combined disturbance, i.e., a combined disturbance can still exist even if CO_2 and HCO_3^- go in the same direction.
- Too much CO_2 is a respiratory acidosis.
- Too little CO_2 is a respiratory alkalosis.

PLASMA ANION GAP (PAG)

The total cation charges in the plasma always equal the total anion charges present. However, only major ions are typically measured in a blood sample and an "anion gap" can be determined (see below and figure IX-1-2).

Cations are estimated as the plasma concentration of the major cation, Na^+. It is not usually the case but some clinicians also include K^+ (normal K^+ is 4 mEq/L and if included, then adjust the normal gap accordingly, i.e., add 4).

Anions are estimated as the plasma Cl^- and HCO_3^-.

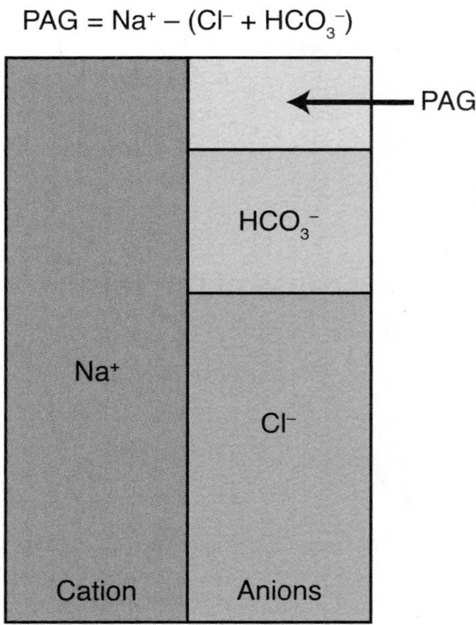

Figure IX-1-2. PAG

Normal values:

Na^+: 140 mEq/L

Cl^-: 104 mEq/L

HCO_3^-: 24 mEq/L

PAG: $Na^+ - (Cl^- + HCO_3^-)$

PAG: 12 ± 2

The anion gap is useful in differentiating the cause of a metabolic acidosis. In most cases, the anion gap increases when the underlying cause involves an organic acid (unmeasured charge is conjugate base of the acid). When the acidosis is the result of bicarbonate loss, e.g., diarrhea, then chloride typically increases resulting in no change in the anion gap. The more common causes of an elevated and non-elevated gap can be remembered using the mnemonics provided below.

Use the following pneumonics to remember **elevated** and **non-elevated gap metabolic acidoses**:

MUDPILES (elevated gap)

M: Methanol

U: Uremia (kidney failure)

D: Diabetic ketoacidosis

P: Paraldehyde

I: Iron; Isoniazid

L: Lactic acidosis

E: Ethylene glycol; ethanol ketoacidosis

S: Salicylates; starvation ketoacidosis; sepsis

HARDUP (non-elevated gap)

H: Hyperchloremia (parental nutrition)

A: Acetazolamide

R: Renal tubular acidosis

D: Diarrhea

U: Ureteral diversion

P: Pancreatic fistula

DIAGNOSIS

Now that we have discussed how the basic reaction responds to respiratory and metabolic disturbances and how the body compensates, let's use the 3 questions to quickly determine acid-base abnormalities.

Question 1: What is the osis?

As indicated above, look at pH.

- If pH <7.35, then it's acidosis.
- If pH >7.45, then it's alkalosis.

Question 2: What is the cause of the osis?

Follow the bicarbonate trail (see also Table IX-1-1).

- If the answer to question 1 is acidosis and HCO_3^- is elevated, then **respiratory acidosis.**
- If the answer to question 1 is acidosis and HCO_3^- is low, then **metabolic acidosis.**
- If the answer to question 1 is alkalosis and HCO_3^- is low, then **respiratory alkalosis.**
- If the answer to question 1 is alkalosis and HCO_3^- is elevated, then **metabolic alkalosis.**

Question 3: Was there compensation?

Respiratory acidosis

Because kidney compensation is slow, it is important to distinguish between **acute (uncompensated)** and **chronic (compensated)** respiratory disturbances.

- If **acute**, there is a 0.1 mEq/L rise in HCO_3^- for every 1 mm Hg increase in $PaCO_2$ (**1:0.1 ratio**).
- If **chronic**, there is a 0.35 mEq/L rise in HCO_3^- for every 1 mm Hg rise in $PaCO_2$ (**1:0.35 ratio**)

For example, a patient has a respiratory acidosis (determined by steps 1 and 2) with $PaCO_2$ 60 mm Hg, which is **20 mm Hg greater than** the normal of 40 mm Hg.

If acute, then bicarbonate will be ~26 ($20 \times 0.1 = 2$; $24 + 2 = 26$). If chronic, then bicarbonate will be ~31 ($20 \times 0.35 = 24 + 7 = 31$).

Metabolic acidosis

The patient's $PaCO_2$ should fall to a level that is ±2 mm Hg of the value computed by Winter's equation:

$$\mathbf{PaCO_2 = (1.5 \times HCO_3^-) + 8}$$

- If the patient's $PaCO_2$ is within 2, then the patient has **metabolic acidosis with respiratory compensation.**
- If it is higher than 2, then the respiratory response is inadequate and the patient has **metabolic and respiratory acidosis.**
- If the patient's $PaCO_2$ is too low, then the patient has a **metabolic acidosis with a respiratory alkalosis.**

For example, a patient has a metabolic acidosis with a HCO_3^- of 10 mEq/L and a $PaCO_2$ of 23 mm Hg. Expected $PaCO_2$ is $(1.5 \times 10) + 8 = 23$ mm Hg, which is what the patient has, thus respiratory compensation is adequate.

Respiratory alkalosis

Again, it is important to distinguish between **acute (uncompensated)** and **chronic (compensated)** respiratory disturbances.

- If **acute,** there is a 0.2 mEq/L fall in HCO_3^- for every 1 mm Hg decrease in $PaCO_2$ (**1:0.2 ratio**).
- If **chronic**, there is a 0.5 mEq/L fall in HCO_3^- for every 1 mm Hg decrease in $PaCO_2$ (**1:0.5 ratio**).

For example, a patient has a respiratory alkalosis (determined by steps 1 and 2) with a $PaCO_2$ of 25 mm Hg, which is **15 mm Hg less than** the normal of 40 mm Hg. If acute, then bicarbonate will be about 21 ($15 \times 0.2 = 3$; $24 - 3 = 21$), but if chronic it will be around 16 ($15 \times 0.5 = 7.5$; $24 - 7.5 = 16.5$).

Note

Chronic ratios/calculations are also provided in the Compensation section above, while acute ratios are provided in Follow the Bicarbonate Trail section.

Metabolic alkalosis

The patient's $PaCO_2$ should rise to a level that is ± 2 the value computed by the following equation (not to exceed 55 mm Hg):

$$\textbf{Expected } PaCO_2 = (0.7 \times \textbf{rise in } HCO_3^-) + 40$$

- If the patient's $PaCO_2$ is within 2, the patient has **metabolic alkalosis with respiratory compensation.**
- If it is higher than 2, then the patient has **metabolic alkalosis and respiratory acidosis.**
- If the patient's $PaCO_2$ is too low, then the patient has a **metabolic and respiratory alkalosis.**

For example, a patient has a metabolic alkalosis with HCO_3^- 34 mEq/L (**10 greater than normal**) and $PaCO_2$ 47 mm Hg. Expected $PaCO_2$ is (10 × 0.7) + 40 = 47 mm Hg, which is what the patient has, thus respiratory compensation is adequate.

Note

Remember to calculate the anion gap to differentiate the possible causes of a metabolic acidosis.

Figure IX-1-3 summarizes the above discussion. This figure can be helpful in remembering the 3 basic steps for analyzing an ABG and come to the correct diagnosis. Some examples follow and you are encouraged to look at the summary figure and apply it to correctly diagnosis the examples provided.

Note

$Paco_2$ is increased in resp acidosis; compensatory increase in metab alkalosis (formula computes compensation value of $Paco_2$)

Note

$Paco_2$ is decreased in resp alkalosis; compensatory decrease in metab acidosis (Winter's determines compensation value of $Paco_2$)

Note

Compute anion gap: [Na⁺ – (Cl⁻ + bicarb)]

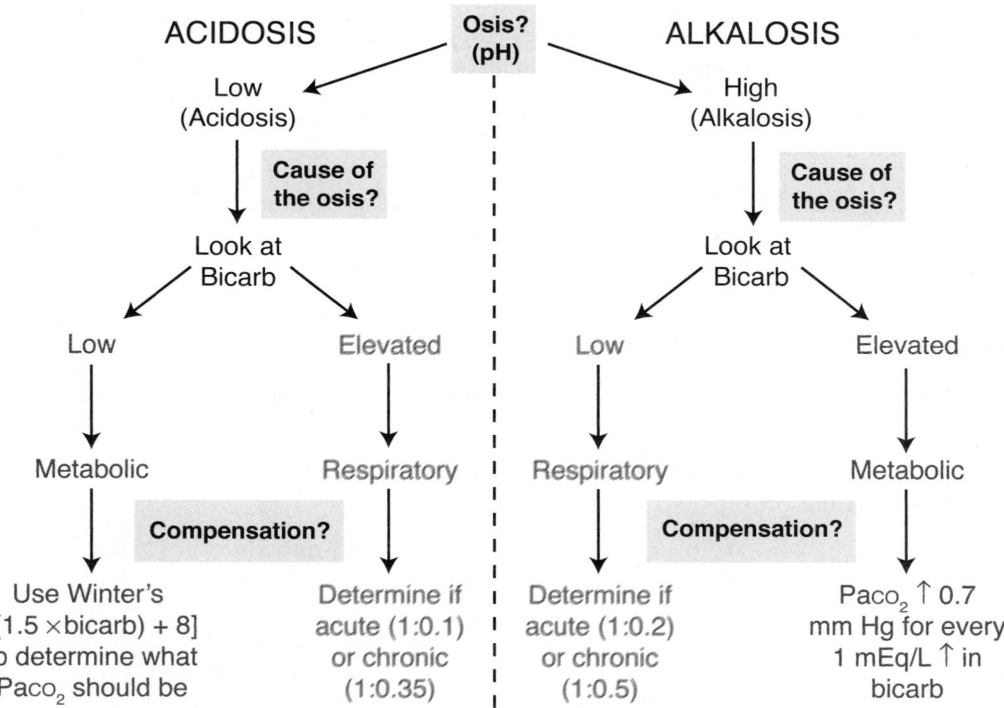

Figure IX-1-3.

Example ABGs Showing Disturbance

Example 1
pH = 7.3
HCO_3^- = 14 mEq/L
PCO_2 = 30 mm Hg
PO_2 = 95 mm Hg

Example 2
pH = 7.6
HCO_3^- = 20 mEq/L
PCO_2 = 20 mm Hg
PO_2 = 95 mm Hg

Example 3
pH = 7.2
HCO_3^- = 30 mEq/L
PCO_2 = 80 mm Hg
PO_2 = 70 mm Hg

Example 4
pH = 7.6
HCO_3^- = 44 mEq/L
PCO_2 = 52 mm Hg
PO_2 = 70 mm Hg

Example 5
HCO3- = 20 mEq/L
PCO_2 = 55 mm Hg

Answers

Example 1

What is the osis? pH is low, so acidosis.

Cause of the osis? HCO_3^- is low, so metabolic acidosis.

Compensation? Use Winter's to compute predicted PCO_2: $(14 \times 1.5) + 8 = 29$. Patient's is 30, which is within 2, thus this is a ***metabolic acidosis with respiratory compensation.***

Example 2

What is the osis? pH is high, so alkalosis.

Cause of the osis? HCO_3^- is low, so respiratory alkalosis.

Compensation? Must determine if acute (uncompensated) or chronic (compensated). PCO_2 is 20 below normal, thus acute: 20 x 0.2 = 4, so HCO_3^- will be around 20 (24 – 4). If chronic, it would be 20 x 0.5 = 10, so HCO_3^- would be around 14 (24 – 10). The measured equals the predicted acute, thus this is an ***acute respiratory alkalosis.***

Example 3

What is the osis? pH is low, so acidosis.

Cause of the osis? HCO_3^- is high, so respiratory acidosis.

Compensation? Must determine if acute (uncompensated) or chronic (compensated). PCO_2 is 40 greater than normal, thus acute: $40 \times 0.1 = 4$, so HCO_3^- will be around 28 (24 + 4). If chronic, it will be $40 \times 0.35 = 14$, so HCO_3^- will be around 38 (24 + 14). The measured is much closer to the predicted acute, thus this is an ***acute respiratory acidosis.***

Example 4

What is the osis? pH is high, so alkalosis.

Cause of the osis? HCO_3^- is high, so metabolic alkalosis.

Compensation? The respiratory compensation is to reduce ventilation, thereby increasing $PaCO_2$. Thus, we need to compute what $PaCO_2$ should be in a patient with this acid-base disorder. Calculation: HCO_3^- is 20 greater than normal of 24, 20 x 0.7 = 14, thus $PaCO_2$ should be 14 mm Hg greater than the normal of 40, thus 40 + 14 = 54 (predicted $PaCO_2$). Patient's is 52, which is within 2, so this is a ***metabolic alkalosis with respiratory compensation.***

Example 5

No pH is given, but we can still figure out the acid-base disorder. HCO_3^- is low, so this must be a metabolic acidosis or respiratory alkalosis (review "follow the bicarbonate trail" above). $PaCO_2$ is well above normal, ruling out a respiratory alkalosis, thus there is a ***mixed metabolic and respiratory acidosis.*** Note that $PaCO_2$ and HCO_3^- went in opposite directions, so we know there is a mixed disturbance. The low HCO_3^- indicates the metabolic acidosis, while the high $PaCO_2$ indicates respiratory acidosis. If this were simply a respiratory acidosis, HCO_3^- would be elevated, not reduced.

GRAPHICAL REPRESENTATION (DAVENPORT PLOT)

The Davenport plot (Figure IX-1-4, panels A–D) provides a graphical representation of the preceding discussion. The pH is on the X-axis, and HCO_3^- is on the Y-axis.

At pH 7.4 and HCO_3^- 24, $PaCO_2$ is 40 (panel A). These represent the normal values indicated above. Knowing either of the 2 measurements allows one to calculate the third, using the Henderson-Hasselbalch equation.

$$pH = pK + \log \frac{[HCO_3^-]}{aPCO_2} \qquad pK = 6.10 \qquad [HCO_3^-] \text{ in mmol/L}$$

$$a = 0.0301 \qquad PCO_2 \text{ in mm Hg}$$

Let's now walk through the 3 questions and see the corresponding values on the Davenport plot.

Question 1: What is the osis?

Splitting the graph at pH 7.4, anything to the left represents an acidosis, while anything to the right represents an alkalosis (Figure X-1-4, panel B)

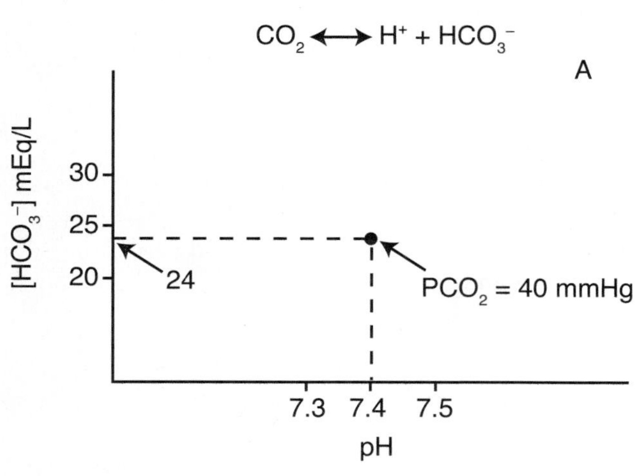

Figure IX-1-4a

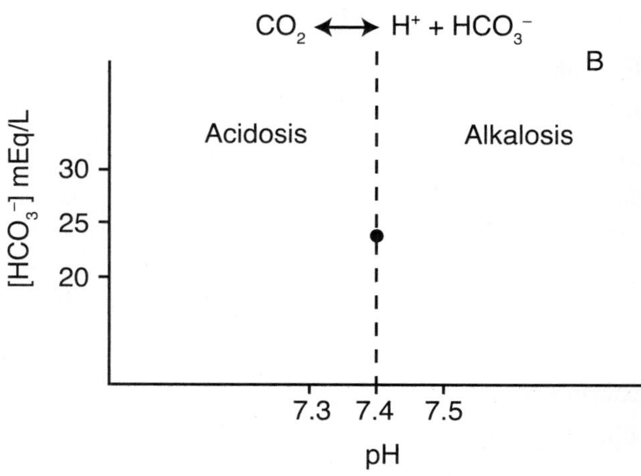

Figure IX-1-4b

Question 2: What is the cause of the osis?

- Respiratory acidosis is characterized by a decrease in pH with concomitant rise in HCO_3^-, while respiratory alkalosis is characterized by a rise in pH with concomitant fall in HCO_3^-. This is denoted by the red line in panel C of Figure X-1-4.
- Metabolic acidosis is a decrease in pH and HCO3-, while metabolic alkalosis is an increase in pH and HCO_3^-. This is denoted by the purple line in panel C of the figure. Note that PCO_2 is the same at all points along the purple line, hence the term *CO_2 isobar.* In other words, the purple line denotes metabolic changes without accompanying CO_2 changes.
- This separates the graph into 4 quadrants (panel C of Figure IX-1-4). Points falling within one of these quadrants with have the respective primary acid-base disturbance.
  - Upper left, respiratory acidosis
  - Lower left, metabolic acidosis
  - Lower right, respiratory alkalosis
  - Upper right, metabolic alkalosis

Question 3: Was there compensation?

- There is no need to be as quantitative when using the Davenport plot to answer this question. Simply determine if the pH moved toward normal (7.4).
- The red respiratory and purple metabolic lines represent buffer lines, thus compensation follows the same plane as it moves toward 7.4.
- The direction the curve shifts if compensation occurred is depicted by the solid black arrows (panel D, Figure IX-1-4).

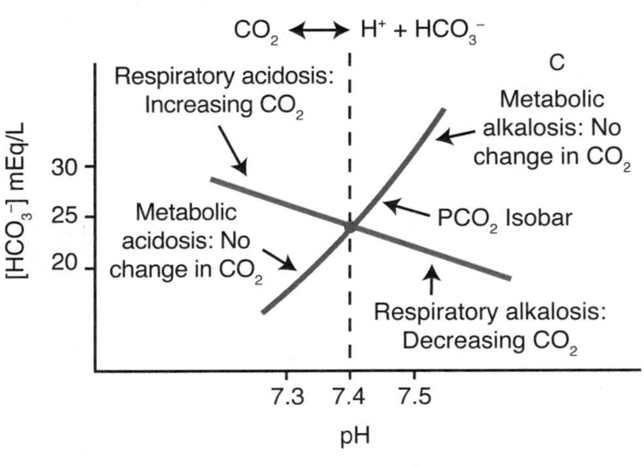

Figure IX-1-4c

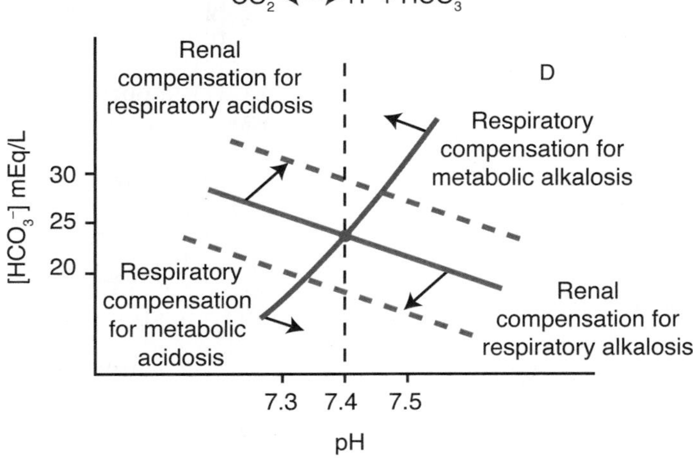

Figure IX-1-4d

A: acute (uncompensated) respiratory acidosis

B: chronic (compensated) respiratory acidosis

C: metabolic alkalosis with respiratory compensation

D: metabolic acidosis with respiratory compensation

E: acute (uncompensated) respiratory alkalosis

F: chronic (compensated) respiratory alkalosis

Assessment using Davenport plot:

Figure IX-1-5 shows unlabelled points on a Davenport plot. The student is encouraged to try and indicate the correct acid-base disturbance depicted by the points. Answers are provided below.

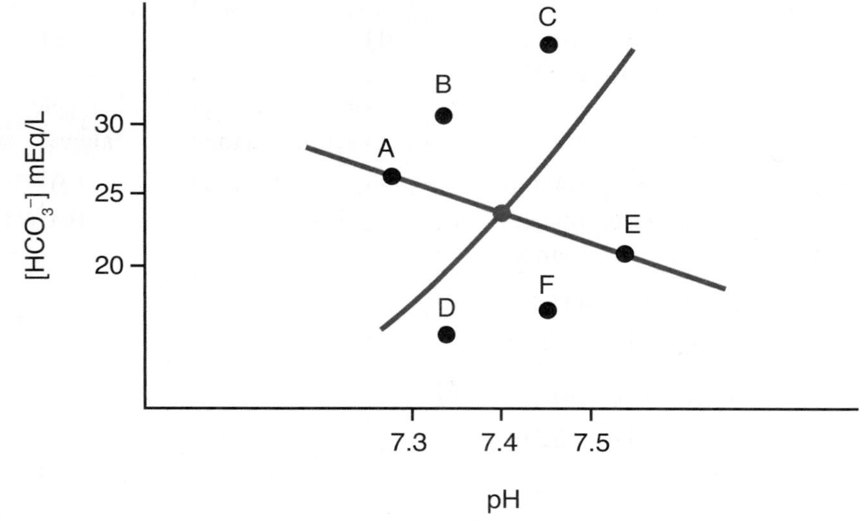

Figure IX-1-5

SUPPLEMENTAL INFORMATION

Respiratory Acidosis

A respiratory acidosis is the result of CO_2 accumulating in the body, which causes an increase in H^+ (or decrease in pH) and an increase in HCO_3^-. Quantitatively, in the acute (uncompensated) state, for every 10 mm Hg rise in $PaCO_2$, HCO_3^- rises about 1 mEq/L and pH falls by 0.08 pH units.

Respiratory acidosis can be caused by the following:

- Respiratory center depression (anesthetics, morphine)
- Pulmonary edema, cardiac arrest
- Airway obstruction
- Muscle relaxants
- Sleep apnea
- Chronic obstructive lung disease
- Neuromuscular defects (multiple sclerosis, muscular dystrophy)
- Obesity hypoventilation syndrome

<u>**Summary**</u>

Cause: increase in $PaCO_2$

Result: decrease in pH, slight increase in HCO_3^-

Metabolic Acidosis

This is caused by a gain in fixed (not of CO_2 origin) acid and/or a loss of base. The increased H^+ drives the reaction to the left, decreasing HCO_3^-. Forcing the reaction to the left produces some CO2, but the hyperventilation evoked by the acidosis eliminates CO_2.

As described above, the possible cause of the acidosis can be narrowed by determining the anion gap (MUDPIILES for elevated; HARDUP if gap is normal).

<u>Summary</u>

Cause: gain in H^+ as fixed acid and/or a loss of HCO_3^- (via GI tract or kidney)

Result: decrease in pH and HCO_3^-; compensatory fall in $PaCO_2$

Respiratory Alkalosis

This is caused by an increase in alveolar ventilation relative to body production of CO_2 (hyperventilation). Quantitatively, in the acute (uncompensated) state, for every 10 mm Hg decrease in $PaCO_2$, HCO_3^- decreases about 2 mEq/L and pH rises 0.08 pH units.

Respiratory alkalosis can be caused by:

- Anxiety
- Fever
- Hypoxemia
- Pneumothorax (in some cases)
- Ventilation–perfusion inequality
- Hypotension
- High altitude

<u>Summary</u>

Cause: decrease in $PaCO_2$

Result: decrease in H^+ (increased pH) and slight decrease in HCO_3^-

Metabolic Alkalosis

This is caused by a loss of fixed acid and/or gain of base. The decreased H^+ forces the reaction to the right, increasing HCO_3^-.

A compensatory rise in $PaCO_2$ is expected because the alkalosis decreases ventilation.

Causes:

- Vomiting or gastric suctioning
- Loop and thiazide diuretic use
- Bartter's, Gitelman's, and Liddle's syndromes
- Intracellular shift of hydrogen ions as in hypokalemia
- Primary hyperaldosteronism
- Loss of bicarbonate-free fluid (contraction alkalosis)

Summary

Cause: loss of H^+ and/or gain in HCO_3^-

Result: increase in pH and HCO_3^-; compensatory rise in $PaCO_2$

Chapter Summary

- There are 4 primary acid–base disturbances.
- The respiratory system regulates CO_2 and provides a rapid, albeit usually incomplete, compensatory mechanism for acid-base alterations.
- The kidneys regulate the body's levels of H^+ and HCO_3^-, and thus play an important role in acid-base regulation. Renal compensation is slow, taking days to fully develop.
- The first step in diagnosing an acid-base disturbance is to determine if it is an acidosis or alkalosis.
- Following the bicarbonate trail allows one to determine the cause of the acid-base disorder and thus diagnosis the primary disturbance.
- The final step in the diagnosis is to determine if the body has compensated. A calculation is required for this final step.
- Compute the anion gap: $Na^+ - (Cl^- + HCO_3^-)$ and remember MUDPILES versus HARDUP.
- The Davenport plot provides a graphical depiction of the interplay of pH, HCO_3^-, and $PaCO_2$ as it relates to acid-base disorders.

SECTION X

Endocrinology

General Aspects of the Endocrine System

1

Learning Objectives

- ❑ Demonstrate understanding of overview of hormones
- ❑ Answer questions about disorders of the endocrine system

OVERVIEW OF HORMONES

Lipid- Versus Water-Soluble Hormones

Figure X-1-1 demonstrates several major differences between the lipid-soluble hormones and the water-soluble hormones.

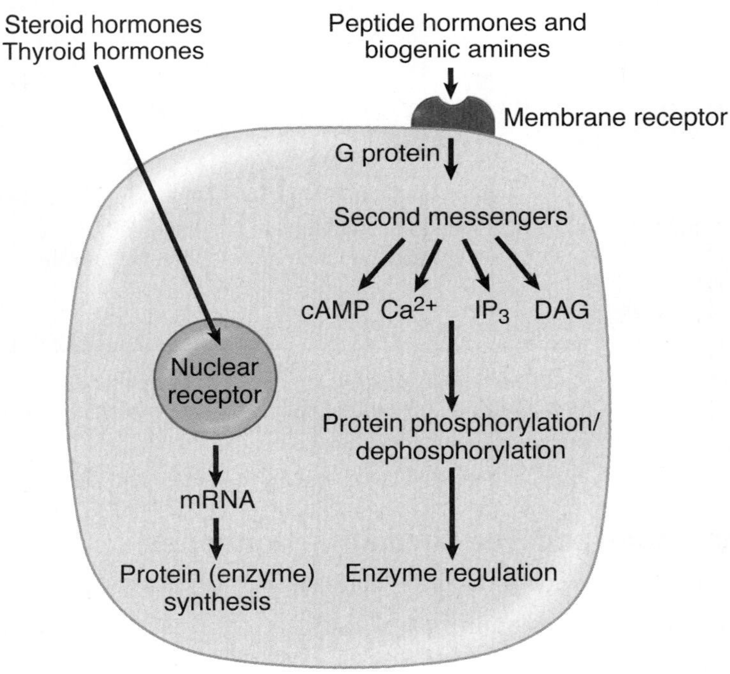

Figure X-1-1. Signal Transduction Mechanisms

IP3: inositol triphosphate

DAG: diacylglycerol

Table X-1-1. Differences Between the 2 Major Classes of Hormones

	Lipid-Soluble Hormones (steroids, thyroid hormones)	**Water-Soluble Hormones** (peptides, proteins)
Receptors	Inside the cell, usually in nucleus	Outer surface of the cell membrane
Intracellular action	Stimulates synthesis of specific new proteins	• Production of second messengers, e.g., cAMP • Insulin does not utilize cAMP, instead activates membrane-bound tyrosine kinase • Second messengers modify action of intracellular proteins (enzymes)
Storage	• Synthesized as needed • Exception: thyroid hormones	• Stored in vesicles • In some cases, prohormone stored in vesicle along with an enzyme that splits off the active hormone Prohormone stored in vesicle Active hormone Inactive peptide
Plasma transport	• Attached to proteins that serve as carriers • Exception: adrenal androgens	Dissolved in plasma (free, unbound)
Half-life	Long (hours, days) $\propto$ to affinity for protein carrier	Short (minutes) $\propto$ to molecular weight

Protein-Bound and Free Circulating Hormones

The liver produces proteins that bind lipid-soluble hormones, e.g.:

- cortisol-binding globulin
- thyroid-binding globulin
- sex hormone-binding globulin (SHBG)

Equilibrium

The lipid-soluble hormone circulating in plasma bound to protein is in equilibrium with a small amount of free hormone. It is the free form that is available to the tissues, and thus the free unbound form normally determines the plasma activity. It is the free form that also creates negative feedback. This equilibrium is shown in Figure X-1-2.

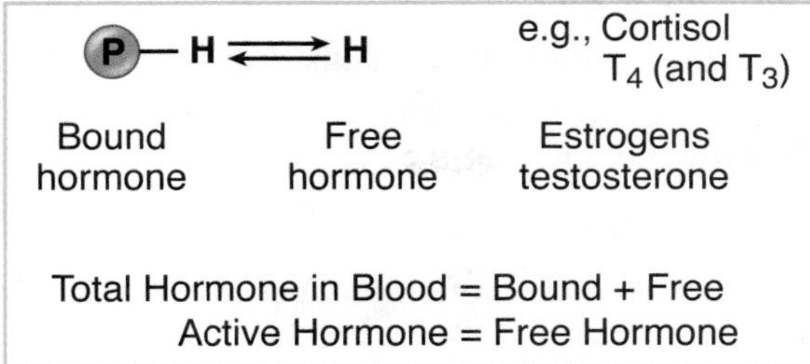

Figure X-1-2. Transport of Lipid-Soluble Hormones

Role of the liver

If the liver changes its production and release of binding proteins, the circulating level of **bound hormone will change.** However, under most conditions the level of **free hormone will remain constant**.

Modulation

Liver dysfunction and androgens can decrease and estrogens can increase the circulating level of binding proteins. For example, a rise in circulating estrogen causes the release of more binding protein by the liver, which binds more free hormone. The transient decrease in free hormone reduces negative feedback to the hormone-secreting tissue. The increased secretion of free hormone quickly returns the plasma free hormone to normal.

This explains why during pregnancy and other states with a rise in estrogen levels:

- Total plasma lipid-soluble hormone increases.
- Free plasma hormone remains constant at a normal level; thus, the individual does not show signs of hyperfunction.

Hormone Receptors

Hormone specificity

A hormone affects only cells that possess receptors specific to that particular hormone.

For example, both adrenocorticotropic hormone (ACTH) and luteinizing hormone (LH) increase the secretion of steroid hormones. However, ACTH does so only in the adrenal cortex and LH only in gonadal tissue.

Hormone activity

Under normal conditions, receptors are not saturated; that is, extra receptors exist. Therefore:

- Normally, the number of hormone receptors is not rate-limiting for hormone action.
- The plasma concentration of free hormone is usually indicative of activity.

Resistance to hormone action

- Abnormalities in receptors or events distal to the ligand-receptor interaction, often due to chronic elevation of circulating hormone (e.g., type II diabetes) or drug therapy.
- Under these conditions receptors are often saturated.
- Reduction of hormone levels often produces some recovery in sensitivity.
- The clinical presentation is often one of normal or elevated hormone levels but with reduced or absent peripheral manifestations of the hormone and a failure of replacement therapy to correct the problem.

Permissive action

A phenomenon in which one type of hormone must be present before another hormone can act; for example, cortisol must be present for glucagon to carry out gluconeogenesis and prevent hypoglycemia.

Measurement of Hormone Levels

Plasma analysis

- Provides information at the time of sampling only and may not reflect the overall secretion rate
- When hormone secretion is episodic, single sampling may reflect peaks (erroneous hyperfunction) or nadirs (erroneous hypofunction). Pulsatile secretion, diurnal and cyclic variation, age, sleep entrainment, and hormone antagonism must all be considered in evaluating circulating levels.
  - Growth hormone is secreted in pulses and mainly at night. This is not reflected in a fasting morning sample. However, growth hormone stimulates the secretion of IGF-I which circulates attached to protein and has a long half-life (20 hours). Plasma IGF-I measured at any time during the day is usually a good index of overall growth hormone secretion.
  - Thyroid is a fairly constant system and T4 has a half-life of about 6–7 days. Thus, a random measurement of total T4 is usually a good estimate of daily plasma levels.

Urine analysis

- Restricted to the measurement of catecholamines, steroid hormones, and water-soluble hormones such as hCG and LH.
- A distinct advantage of urine analysis is that it provides an integrated sample.
  - A "24-hour urine free cortisol" is often necessary to pick up a low-level Cushing's syndrome and to eliminate the highs and lows of the normal circadian rhythm.

DISORDERS OF THE ENDOCRINE SYSTEM

Primary versus Secondary Disorders

- A primary disorder means dysfunction originating in the endocrine gland itself, either hyper- or hypo-function. Examples of a primary disorder include:
  - excess cortisol from an adrenal adenoma (Cushing syndrome)
  - decreased thyroid secretion (Hashimoto's thyroiditis)
  - reduced ADH secretion (central diabetes insipidus)
- A secondary disorder indicates that a disturbance has occurred causing the gland secrete more or less of the hormone. Examples of a secondary disorder include:
  - Cushing disease (pituitary adenoma secreting ACTH) resulting in hypercortisolism
  - a dehydrated patient with elevated plasma osmolality causing high ADH levels

Hypofunction

- Can be caused by autoimmune disease (e.g., type I diabetes, hypothyroidism, primary adrenal insufficiency, gonadal failure), tumors, hemorrhage, infection, damage by neoplasms
- Evaluated by a stimulation test
  - Hypothalamic hormones test anterior pituitary reserve
  - Injection of the pituitary trophic hormone (e.g., ACTH) tests target gland reserve.
  - Failure of growth hormone release after arginine injection

Hyperfunction

- Caused by hormone-secreting tumors, hyperplasia, autoimmune stimulation, ectopically produced peptide hormones (e.g., ACTH, ADH)
- Evaluated by a suppression test
  - Failure of glucose to suppress growth hormone diagnostic for acromegaly
  - Failure of dexamethasone (low dose) to suppress cortisol diagnostic for hypercortisolism
  - Multiple endocrine neoplasia (MEN) represents a group of inheritable syndromes characterized by multiple benign or malignant tumors.
    - MEN 1: hyperparathyroidism, endocrine pancreas, and pituitary edenomas
    - MEN 2A: medullary carcinoma of the thyroid, pheochromocytoma, hyperparathyroidism
    - MEN 2B: medullary carcinoma of the thyroid, pheochromocytoma, hyperparathyroidism typically absent.

Gland Structure and Size

- When an endocrine gland does not receive its normal stimulus, it generally undergoes a reversible atrophy.
  - Long-term high doses of glucocorticoids suppress the ACTH-adrenal axis. Withdrawal of therapy can require up to a year for complete recovery.
- Overstimulation of endocrine tissue can cause cell proliferation or hypertrophy in addition to hormone overproduction.
  - In Graves' disease, overstimulation of the thyroid tissues causes cell proliferation and this polyclonal expansion creates a goiter in addition to hyperthyroidism.
- Tumors, which are generally monoclonal expansions, may also create a hyperfunction. Others produce little if any hormone but are still disease-producing because of the compressive (mass) effect of the additional tissue.

Chapter Summary

- Lipid-soluble endocrine hormones: Receptors are inside cells. Because they must be synthesized as needed and must generate new proteins to carry out their actions, they represent slow-acting systems. The total plasma level does not necessarily provide an index of activity because most is bound. It is the free hormone that determines activity.
- Water-soluble hormones: Receptors are on the membrane surface. Second messengers carry out intracellular action. Because they are stored in vesicles and need only modify proteins to carry out their actions, they are fast-acting systems.
- Normally, receptors are not saturated. It is the plasma level of free hormone that determines activity.
- Tissue resistance elevates plasma hormone levels but reduces peripheral effects.
- Plasma hormonal analysis may not reflect overall secretion rate.
- Urine analysis provides an integrated sample for catecholamines and some steroid hormones.
- Hypofunction is evaluated by a stimulation test.
- Hyperfunction is evaluated by a suppression test.
- Lack of glandular stimulation causes a reversible atrophy.
- Overstimulation of a gland can cause hypertrophy or hyperplasia.

Hypothalamic–Anterior Pituitary System 2

Learning Objectives

- ❑ Solve problems concerning hypothalamic–anterior pituitary axis
- ❑ Solve problems concerning disorders of the hypothalamic–anterior pituitary axis

HYPOTHALAMIC–ANTERIOR PITUITARY AXIS

- The hormones in this system are all water-soluble.
- The hypothalamic hormones are synthesized in the neuron cell body, packaged in vesicles, and transported down the axon to be stored and released from the nerve terminals.
- Pituitary is located in the bony sella turcica at the base of the skull. It hangs from the hypothalamus by a stalk (the infundibulum) and is controlled by the hypothalamus. The dura membrane (diaphragm sellae) separates it from and prevents cerebrospinal fluid from entering the sella turcica.
- Optic chiasm is 5–10 mm above this diaphragm.
- In the hypothalamic–anterior pituitary system, hormonal release is mainly pulsatile. A possible exception is the thyroid system.
- The pulsatile release of GnRH prevents downregulation of its receptors on the gonadotrophs of the anterior pituitary. A constant infusion of GnRH will cause a decrease in the release of both LH and FSH.

The hypothalamic–anterior pituitary system is summarized in Figure X-2-1.

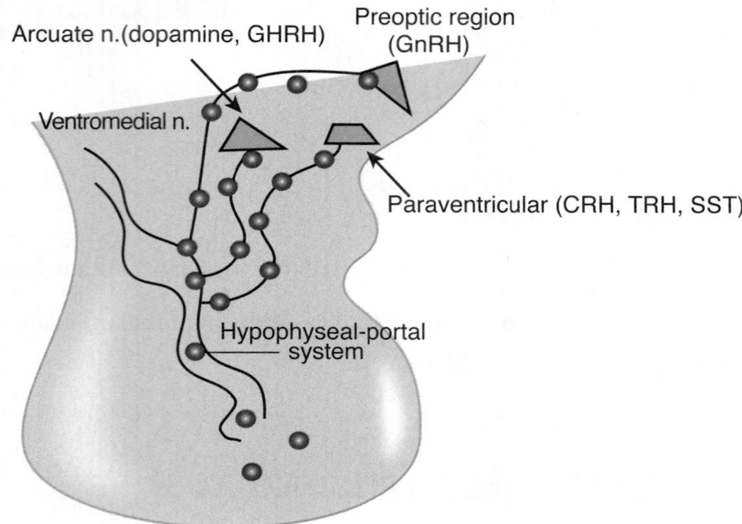

Figure X-2-1. Hypothalamic–Anterior Pituitary Axis

- The hypothalamic hormones, thyrotropin-releasing hormone (TRH), corticotropin-releasing hormone (CRH), growth hormone–releasing hormone (GHRH), somatostatin (SST), and dopamine are synthesized in neuronal cell bodies in the arcuate and paraventricular nuclei; gonadotropin-releasing hormone (GnRH) is synthesized in the preoptic nucleus.
- The nerve endings all come together in the median eminence region of the hypothalamus. The hormones are then secreted into the hypophyseal-portal system and transported to the anterior pituitary.
- Hypothalamic hormones bind to receptors on cells of the anterior pituitary and modify the secretion of thyroid-stimulating hormone (TSH) (thyrotropin), corticotropin (ACTH), luteinizing hormone (LH), follicle-stimulating hormone (FSH), growth hormone (GH), and prolactin.

Effect of Each Hypothalamic Hormone on Anterior Pituitary

Hypothalamus		Pituitary Target	Secretion
TRH	+ →	Thyrotrophs (10%)	TSH
CRH	+ →	Corticotrophs (10–25%)	ACTH
GnRH*	+ →	Gonadotrophs (10–15%)	LH, FSH
GHRH**	+ →	Somatotrophs (50%)	GH
SST	– →		
Dopamine***	– →	Lactotrophs (10–15%)	Prolactin
TRH (elevated)	+ →		

*High frequency pulses favor LH, low frequency pulses favor FSH

**The fact that eliminating hypothalamic input causes a decrease in growth hormone secretion indicates that GHRH is the main controlling factor.

***When the connection between the hypothalamus and the anterior pituitary is severed (e.g., there is damage to the pituitary stalk), secretion of all anterior pituitary hormones decreases, except prolactin, which increases. The secretion of prolactin increases because a chronic source of inhibition (dopamine) has been removed.

Figure X-2-2. Control of the Anterior Pituitary

+ = releaser
– = inhibitor

TRH:	thyrotropin-releasing hormone
TSH:	thyroid-stimulating hormone or thyrotropin
CRH:	corticotropin-releasing hormone
ACTH:	adrenocorticotropic hormone or corticotropin
GnRH:	gonadotropin-releasing hormone
LH:	luteinizing hormone
FSH:	follicle-stimulating hormone
GHRH:	growth hormone–releasing hormone
GH:	growth hormone
SST:	somatostatin

DISORDERS OF THE HYPOTHALAMIC–ANTERIOR PITUITARY AXIS

Hypopituitarism

- Can be inherited but other causes include head trauma (most common), mass effects of tumors, inflammation, or vascular damage
- Characteristic sequential loss of function: growth hormone and gonadotropin, followed by TSH then ACTH and finally prolactin.
- Isolated deficiency:

  Growth hormone: sporadic or familial

  Gonadotropins: Kallman syndrome – (tertiary) defective GnRH synthesis; ↓ LH ↓ FSH ↓ sex steroids

  ACTH, TSH, and prolactin extremely rare deficiencies, usually a sign of panhypopituitarism
- Craniopharyngioma is the most common tumor affecting the hypothalamic–pituitary system in children (pituitary adenomas rare).
- Although one would predict the trophic hormones to be low, this is not often the case. Typically, they are in the normal range, but their level is inadequate to stimulate peripheral glands adequately.
- From an academic perspective, stimulation tests include: GnRH → LH, FSH; TRH → TSH, prolactin; insulin infusion → GH, ACTH

Sheehan syndrome

The pituitary in pregnancy is enlarged and therefore more vulnerable to infarction. Sometimes when delivery is associated with severe blood loss, the ensuing shock causes arteriolar spasm in the pituitary with subsequent ischemic necrosis. Some degree of hypopituitarism has been reported in 32% of women with severe postpartum hemorrhage. Symptoms vary, depending on the extent and location of pituitary damage, but failure to lactate for days following birth is a strong sign of pituitary damage.

Pituitary Adenomas

- Most common cause of hypothalamic–pituitary dysfunction
- Microadenomas (< 1 cm. dia.): characterized by hormonal excess, no panhypopituitarism, treatable, e.g., ACTH (Cushing disease)
- Hypogonadism is the most common manifestation.
- Usually benign and can autonomously secrete hormone leading to hyperprolactinemia (60%), acromegaly (growth hormone 20%), and Cushing disease (ACTH 10%).
- Prolactinomas associated with hypogonadism and galactorrhea
- MEN 1 association
- Macroadenomas (> 1 cm. dia): mass effect, larger tumors with suprasellar extension, associated with panhypopituitarism and visual loss

Chapter Summary

- Hypothalamic hormones affecting the pituitary are synthesized in the ventromedial, arcuate, and preoptic nuclei but are stored and released from the median eminence.
- Pulsatile system and the pulsatile release of GnRH prevents downregulation of gonadotroph receptors.
- Anterior pituitary hormones are regulated primarily by hypothalamic releasing hormones, except prolactin, which is mainly under the influence of dopamine, an inhibiting hormone.
- Damage to the pituitary stalk causes a decrease in all anterior pituitary hormones except prolactin, which increases.
- Pituitary adenomas are the most common cause of anterior pituitary dysfunction.
- The mass effect causes sequential loss of GH and gonadotropin followed by TSH, ACTH, and finally prolactin.
- Prolactinomas are the most common tumor, and hypogonadism is the most common manifestation.

Posterior Pituitary 3

Learning Objectives

- ❑ Answer questions about hormones of the posterior pituitary
- ❑ Explain information related to regulation of ECF volume and osmolarity
- ❑ Answer questions about pathophysiologic changes in ADH secretion
- ❑ Use knowledge of hyponatremia

HORMONES OF THE POSTERIOR PITUITARY

- Made up of distal neuron terminals
- Secreted hormones; arginine vasopressin (ADH), oxytocin (see chapter 11)—both are peptide hormones.
- Cell bodies located in the supraoptic nucleus and paraventricular nucleus of the hypothalamus.
- ADH is a major controller of water excretion and regulator of extracellular osmolarity.
- The osmoreceptor neurons in the hypothalamus are extremely sensitive and are able to maintain ECF osmolarity within a very narrow range.
- There is a downward shift in plasma osmolarity regulation in pregnancy, the menstrual cycle, and with volume depletion. In the latter case osmoregulation is secondary to volume regulation; a return of circulating volume occurs even though osmolarity decreases.
- Volume receptors are less sensitive than osmoreceptors and a change of 10–15% in volume is required to produce a measurable change in ADH.
- Angiotensin II and CRH can stimulate the release of ADH.

Figure X-3-1 illustrates the neural control mechanisms that regulate secretion of ADH by the posterior pituitary. The principal inputs are inhibition by baroreceptor and cardiopulmonary mechanoreceptors (see Section V, Chapter 1) and stimulation by osmoreceptors.

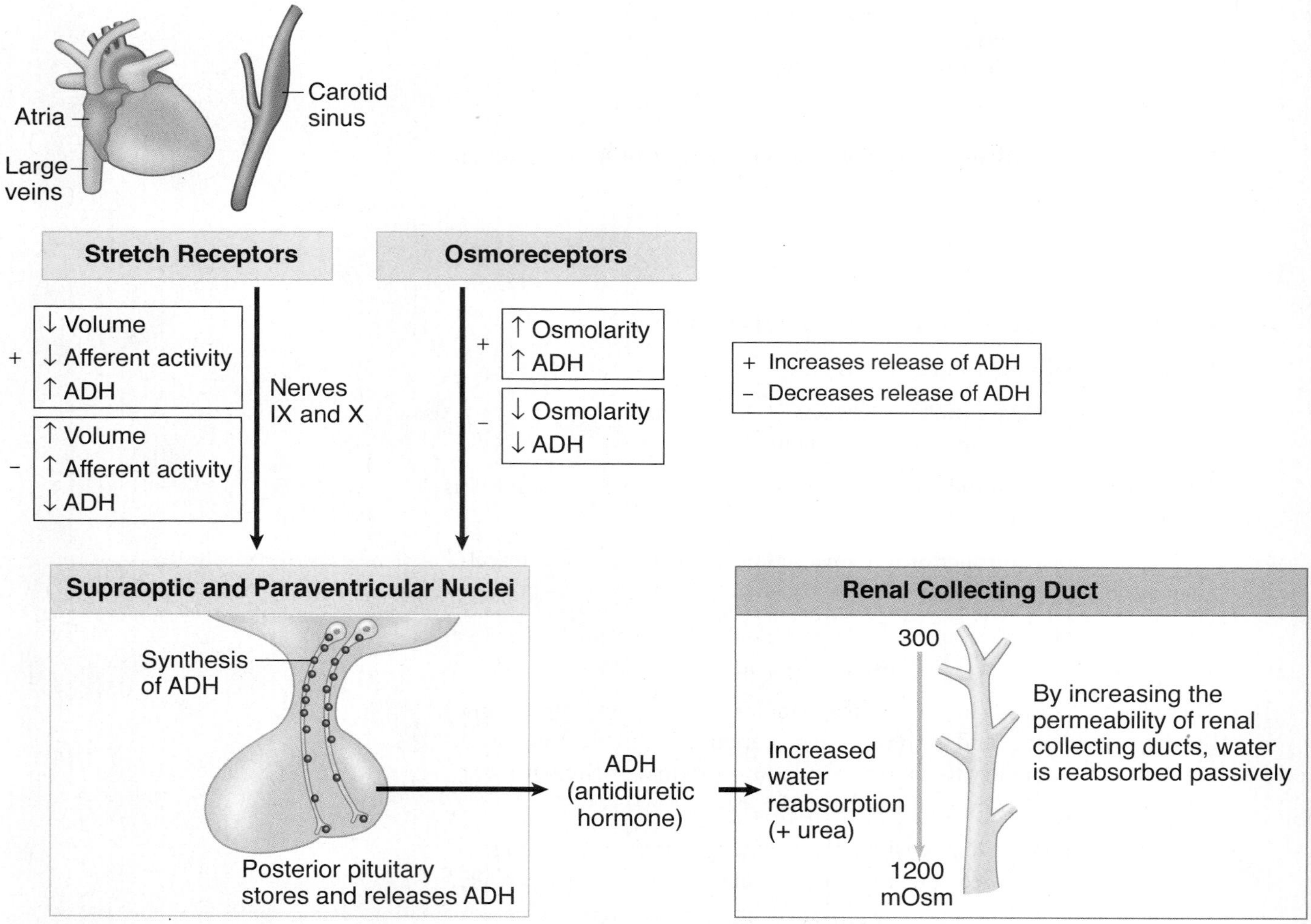

Atria
Large veins
Carotid sinus

Stretch Receptors

+ ↓ Volume, ↓ Afferent activity, ↑ ADH

– ↑ Volume, ↑ Afferent activity, ↓ ADH

Nerves IX and X

Osmoreceptors

+ ↑ Osmolarity, ↑ ADH

– ↓ Osmolarity, ↓ ADH

+ Increases release of ADH
– Decreases release of ADH

Supraoptic and Paraventricular Nuclei

Synthesis of ADH

Posterior pituitary stores and releases ADH

ADH (antidiuretic hormone)

Renal Collecting Duct

300

Increased water reabsorption (+ urea)

1200 mOsm

By increasing the permeability of renal collecting ducts, water is reabsorbed passively

Figure X-3-1. Neural Control Mechanism

Synthesis and Release of ADH

- ADH is synthesized in the supraoptic (SO) and paraventricular (PVN) nuclei of the hypothalamus; it is stored and released from the posterior pituitary.
- Osmoreceptors are neurons that respond to increased plasma osmolarity, principally plasma sodium concentration. They synapse with neurons of the SO and PVN and stimulate them to secrete ADH from the posterior pituitary. They also stimulate consumption of water through hypothalamic centers that regulate thirst.
- The SO and PVN also receive input from cardiopulmonary mechanoreceptors, as well as arterial baroreceptors. High blood volume or blood pressure tends to inhibit secretion of ADH.
- Secretion of ADH is most sensitive to plasma osmolarity (1%); however, if blood volume decreases by 10% (such as hemorrhage) or cardiac output falls, high levels of ADH are secreted even if it causes abnormal plasma osmolarity.

Note

ADH is also stimulated by Ang II and CRH.

Action of ADH

- The main target tissue is the renal collecting duct (V2 receptors).
- ADH increases the permeability of the duct to water by placing water channels (aquaporins) in the luminal membrane.
- ADH, acting via the V1 receptor, contracts vascular smooth muscle.

REGULATION OF ECF VOLUME AND OSMOLARITY

Osmoregulation

- An increase of only 1% in the osmolality of the ECF bathing the hypothalamic osmoreceptors evokes an increase in ADH secretion.
- A similarly sized decrease in osmolality decreases ADH secretion.
- In this manner, ECF osmolality is kept very close to 285 mOsm/Kg.

Volume Regulation

- Stimuli arising from stretch receptors act to chronically inhibit ADH secretion.
- Decreases in blood volume cause venous and arterial stretch receptors to send fewer signals to the CNS, decreasing chronic inhibition of ADH secretion.
- This mechanism is especially important for restoring ECF volume following a hemorrhage.

Effect of Alcohol and Weightlessness on ADH Secretion

Ingesting ethyl alcohol or being in a weightless environment suppresses ADH secretion. In weightlessness, there is a net shift of blood from the limbs to the abdomen and chest. This results in greater stretch of the volume receptors in the large veins and atria, thus suppressing ADH secretion.

Atrial Natriuretic Peptide (ANP)

ANP is the hormone secreted by the heart. ANP is found throughout the heart but mainly in the right atrium. The stimuli that release ANP (two peptides are released) are:

- Stretch, an action independent of nervous involvement
- CHF and all fluid overload states

ANP increases sodium loss (natriuresis) and water loss by the kidney because of, in part, an increase in glomerular filtration rate due to:

- ANP-mediated dilation of the afferent arteriole
- ANP-mediated constriction of the efferent arteriole

ANP also increases sodium loss (natriuresis) and water loss (diuresis) by the kidney because it inhibits aldosterone release as well as the reabsorption of sodium and water in the collecting duct.

Clinical Correlate

Circulating levels of brain natriuretic peptide (BNP) correlate well with the degree of heart failure. Although very little BNP is synthesized and released in the normal heart, there is a marked elevation as the ventricle dilates, hence the correlation. The functional or pathologic significance is still unknown, but there is a strong correlation.

The physiologic importance of ANP is not known because it has not been possible to identify or produce a specific deficiency state in humans. However, ANP secretion increases in weightlessness and submersion to the neck in water, while renin, aldosterone, and ADH secretion decrease. It may play a role in normal regulation of the ECF osmolality and volume.

ANP tends to antagonize the effects of aldosterone and ADH.

A normal ANP level is used to exclude CHF as a cause of dyspnea.

PATHOPHYSIOLOGIC CHANGES IN ADH SECRETION

Diabetes Insipidus

The consequences can be explained on the basis of the lack of an effect of ADH on the renal collecting ducts.

Central diabetes insipidus (CDI)

- Sufficient ADH is not available to affect the renal collecting ducts.
- Causes include familial, tumors (craniopharyngioma), autoimmune, trauma
- Pituitary trauma – transient diabetes insipidus
- Sectioning of pituitary stalk – triphasic response: diabetes insipidus, followed by SIADH, followed by a return of diabetes insipidus

- Destruction of the hypothalamus from any cause can lead to diabetes insipidus. Forms of hypothalamic destruction are stroke, hypoxia, head trauma, infection, cancer or mass lesions.
- CDI = ADH deficiency. CDI is treated with replacing ADH as vasopressin or DDAVP (desmopressin).

Nephrogenic diabetes insipidus

- Due to inability of the kidneys to respond to ADH
- Causes include familial, acquired, drugs (lithium)
- Hypokalemia
- Hypercalcemia

Lithium, low potassium, and high calcium all diminish ADH's effectiveness on principal cells. The precise mechanism is still unclear, but it may involve disruption in the ability to traffic aquaporins to the luminal membrane of principal cells of the kidney.

Table X-3-1. Differential Diagnosis Following Water Deprivation

	Plasma Osm	Urine Osm	Plasma ADH	Urine Osm Post Desmopressin
Normal	297	814	↑	815
Central DI*	342	102	↓	622
Nephrogenic	327	106	↑	118

*Patients with partial central DI will concentrate their urine somewhat but will achieve an additional boost following desmopressin.

Syndrome of Inappropriate ADH Secretion (SIADH)

Excessive secretion of ADH causes an inappropriate increased reabsorption of water in the renal collecting duct.

Causes

- Ectopic production of ADH (any CNS or small cell lung pathology)
- Drug induced: SSRI, carbamazepine
- Lesions in the pathway of the baroreceptor system

Pathophysiology

- Increased water retention, hyponatremia, but clinically euvolumic
- Inappropriate concentration of urine, often greater than plasma osmolarity
- With hyponatremia, a normal person should have urine sodium and osmolarity that are low. In SIADH, it is a disease because urine sodium and osmolarity are inappropriately high.

Treatment

- Fluid restriction but not salt restriction
- Sodium disorders cause neurological symptoms.
- Only mild hyponatremia from SIADH can be managed with fluid restriction.
- Severe disease needs 3% hypertonic saline or V2 receptor antagonists.
- Conivaptan and tolvaptan are V2 receptor antagonists; they stop ADH effect on kidney tubule.

Summary of Changes

Table X-3-2. The Effects of Diabetes Insipidus, Dehydration, SIADH, and Primary Polydipsia

	Diabetes Insipidus	Dehydration	SIADH	Primary Polydipsia
1. Permeability of collecting ducts to H_2O	↓	↑	↑	↓
2. Urine flow	↑	↓	↓	↑
3. Urine osmolarity	↓	↑	↑	↓
4. ECF volume	↓	↓	↑	↑
5. ECF osmolarity* (Na concentration)	↑	↑	↓	↓
6. ICF volume	↓	↓	↑	↑
7. ICF osmolarity	↑	↑	↓	↓

*Overt physical and laboratory signs of dehydration do not necessarily develop unless there is a defect in thirst stimulation.

HYPONATREMIA

General Features

- One of the most common disorders of fluid and electrolyte balance in hospitalized patients
- Is usually equivalent to a hypo-osmolar state (exception hyperglycemia)
- Involves both solute depletion and water retention but water retention is usually the more important factor
- Solute depletion can occur from any significant loss of ECF fluid. The hyponatremia is the result of replacement by more hypotonic fluids.
- When it develops rapidly (< 48 hours) and is severe (Na < 120 mEq/L), patient is at risk for seizures and respiratory arrest. Often treated aggressively with hypertonic saline (3%) and diuretics or ADH antagonists.
- When it develops more slowly, it appears to be well-tolerated and patient is asymptomatic. Aggressive treatment may result in "central pontine myelinolysis." General recommendation is to slowly raise Na concentration over a period of days.

Subgroups

Hypervolemia

Caused by marked reduction in water excretion and/or increased rate of water ingestion. Would include congestive heart failure and cirrhosis

Hypovolemia

Indicates solute depletion. Would include mineralocorticoid deficiency, diuretic abuse, renal disease, diarrhea, and hemorrhage

Clinical euvolemia

Would include SIADH and primary (psychogenic) polydipsia. A clinically equivalent presentation may occur in glucocorticoid deficiency or hypothyroidism.

Chapter Summary

- ADH is synthesized in the hypothalamus but is stored and released from the posterior pituitary.
- The major action of ADH is the reabsorption of water and urea, but not electrolytes, in the renal collecting duct.
- Osmoreceptors are very sensitive and normally maintain osmolarity in a very narrow range.
- Reduced input from the low-pressure stretch receptors is a strong stimulus for the release of ADH.
- ANP, found mainly in the tissue of the right atrium, is released in response to stretch. The major action of ANP is diuresis and natriuresis.
- In diabetes insipidus, central form has low plasma ADH, nephrogenic form has high plasma ADH.
- Easily separated by measuring plasma ADH or injection of desmopressin
- SIADH: Inappropriately elevated secretion of ADH. Characterized by euvolemia but hyponatremia.
- Acute hyponatremia is life threatening if severe. Treated aggressively.
- Chronic hyponatremia is usually well-tolerated. Aggressive treatment is associated with central pontine myelinolysis.

Adrenal Cortex 4

Learning Objectives

- ❑ Use knowledge of functional regions of the adrenal gland
- ❑ Demonstrate understanding of biosynthetic pathways of steroid hormone synthesis
- ❑ Interpret scenarios on physiologic actions of glucocorticoids
- ❑ Solve problems concerning control of adrenocorticotropin and cortisol secretion
- ❑ Demonstrate understanding of physiologic actions of aldosterone
- ❑ Explain information related to control of aldosterone secretion
- ❑ Explain information related to glucocorticoid disorders
- ❑ Explain information related to mineralocorticoid disorders
- ❑ Explain information related to enzyme deficiencies

FUNCTIONAL REGIONS OF THE ADRENAL GLAND

Figure X-4-1 summarizes each adrenal region.

- ACTH controls the release of both cortisol and adrenal androgens.
- Aldosterone is stimulated by a rise in angiotensin II and/or K^+.

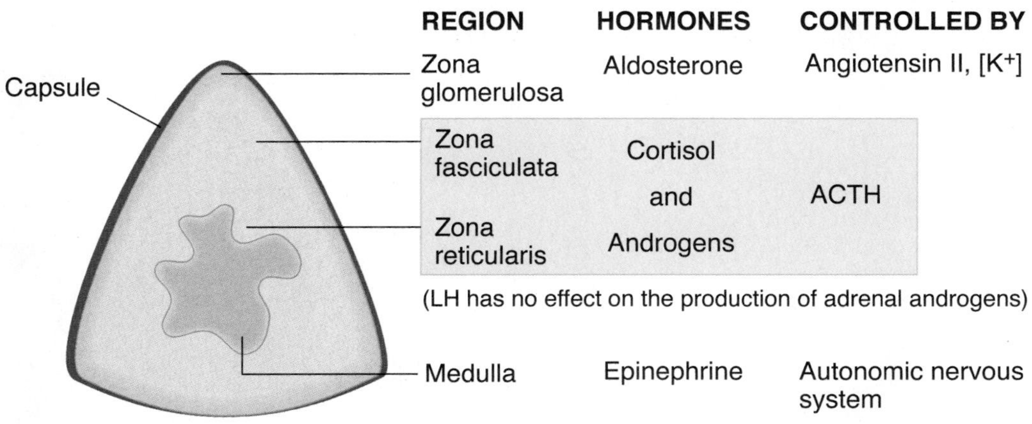

Figure X-4-1. Adrenal Cortex Regions

Consequences of the Loss of Regional Adrenal Function

Zona glomerulosa: The **absence of the mineralocorticoid, aldosterone**, results in:

- Loss of Na^+
- Decreased volume of the ECF
- Low blood pressure
- Circulatory shock
- Death

Zona fasciculata, zona reticularis: The **absence of the glucocorticoid, cortisol,** contributes to:

- Circulatory failure, because without cortisol, catecholamines do not exert their normal vasoconstrictive action.
- An inability to readily mobilize energy sources (glucose and free fatty acids) from glycogen or fat. Under normal living conditions, this is not life-threatening; however, under stressful situations, severe problems can arise. For example, fasting can result in fatal hypoglycemia.

If problems develop with anterior pituitary secretion, glucocorticoid secretion may be affected, but the mineralocorticoid system remains intact.

BIOSYNTHETIC PATHWAYS OF STEROID HORMONE SYNTHESIS

Synthetic Pathways

Figure X-4-2 shows a composite of the synthetic pathways in all steroid hormone-producing tissues. A single tissue has only the pathways necessary to produce the hormones normally secreted by that particular tissue. For example, the zona glomerulosa has only the pathways of the first column because the main output of the zona glomerulosa is aldosterone. Cholesterol is pulled off circulating LDL or made de novo by acetate.

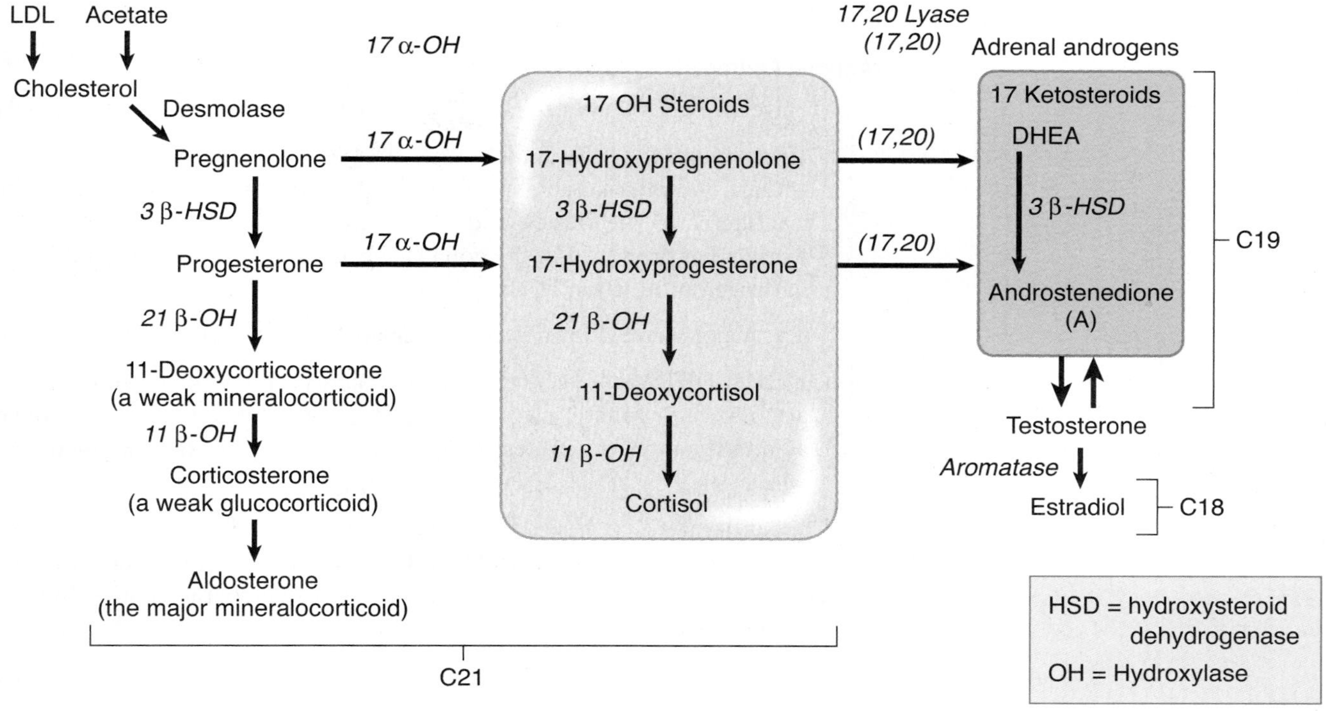

Figure X-4-2. Pathways of Adrenal Steroid Synthesis

C21 steroids (21 carbon atoms)

C21 steroids with an OH at position 17 are called 17-hydroxysteroids. The only 17 OH steroid with hormonal activity is cortisol.

The lipid-soluble 17 OH steroids are metabolized to water-soluble compounds before they are filtered and excreted in the urine. The pathway for cortisol is shown in Figure X-4-3.

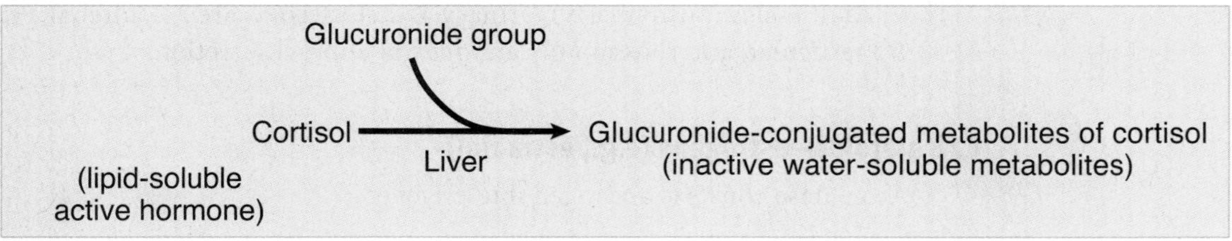

Figure X-4-3. Metabolism of Cortisol

Urinary 17 OH steroids have in the past been measured as an index of cortisol secretion. This has been replaced by the measurement of the 24-hour urine-free cortisol.

C19 steroids (19 carbon atoms)

Adrenal Androgens

- Have a keto group at position 17 and are therefore called 17-ketosteroids.
- Are conjugated with sulfate in the adrenal cortex, making them water soluble. As water-soluble metabolites, they circulate in the bloodstream, are filtered by the kidney, and are excreted in the urine. The sulfated form is not produced in the gonads and is thus considered an index of androgen production by the adrenals.
- The major secreted form is dehydroepiandrosterone (DHEA).
- DHEA, DHEA sulfate, and androstenedione have very low androgenic activity. They function primarily as precursors for the peripheral conversion to the more potent testosterone and dihydrotestosterone (men and women).
- In adult males, excessive production of adrenal androgens has no clinical consequences. In prepubertal males it causes premature penile enlargement and early development of secondary sexual characteristics. In women excessive adrenal androgens cause hirsutism and virilization.

Testosterone

- Produced mainly by the Leydig cells of testes
- The active hormone is lipid-soluble and not a 17-ketosteroid.
- When metabolized, it is converted to a 17-ketosteroid and conjugated to become water soluble. In this form, it is filtered and excreted by the kidney.

Urinary Excretion

- Urinary 17-ketosteroids are an index of all androgens, adrenal and testicular.
- In females and prepubertal males, urinary 17-ketosteroids are an index of adrenal androgen secretion.
- In adult males (postpuberty), urinary 17-ketosteroids are 2/3 adrenal and 1/3 testicular, and thus mainly an index of adrenal secretion.

C18 steroids—estrogens (e.g., estradiol)

- Aromatase converts androgen into estrogen.

Regional Synthesis

Conversion of cholesterol to pregnenolone

The starting point in the synthesis of all steroid hormones is the transport of cholesterol into the mitochondria by steroidogenic acute regulatory protein (StAR). This is the rate-limiting step.

The enzyme catalyzing the conversion of cholesterol to pregnenolone is side-chain cleavage enzyme (SCC, also called desmolase).

Synthesis in the zona glomerulosa

Figure X-4-4 represents the pathways present in the zona glomerulosa. Angiotensin II is the main stimulus to the zona glomerulosa, which produces aldosterone, the major mineralocorticoid.

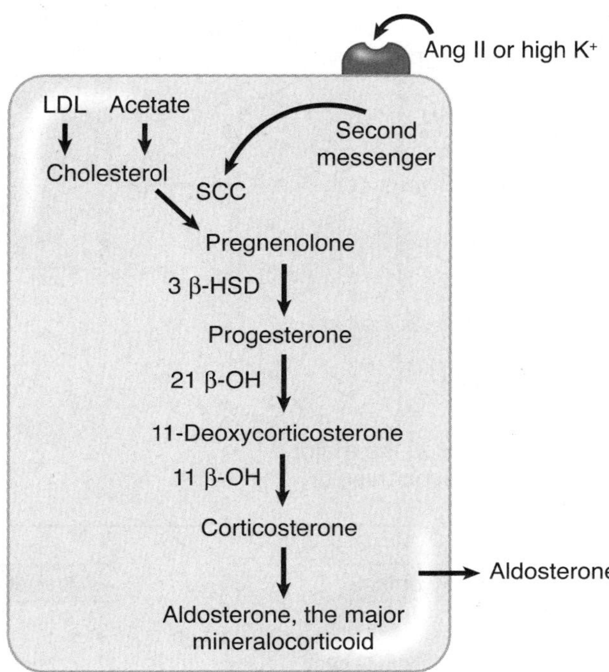

Figure X-4-4. Pathway to Aldosterone Synthesis

Synthesis in the zona fasciculata and the zona reticularis

Normal hormonal output of the zona fasciculata and zona glomerulosa consists of the following:

- 11-Deoxycorticosterone: Under normal conditions, this weak mineralocorticoid is not important. Almost all mineralocorticoid activity is due to aldosterone.
- Corticosterone: Also not important under normal conditions. Almost all glucocorticoid activity is due to cortisol.
- Cortisol: Main glucocorticoid secreted by the adrenal cortex, responsible for most of the hypothalamic and anterior pituitary negative feedback control of ACTH secretion.

Normal hormonal output of the zona reticularis consists of the following:

- Adrenal androgens: These weak water-soluble androgens represent a significant secretion; however, they produce masculinizing characteristics only in women and prepubertal males when secretion is excessive.

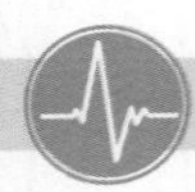

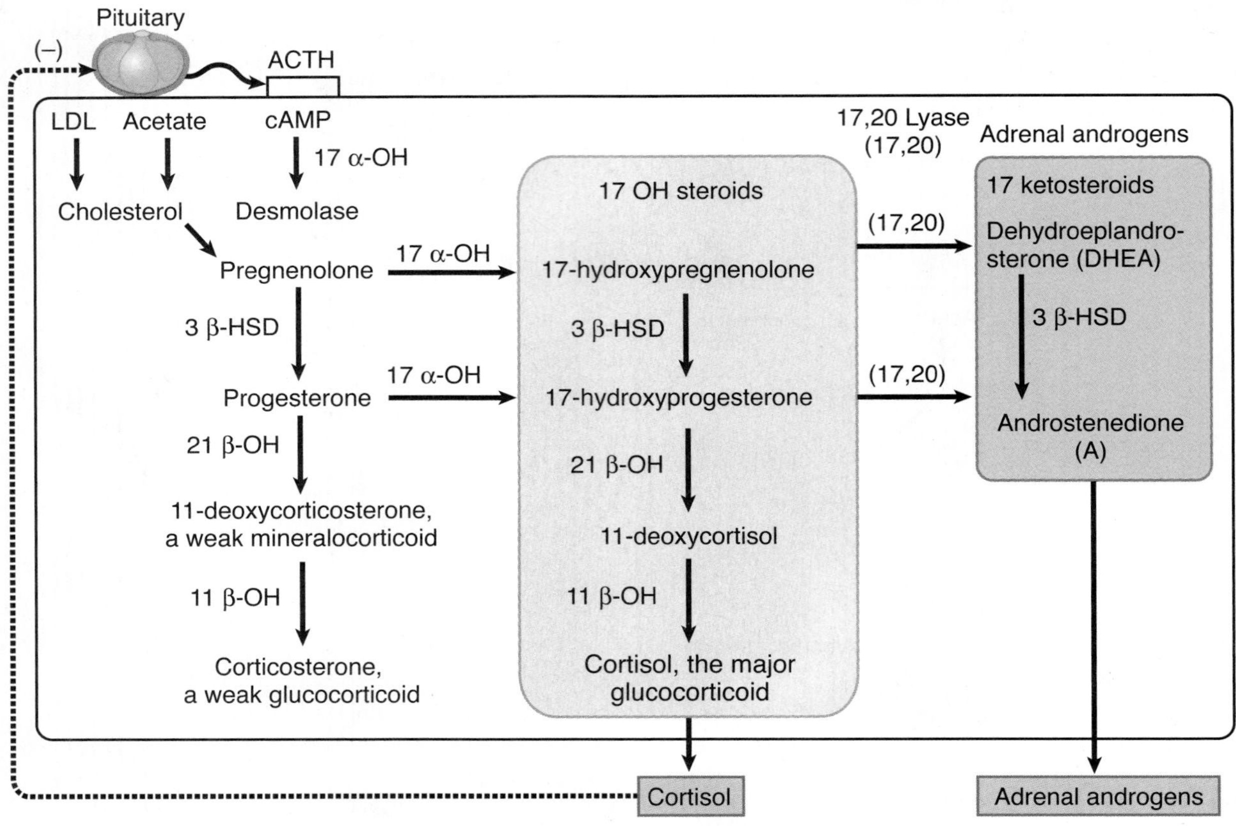

Figure X-4-5. Control of Steroid Hormone Synthesis in the Zonas Fasciculata and Reticularis

PHYSIOLOGIC ACTIONS OF GLUCOCORTICOIDS

Stress

Stress includes states such as trauma, exposure to cold, illness, starvation, and exercise. The capacity to withstand stress is dependent on adequate secretion of the glucocorticoids.

Stress hormones usually act to mobilize energy stores. The stress hormones are:

- **Growth hormone:** mobilizes fatty acids by increasing lipolysis in adipose tissue
- **Glucagon:** mobilizes glucose by increasing liver glycogenolysis
- **Cortisol:** mobilizes fat, protein, carbohydrate (see below)
- **Epinephrine,** in some forms of stress such as exercise: mobilizes glucose via glycogenolysis and fat via lipolysis

All stress hormones raise plasma glucose. Severe hypoglycemia is a crisis and causes a rapid increase in all stress hormones. By definition, because these hormones raise plasma glucose, they are referred to as counterregulatory hormones (opposite to insulin).

A deficiency in a stress hormone may cause hypoglycemia.

Metabolic Actions of Cortisol

Cortisol promotes the mobilization of energy stores, specifically:

- **Protein:** Cortisol promotes degradation and increased delivery of hepatic gluconeogenic precursors.
- **Lipids:** Cortisol promotes lipolysis and increased delivery of free fatty acids and glycerol.
- **Carbohydrate:** Cortisol raises blood glucose, making more glucose available for nervous tissue. Two mechanisms are involved:
  - Cortisol counteracts insulin's action in most tissues (muscle, lymphoid, and fat).
  - Cortisol increases hepatic output of glucose by regulating the enzymes involved in gluconeogenesis, particularly phosphoenolpyruvate carboxykinase (PEPCK) (not from liver glycogenolysis).

Permissive Actions of Cortisol

Cortisol enhances the capacity of glucagon and catecholamines, hence the adjective *permissive* aptly describes many of the actions of cortisol.

Glucagon

Promotes glycogenolysis in the liver (some lipolysis from adipocytes as well). Without cortisol, fasting hypoglycemia rapidly develops. Cortisol permits glucagon to raise blood glucose.

Catecholamines

Promotes both alpha and beta receptor expression. Beta receptor function involves glucose regulation, lipolysis (see next chapter), and bronchodilation. Alpha receptor function is pivotal for blood pressure regulation. Without cortisol, blood pressure decreases.

CRH = hypothalamic corticotropin-releasing hormone

CONTROL OF ADRENOCORTICOTROPIN (ACTH) AND CORTISOL SECRETION

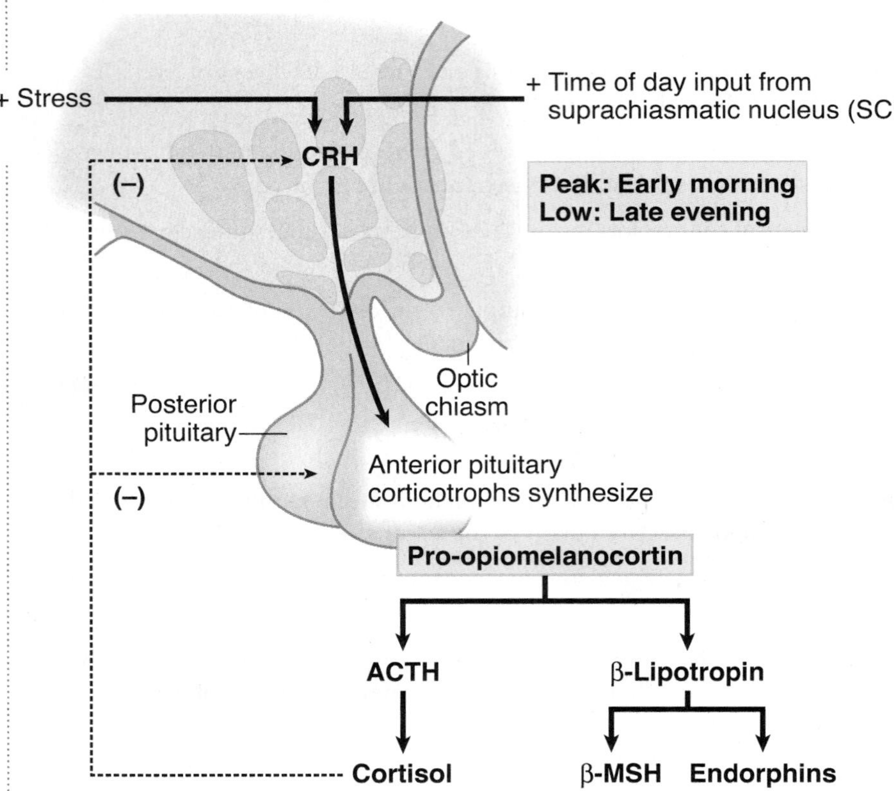

Figure X-4-6. Control of ACTH and Cortisol

Role of the Specific Modulators

Corticotropin-releasing hormone (CRH)

Secretion of CRH increases in response to stress and in the early morning:

- Peak cortisol secretion occurs early in the morning between the 6th and 8th hours of sleep. Secretion then declines slowly during the day and reaches a low point late in the evening.
- Increased AM CRH = increased AM cortisol
- Increased AM cortisol = increased AM blood sugar and lipid levels
- Increased AM sugar and lipid levels help get you out of bed

ACTH

Stimulates the secretion of cortisol (and adrenal androgens) of adrenal cortex. Cortisol suppresses the release of ACTH by acting on the hypothalamus and anterior pituitary.

Excessive secretion of ACTH (e.g., primary adrenal insufficiency) causes darkening of the skin. This is due to the melanocyte-stimulating hormone (α-MSH) sequence within the ACTH molecule, and the β-MSH activity of β-lipotropin.

β-Lipotropin

- Role not well understood
- Precursor to β-MSH and endorphins. Endorphins modulate the perception of pain.

PHYSIOLOGIC ACTIONS OF ALDOSTERONE

The primary target tissue for aldosterone is the kidney, where it increases Na^+ reabsorption by the principal cells of the kidney's collecting ducts. Because water is reabsorbed along with the Na^+, aldosterone can be considered to control the amount of Na^+ rather than the concentration of Na^+ in the ECF.

Aldosterone also promotes the secretion of H^+ by the intercalated cells of the collecting duct, and K^+ secretion by the principal cells. The Na^+-conserving action of aldosterone is also seen in salivary ducts, sweat glands, and the distal colon.

Figure X-4-7 shows the overall effects of aldosterone. This is a generalized representation of the effect of aldosterone on the renal distal tubule/collecting duct region.

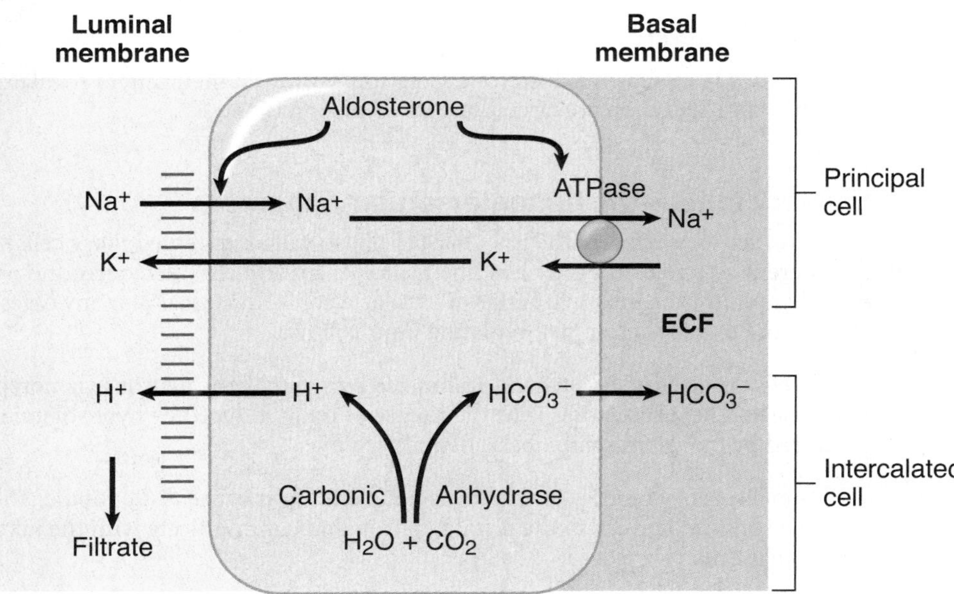

Figure X-4-7. Late Distal Tubule and Collecting Duct

Specific Actions of Aldosterone

Aldosterone promotes the activity of Na/K-ATPase–dependent pump that moves Na^+ into the renal ECF in exchange for K^+. In addition, aldosterone enhances epithelial Na^+ channels (ENaC) in the luminal membrane of principal cells. The net effect is to increase Na^+ reabsorption, which in turn increases water reabsorption. Aldosterone regulates Na^+ to regulate extracellular volume.

The reabsorption of Na^+ creates a negative luminal potential promoting K^+ excretion.

Aldosterone stimulates H^+ secretion by intercalated cells. Thus, excess aldosterone causes alkalosis, while insufficient aldosterone causes acidosis (type IV RTA).

Table X-4-1. Actions of Aldosterone

	Renal	
Na^+	reabsorption	↑ total body Na^+
K^+	secretion	↓ plasma $[K^+]$
H^+	secretion	promotes metabolic alkalosis
HCO_3^-	production	promotes metabolic alkalosis
H_2O	reabsorption	volume expansion

CONTROL OF ALDOSTERONE SECRETION

Controlling Factors

Acutely, ACTH increases aldosterone secretion. However, the primary regulators of aldosterone secretion are circulating levels of Ang II and K^+.

Sensory Input—the Juxtaglomerular Apparatus

The main sensory cells are the granular cells (also called juxtamedullary cells) of the afferent arteriole. They are modified smooth-muscle cells that surround and directly monitor the pressure in the afferent arteriole. This signal in many cases is in response to a reduction in circulating fluid volume.

These cells are also innervated and stimulated by sympathetic neurons via norepinephrine and beta receptors. Thus the release of renin induced by hypovolemia is enhanced by increased sympathetic neural activity.

Additional sensory input is from the macula densa cells of the distal tubule. They perceive sodium delivery to the distal nephron and communicate with the juxtaglomerular cells.

The juxtaglomerular apparatus is represented in Figure X-4-8.

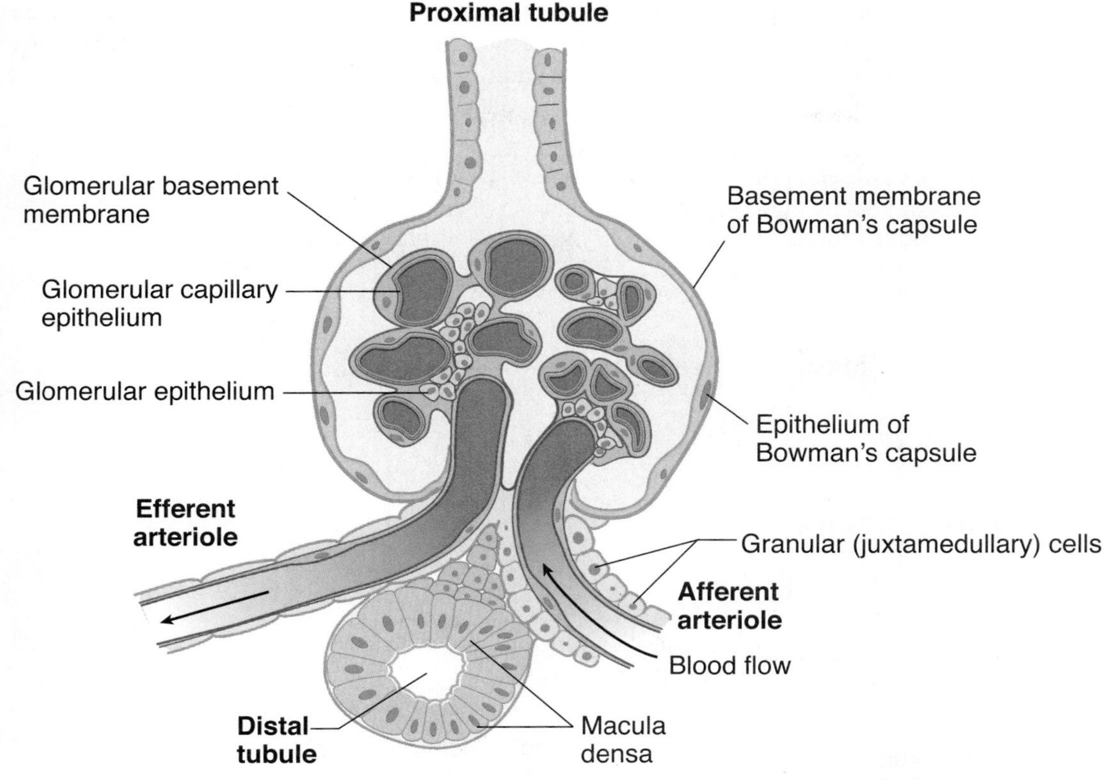

Figure X-4-8. Renal Corpuscle and Juxtaglomerular Apparatus

Long-Term Regulation of Blood Pressure and Cardiac Output by the Renin-Angiotensin-Aldosterone System

Long-term regulation of blood pressure and cardiac output is accomplished by the renin-angiotensin-aldosterone system.

Blood pressure is monitored by the juxtaglomerular apparatus. When renal perfusion pressure decreases, secretion of renin increases; conversely, when pressure increases, renin secretion is suppressed. Renin is an enzyme that converts a circulating protein produced in the liver, **angiotensinogen** into **angiotensin I**. Angiotensin converting enzyme (ACE), found mainly in endothelial cells of pulmonary vessels, converts angiotensin I into **angiotensin II**. Angiotensin II has potent effects to stimulate secretion of aldosterone and to cause arteriolar vasoconstriction. It also directly stimulates reabsorption of sodium in the proximal tubule.

$$\mathbf{MAP = CO \times TPR}$$

This system regulates both resistance, via vasoconstriction, and cardiac output, via preload. Since aldosterone also causes increased renal excretion of potassium, it affects plasma potassium concentration. Plasma potassium strongly stimulates secretion of aldosterone , so this constitutes a negative-feedback control system for plasma potassium concentration.

Volume-depleted states tend to produce metabolic alkalosis, in part because aldosterone increases to compensate for the volume loss; the aldosterone increase stimulates excretion of acid and addition of bicarbonate to the plasma.

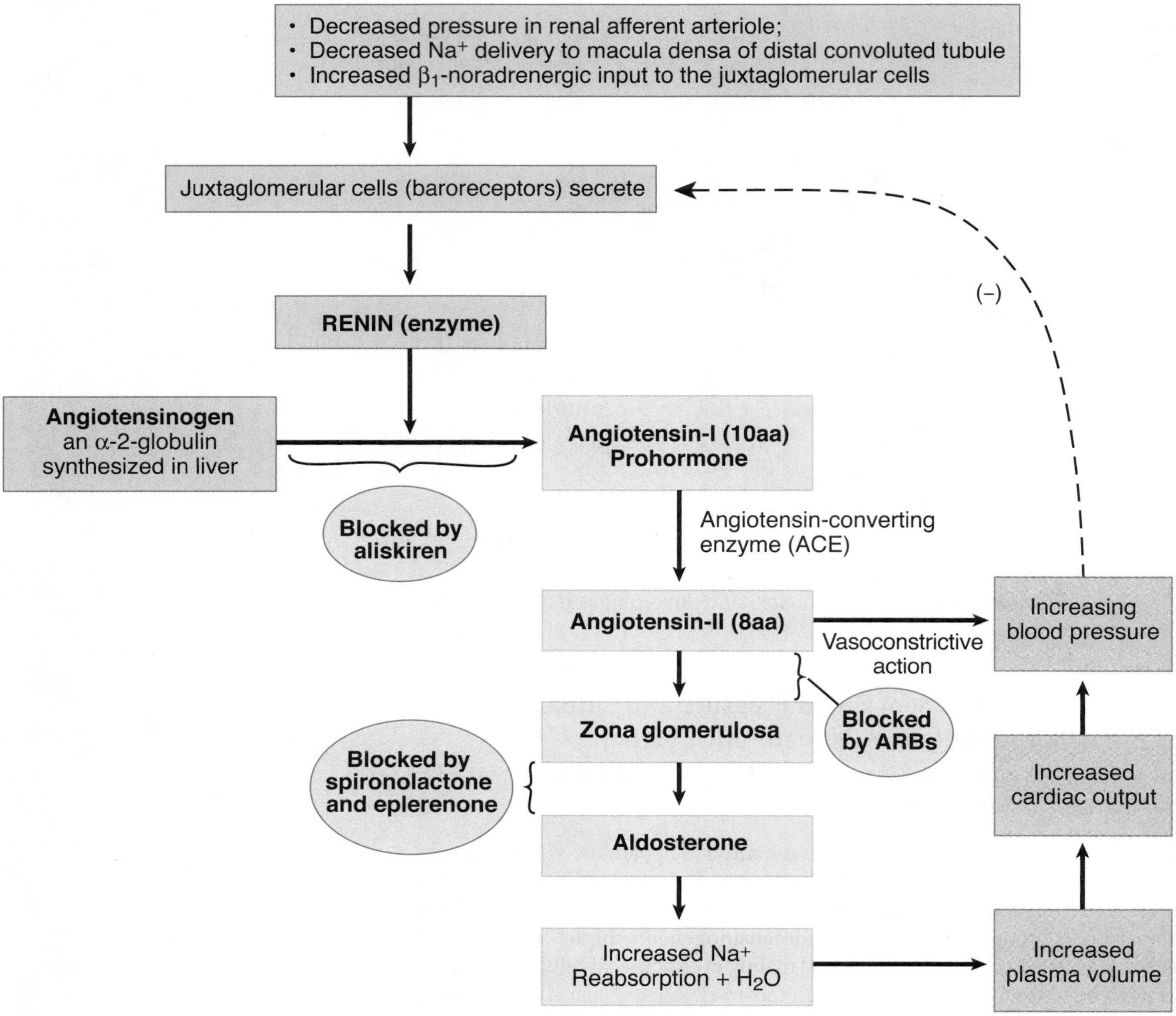

- Decreased pressure in renal afferent arteriole;
- Decreased Na^+ delivery to macula densa of distal convoluted tubule
- Increased β_1-noradrenergic input to the juxtaglomerular cells

Juxtaglomerular cells (baroreceptors) secrete

RENIN (enzyme)

Angiotensinogen
an α-2-globulin
synthesized in liver

Blocked by aliskiren

Angiotensin-I (10aa)
Prohormone

Angiotensin-converting enzyme (ACE)

Angiotensin-II (8aa)

Vasoconstrictive action

Blocked by ARBs

Zona glomerulosa

Blocked by spironolactone and eplerenone

Aldosterone

Increased Na^+ Reabsorption + H_2O

Increased plasma volume

Increased cardiac output

Increasing blood pressure

(–)

Figure X-4-9. Feedback Control of Blood Pressure by Renin-Angiotensin-Aldosterone System

Any of the 3 stimuli listed at the top of the figure produces an increase in the secretion of renin and circulating angiotensin II. Angiotensin II raises blood pressure by 2 independent actions:

- The direct vasoconstrictive effects of angiotensin II increase total peripheral resistance.
- It stimulates the adrenal cortex to secrete aldosterone, resulting in increased reabsorption of Na^+.

As Na^+ reabsorption is increased, so is water. This increases the volume of the ECF, thus raising cardiac output and blood pressure.

An increase in blood pressure suppresses the renin-angiotensin-aldosterone system (RAAS). This decrease in angiotensin II reduces total peripheral resistance. Reduced activity of aldosterone causes a urinary loss of sodium and water, lowering cardiac output.

In addition to its effects to serve as a direct vasoconstrictor and increase aldosterone secretion, angiotensin II also:

- Increases ADH release from posterior pituitary
- Increases thirst
- Increases sodium reabsorption in proximal tubule

Potassium Effect

Any condition that decreases arterial blood pressure (e.g., hemorrhage, prolonged sweating) reduces perfusion pressure to the kidney and activates RAAS. In addition, it activates the sympathetic nervous system, which also stimulates RAAS. Sympathetic and RAAS activation work to restore arterial blood pressure.

Physiologic Changes in Aldosterone Secretion

Increased aldosterone secretion

Increased aldosterone secretion is any condition that activates the renin-angiotensin system, such as decreased perfusion pressure to glomeruli and/or activation of the sympathetic nervous system (e.g., hemorrhage, prolonged sweating). In turn, aldosterone works to return blood pressure back toward normal.

Decreased aldosterone secretion

Decreased aldosterone secretion is any condition that increases blood pressure in the renal artery. This includes weightlessness, because blood no longer pools in the extremities when the individual is standing or sitting. A large portion of the redistributed blood ends up in the atria and large veins of the chest and abdomen. The increased distention of these vessels stimulates baroreceptors located there. Signals from these baroreceptors reach the vasomotor center, where they inhibit sympathetic output, including sympathetic signals that normally promote renin secretion by the juxtaglomerular cells. As a result, less renin, angiotensin II, and aldosterone are secreted, causing individuals to lose Na^+ and ECF volume.

GLUCOCORTICOID DISORDERS

Definitions

Cushing syndrome: hypercortisolism regardless of origin, including chronic glucocorticoid therapy

Cushing disease: hypercortisolism due to an adenoma of the anterior pituitary (microadenoma)

The first step in the evaluation of possible hypercortisolism is to establish that the cortisol level is truly elevated. Once this is done, the ACTH level and high-dose dexamethasone suppression tests are used to determine the source or etiology of the hypercortisolism.

Establishing the Presence of Hypercortisolism

First do a 24-hour urine-free-cortisol or 1 mg overnight dexamethasone suppression test. A single random cortisol level should not be used to diagnose hypercortisolism.

24-hour urine-free-cortisol is harder to do but it has fewer falsely positive tests.

1-mg overnight dexamethasone suppression test

- For the presence of Cushing syndrome regardless of the cause
- Normal; cortisol decreases
- Hypercortisolism; cortisol not suppressed
- False-positives from depression or alcoholism

High-dose dexamethasone

- To differentiate pituitary adenoma from ectopic ACTH secretion and adrenal tumors
- Pituitary source; cortisol decreases
- Ectopic ACTH, adrenal tumor; cortisol not suppressed

Note

Hypercortisolism and an ACTH that is in the normal range or high is a secondary condition. Via negative feedback, a high corstisol should produce a low ACTH. If ACTH is in the "normal" range, then it is "inappropriately" normal (meaning it is too high) and is thus the cause of the hypercortisolism.

ACTH level

- Used after 24 hour urine cortisol establishes presence of hypercortisolism
- ACTH levels establish etiology of hypercortsolism
- Low ACTH = Adrenal source of cortisol overproduction
- Normal or high ACTH = Pituitary or Ectopic source
- High dose dexamethasone distinguishes Pituitary vs Ectopic source

Stimulation Tests

ACTH stimulation test diagnoses adrenal insufficiency.

- To diagnose atrophied adrenal nonresponsive
- **Normal;** cortisol increases after ACTH
- Adrenal insufficiency: no change in cortisol level

Hypercortisolism

Primary hypercortisolism (adrenal source)

- ACTH independent
- Cortisol elevated, ACTH depressed
- Most are benign adrenocorticol adenomas
- Adrenal adenoma usually unilateral and secretes only cortisol; decreased adrenal androgen and deoxycorticosterone (hirsutism absent)
- Presence of androgen or mineralocorticoid excess suggests a carcinoma.

Secondary hypercortisolism (pituitary vs. ectopic source)

- ACTH dependent
- Hypersecretion of ACTH results in bilateral hyperplasia of the adrenal zona fasciculata and reticularis
- Elevated ACTH, cortisol, adrenal androgen, deoxycorticosterone
- Two main subcategories:
  - Pituitary adenoma, usually a microadenoma (< 1 cm dia.)
    - This is Cushing disease
    - Increased ACTH not sufficient to cause hyperpigmentation
    - Dexamethasone suppressible
  - Ectopic ACTH syndrome:
    - Most frequently in patients with small cell carcinoma of the lung
    - Greater secretion of ACTH than in Cushing disease and hyperpigmentation often present
    - Ectopic site nonsupressible with dexamethasone

Differential diagnosis

- Hypercortisolism established by lack of cortisol suppression to 1 mg overnight dexamethasone and/or elevated 24-hour urine free cortisol
- Decreased plasma ACTH: Adrenal is source (primary hypercortisolism)
- High-dose dexamethasone
  - ACTH suppressed = Cushing disease (pituitary source)
  - ACTH not suppressed = ectopic ACTH syndrome

Characteristics of Cushing syndrome

- Obesity because of hyperphagia, classically central affecting mainly the face, neck, trunk, and abdomen: "moon facies" and "buffalo hump"
- Protein depletion as a result of excessive protein catabolism
- Inhibition of inflammatory response and poor wound healing
- Hyperglycemia leads to hyperinsulinemia and insulin resistance.
- Hyperlipidemia
- Bone breakdown and osteoporosis
- Thinning of the skin with wide purple striae located around abdomen and hips

Clinical Correlate

Metyrapone testing is no longer performed.

- Metyrapone is no longer manufactured
- Simulates 11 beta-hydroxylase deficiency
  - Normal = ACTH **goes up**
  - Pituitary insufficiency = ACTH **fails to rise**

- Increased adrenal androgens, when present in women, can result in acne, mild hirsutism, and amenorrhea. In men, decreased libido and impotence
- Mineralocorticoid effects of the high level of glucocorticoid and deoxycorticosteroid lead to salt and water retention (hypertension), potassium depletion, and a hypokalemic alkalosis.
- Increased thirst and polyuria
- Anxiety, depression, and other emotional disorders may be present.

Hypocortisolism

Primary hypocortisolism (in primary adrenal insufficiency, Addison's disease)

Cortisol deficiency leads to weakness, fatigue, anorexia, weight loss, hypotension, hyponatremia, hypoglycemia. Increases in ACTH result in hyperpigmentation of skin and mucous membranes.

Aldosterone deficiency leads to sodium wasting and hyponatremia, potassium retention and hyperkalemia, dehydration, hypotension, and acidosis

- Autoimmune origin with slow onset in about 80% of cases
- Loss of 90% of both adrenals required before obvious clinical manifestations
- With gradual adrenal destruction, basal secretion is normal but secretion does not respond to stress, which may initiate an adrenal crisis.
- Bilateral hemorrhage as the origin results in an adrenal crisis. Hyperpigmentation, hyponatremia, and hyperkalemia usually absent
- Orthostatic intolerance due to diminished alpha-receptor function and low blood volume.
- Abnormalities in GI function
- Loss of axillary and pubic hair in women due to loss of androgens, amenorrhea
- Insufficient glucocorticoids leads to hypoglycemia and an inability of the kidney to excrete a water load
- Severe hypoglycemia in children but rare in adults

Secondary hypocortisolism (secondary adrenal insufficiency)

- Most commonly due to sudden withdrawal of exogenous glucocorticoid therapy
- Trauma, infection, and infarction most common natural origin of ACTH deficiency
- In the early stages baseline hormone values are normal but ACTH reserve compromised and stress response subnormal (glucocorticoids administered presurgery)
- May be associated with the loss of other anterior pituitary hormones (panhypopituitarism) or adenomas secreting prolactin or growth hormone
- Atrophy of the zona fasciculata and zona reticularis
- Zona glomerulosa and aldosterone normal; no manifestations of mineralocorticoid deficiency
- Consequences as stated for cortisol deficiency
- Severe hypoglycemia and severe hypotension unusual (RAAS is still intact)
- Hyponatremia due to water retention

Differential diagnosis

- Rapid ACTH stimulation test: initial procedure in the assessment of adrenal insufficiency, both primary and secondary.
  - Normal: ↑ cortisol
  - Hypocortisolism: diminished ↑ cortisol
- Normal responsiveness of ACTH test does not exclude decreased pituitary reserve and decreased response to stress (insulin infusion)
- In same sample, a normal aldosterone would be evidence of a secondary problem
- Definitive test for primary vs. secondary is ACTH: ↑ primary hypocortisolism (Addison's); inappropriately low in secondary hypocortisolism

Summary

Table X-4-2. Primary and Secondary Disorders of Cortisol Secretion

Disorder	Plasma Cortisol	Plasma ACTH	Hyperpigmentation
Primary hypercortisolism	↑	↓	no
Secondary hypercortisolism			
Cushing disease	↑	normal or ↑	no
Ectopic ACTH	↑	↑	yes (maybe)
Primary hypocortisolism	↓	↑	yes
Secondary hypocortisolism	↓	↓	no

MINERALOCORTICOID DISORDERS

Hyperaldosteronism with Hypertension

Primary hyperaldosteronism (Conn's syndrome)

- Most common cause is a small unilateral adenoma, on either side
- Remainder mostly bilateral adrenal hyperplasia (idiopathic hyperaldosteronism)
- Rarely due to adrenal carcinoma
- Increased whole body sodium, fluid, and circulating blood volume
- Hypernatremia is infrequent
- Increased peripheral vasoconstriction and TPR
- Blood pressure from borderline to severe hypertension
- Edema rare (sodium escape*)
- Modest left ventricular hypertrophy

*A major increase in sodium and water retention is prevented by "sodium escape" in primary hyperaldosteronism. The mechanism for this escape is still unclear.

- Potassium depletion and hypokalemia create symptoms of weakness and fatigue.
- Detection of hypertension with hypokalemia is often the initial clue for Conn's syndrome
- Increased hydrogen ion excretion and new bicarbonate create metabolic alkalosis.
- A positive Chvostek or Trousseau's sign is suggestive of alkalosis leading to low calcium levels.
- Cortisol is normal.
- Suppression of renin a major feature

Secondary hyperaldosteronism refers to a state in which there is an appropriate increase in aldosterone in response to activation of the renin-angiotensin system.

Secondary hyperaldosteronism with hypertension

- In most cases a primary over-secretion of renin secondary to a decrease in renal blood flow and/or pressure
- Renal arterial stenosis, narrowing via atherosclerosis, fibromuscular hyperplasia.
- Renin-secreting tumor rare
- Modest to highly elevated renin
- Modest to highly elevated aldosterone
- Hypokalemia and metabolic alkalosis

Differential diagnosis

- Hypokalemia in a hypertensive patient not taking diuretics
- Hyposecretion of renin with elevated aldosterone that fails to respond to a volume contraction: Conn's syndrome
- Hypersecretion of renin with elevated aldosterone: renal vascular

Hyperaldosteronism with Hypotension

Secondary hyperaldosteronism with hypotension

Sequestration of blood on the venous side of the systemic circulation is a common cause of secondary hyperaldosteronism. This results in decreased cardiac output and thus decreased blood flow and pressure in the renal artery. The following conditions produce secondary hyperaldosteronism through this mechanism:

- Congestive heart failure
- Constriction of the vena cava
- Hepatic cirrhosis

Table X-4-3. Summary of Secondary Hyperaldosteronism

The cause in all cases is a **decrease** in blood pressure.	
1. Plasma renin and angiotensin II activity: The increased angiotensin II activity will drive the secondary hyperaldosteronism.	↑
2. Total body sodium:	↑
3. ECF volume:	↑
4. Plasma volume:	↑
5. Edema*:	yes

*Na^+ escape prevents peripheral edema in primary but not secondary hyperaldosteronism. Also note that the increased ECF volume remains mainly on the venous side of the circulation, accentuating the venous congestion and preventing a return of circulating blood volume to normal.

ENZYME DEFICIENCIES

Single enzyme defects can occur as congenital "inborn errors of metabolism." Congenital defects in any of the enzymes lead to **deficient cortisol secretion** and the syndrome called *congenital adrenal hyperplasia.* Hyperplasia is caused by the excessive secretion of ACTH that results from the loss of the negative feedback action of cortisol. In all of the following examples, assume the deficiency is significant to the extent that it affects normal hormonal production but not a complete blockade.

A useful summary of enzyme deficiency conditions is that a horizontal cut of the pathway causes decreased production of all substances below the cut and increased secretion of substances above the cut. A vertical cut causes decrease of substances to the right of the cut and increase of substances to the left of the cut.

21 β-Hydroxylase Deficiency

Tissues affected: zona glomerulosa, zona fasciculata, zona reticularis

21 β-hydroxylase deficiency is the most common of the congenital enzyme deficiencies.

Effect in the zona glomerulosa

Blockade Point

Figure X-4-10 illustrates the blockade point in the zona glomerulosa.

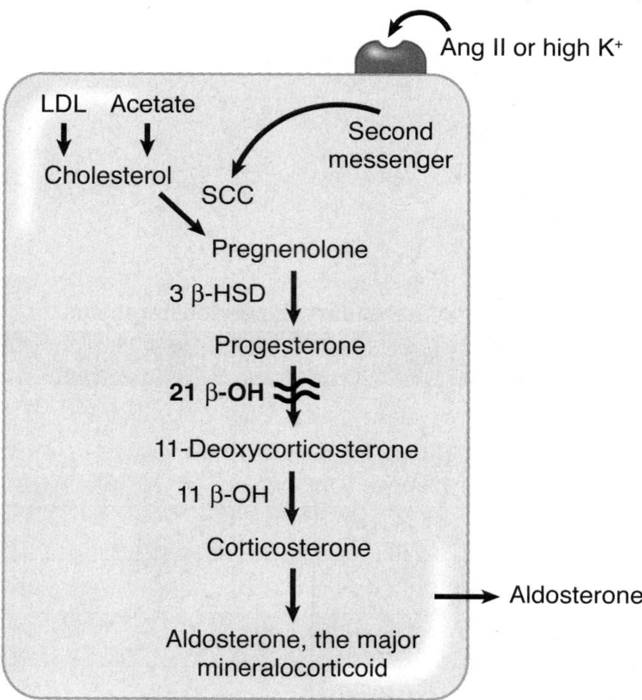

Figure X-4-10. 21-β Enzyme Deficiency in the Zona Glomerulosa

Consequence: Result is a decreased production of aldosterone, the main mineralocorticoid.

Cholesterol can be made "de novo" from acetate if there is nutritional deficiency.

Effect in the zona fasciculata and zona reticularis

Blockade Points

Figure X-4-11 shows the two blockade points (wavy lines) in the zona fasciculata and zona reticularis.

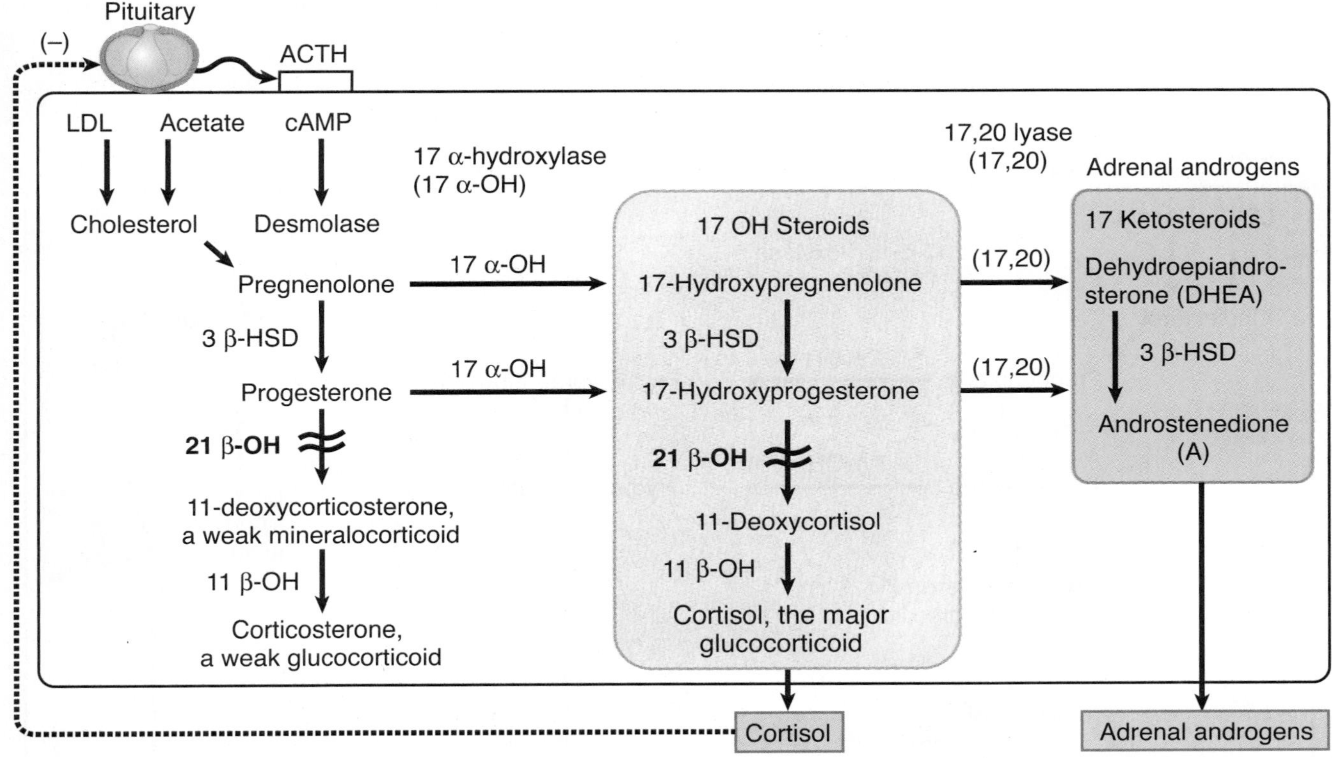

Figure X-4-11. 21-β Enzyme Deficiency in the Zona Fasciculata and Zona Reticularis

Summary of overall pathway changes:

- Zona glomerulosa: decreased aldosterone
- Zona fasciculata, reticularis: decreased production of 11-deoxycorticosterone, a weak mineralocorticoid.
- Therefore, a mineralocorticoid deficiency, loss of Na^+, volume and a hypotensive state (salt-wasting state).
- Increased renin secretion and increased circulating angiotensin II.
- Decreased production of corticosterone, a weak glucocorticoid, and cortisol.
- Therefore, glucocorticoid deficiency and increased ACTH, which drive increases in adrenal androgen secretion

11 β-Hydroxylase Deficiency

Tissues affected: zona fasciculata, zona reticularis, zona glomerulosa

Effect in the zona fasciculata and zona reticularis

Blockade

Figure X-4-12 illustrates the blockade in the zona fasciculata and zona reticularis.

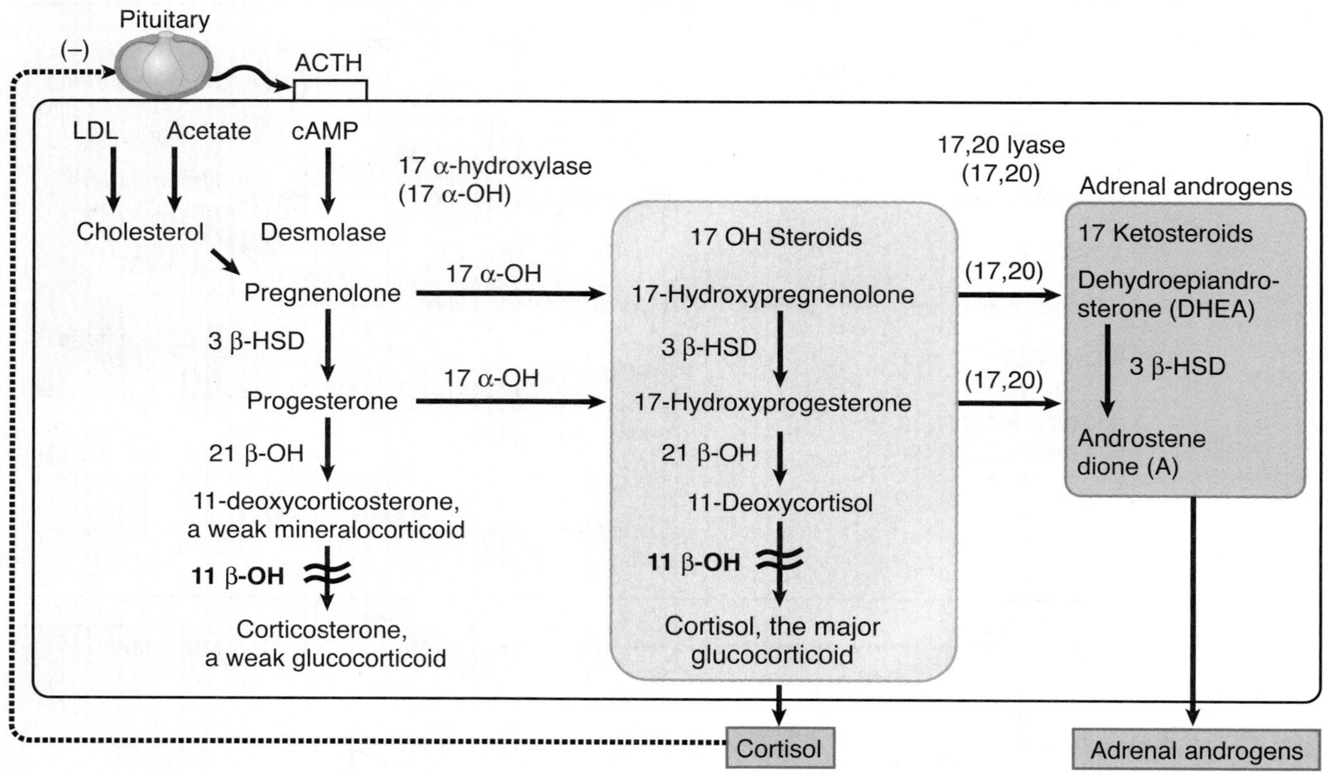

Figure X-4-12. 11-β-Hydroxylase Deficiency in the Zona Fasciculata and Zona Reticularis

Deoxycorticosterone increases blood pressure. Only cortisol is feedback inhibition of the pituitary for ACTH.

Effect in the zona glomerulosa

Figure X-4-13 illustrates the effect on the zona glomerulosa.

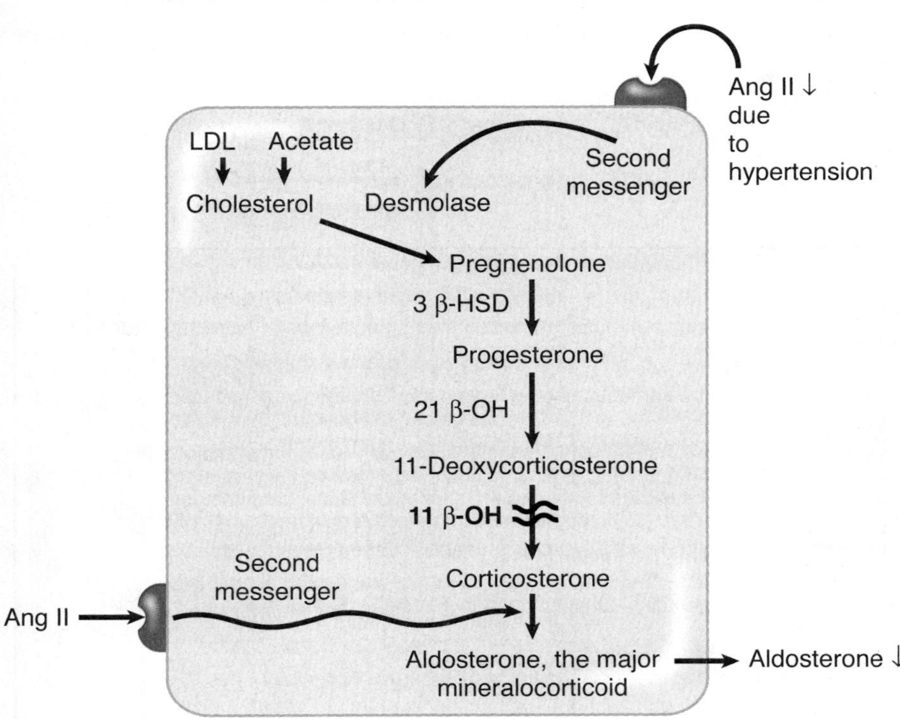

Figure X-4-13. 11-β-Hydroxylase Deficiency in the Zona Glomerulosa

Summary of overall pathway changes:

- Zona fasciculata, reticularis: decreased corticosterone and cortisol, increased ACTH and overproduction of steroids above the blockade, including:
  - Androgens and the consequences in women and prepubertal males
  - 11-deoxycorticosterone, a mineralocorticoid that leads to hypertension and a decrease in circulating angiotensin II
- Zona glomerulosa: decreased aldosterone because of loss of necessary enzyme and low angiotensin II

17 α-Hydroxylase Deficiency

Tissues affected: zona fasciculata, zona reticularis, testis, ovary

Blockade in the adrenal zona fasciculata and the zona reticularis

Figure X-4-14 illustrates the blockade points in the zona fasciculata and zona reticularis.

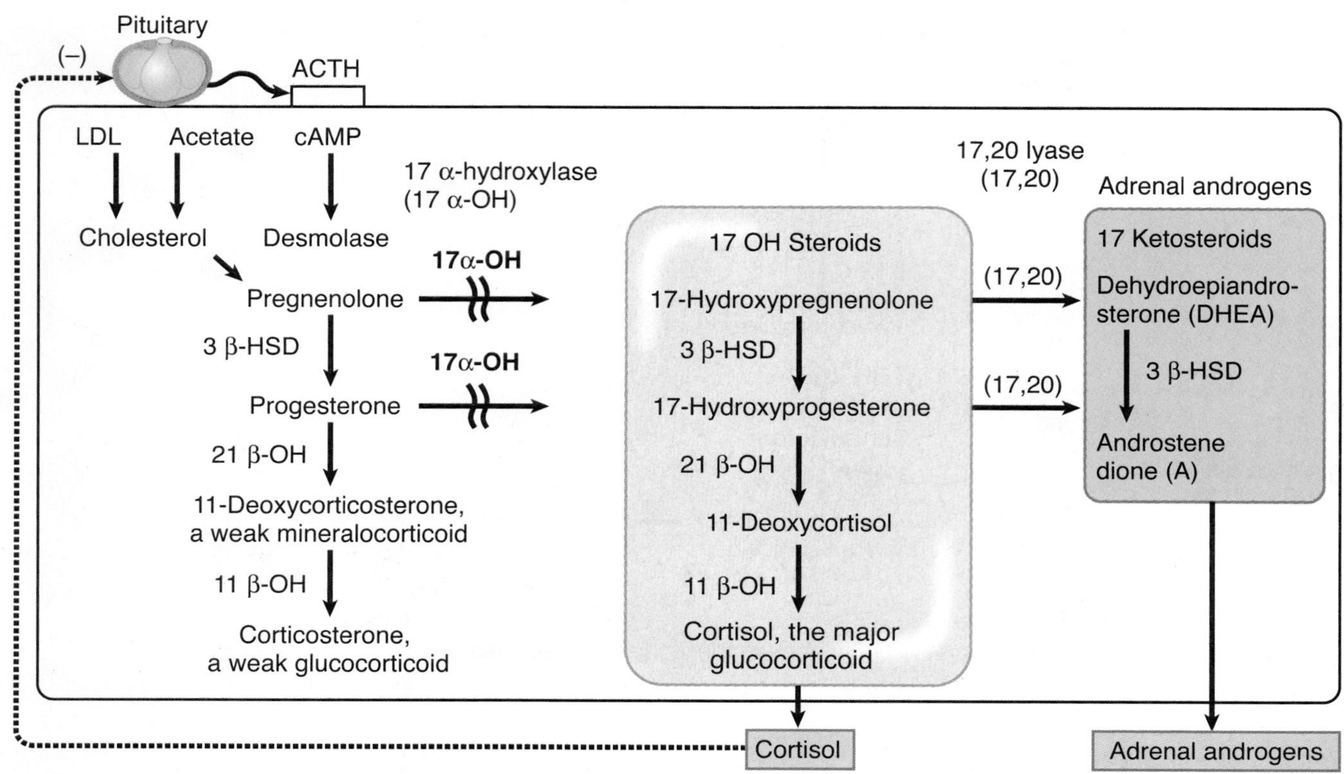

Figure X-4-14. 17 α-Hydroxylase Deficiency

Summary of overall pathway changes:

- Zona fasciculata, reticularis: decreased adrenal androgens, decreased cortisol, and increased ACTH. Increased 11-deoxycorticosterone leading to hypertension. The reduced circulating angiotensin II reduces stimulation of zona glomerulosa and aldosterone secretion.

Effect in the testes

Figure X-4-15 illustrates the blockade points in the testes.

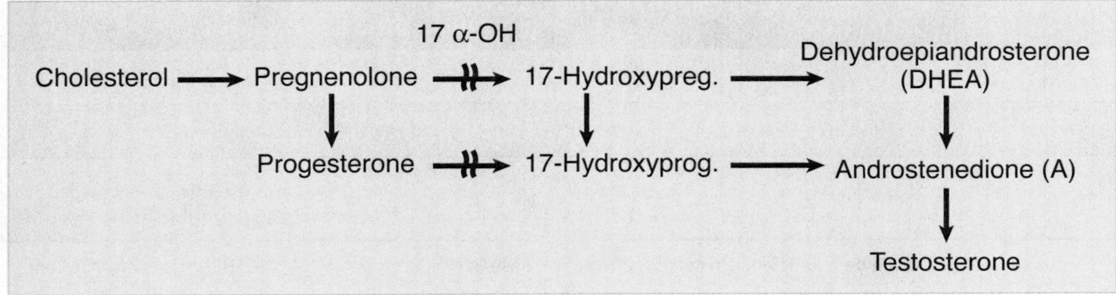

Figure X-4-15. Testicular 17 α-OH Deficiency

Summary

Decreased production of all androgens including testosterone

Effect in the ovaries

Figure X-4-16 illustrates the blockade points in the ovaries.

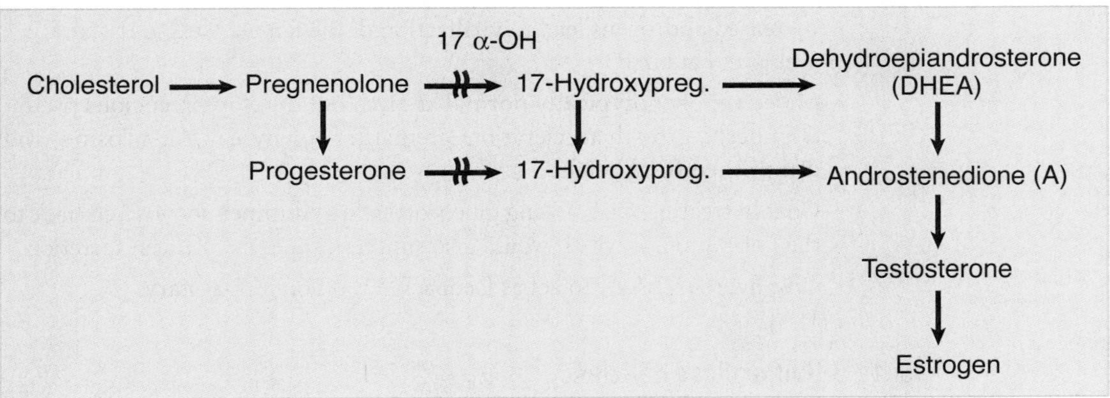

Figure X-4-16. Ovarian 17 α-OH Deficiency

Summary

Decreased production of estrogens and androgens

Summary

Table X-4-4. Summary of Enzyme Deficiencies

Deficiency	Glucocorticoid	ACTH	Blood Pressure	Mineralocorticoid Aldo	Mineralocorticoid DOC	Androgen	Estrogen
21 β-OH	↓	↑	↓	↓	↓	↑ adrenal	–
11 β-OH	↓	↑	↑	↓	↑	↑ adrenal	–
17 α-OH	↓	↑	↑	↓	↑	↓ adrenal & testicular	↓

Note: In all three disorders, there will be a deficiency in cortisol and an increase in circulating ACTH. The ACTH is responsible for the adrenal hyperplasia.

Consequences of Congential Adrenal Hyperplasia

21 β-Hydroxylase deficiency

- Accounts for about 90% of the cases
- 75% of the cases have mineralocorticoid deficiency
- Neonates may present with a salt-wasting crisis.
- Salt wasters tend to have hyponatremia, hyperkalemia, and raised plasma renin.
- 17-hydroxyprogesterone is elevated.
- Increased androgens lead to virilization of the female fetus and sexual ambiguity at birth
- Males are phenotypically normal at birth but develop precocious pseudopuberty, growth acceleration, premature epiphyseal plate closure, and diminished final height.
- Goal in treatment is to bring glucocorticoid and mineralocorticoid back to the normal range which would also suppress adrenal androgen secretion.
- Give hydrocortisone to act as feedback inhibition on pituitary.

11 β-Hydroxylase deficiency

- Clinical features of increased androgens similar to the preceding form, including virilization of female fetus.
- The principal difference with this form is the hypertension produced by 11-deoxycorticosterone, along with hypokalemia and suppressed renin secretion.
- Treatment for all forms of CAH is glucocorticoids such as hydrocortisone and dexamethasone.

17 α-Hydroxytlase deficiency

- Extremely rare
- Usually diagnosed at the time of puberty when the patient presents with hypertension, hypokalemia, and hypogonadism
- Individuals have eunuchoid characteristics.

Chapter Summary

- Loss of mineralocorticoid function causes severe hypotension and can be fatal. Lack of glucocorticoids is not life-threatening under normal conditions, but stressful situations can cause severe problems.
- Loss of pituitary function causes loss of glucocorticoids but not mineralocorticoids.
- Cortisol, aldosterone, and adrenal androgens can be easily measured in plasma and urine.
- Sulfated androgen is specific to synthesis in the adrenals.
- Zona glomerulosa is stimulated by angiotensin II and K^+, and secretion is aldosterone.
- Zona fasciculata and reticularis main stimulus is ACTH and main secretions are cortisol and androgens. Weak mineralocorticoid and glucocorticoid normally unimportant.
- Cortisol is a stress hormone that mobilizes carbohydrate, protein and lipid. Other stress hormones include growth hormone, glucagon, and epinephrine.
- Stress hormones are counter-regulatory because they raise plasma glucose.
- Aldosterone's main action is to increase sodium reabsorption in the kidney. Because the water follows the sodium, aldosterone does not affect sodium concentration.
- Aldosterone also increases potassium and hydrogen loss by the kidney.
- The renin-angiotensin-aldosterone system represents the long-term regulation of blood pressure. Activation is a decrease in blood pressure inside the kidney.
- Cushing syndrome is hypercortisolism.
- Primary hypercortisolism is usually an adrenal adenoma secreting cortisol. ACTH, adrenal androgens decrease.
- Secondary hypercortisolism is due to an increase in ACTH. If the source is the anterior pituitary it is Cushing disease. Ectopic ACTH hypersecretion is most often due to small cell carcinoma of the lung.
- Primary hypocortisolism is usually associated with Addison's disease and a concurrent loss of mineralocorticoid, increased ACTH, renin and hyperpigmentation.
- Secondary hypocortisolism is due to withdrawal of glucocorticoid therapy or an anterior pituitary mass with the loss of ACTH.
- Primary hyperaldosteronism (Conn's) due to an adenoma or hyperplasia of the zona glomerulosa. Hypertension, hypokalemia, alkalosis, low renin, and no edema (sodium escape).
- Secondary hyperaldosteronism with hypertension usually has a renal vascular origin. Hypertension, hypokalemia, and high renin.
- Secondary hyperaldosteronism with hypotension is usually due to a low cardiac output. Low blood pressure, hyponatremia, and edema (no sodium escape).
- In congenital adrenal hyperplasia, decreased cortisol synthesis causes increased ACTH.

(Continued)

Chapter Summary (*Cont'd*)

- In 21 β-hydroxylase deficiency there is mineralocorticoid deficiency, salt wasting and hypotension, androgen excess, and female virilization.
- In 11 β-hydroxylase deficiency there is mineralocorticoid excess, salt retention and hypertension, and androgen excess as in the preceding.
- In 17 α-hydroxylase deficiency there is mineralocorticoid excess, adrenal androgen deficiency, and hypertension with gonadal steroid deficiency and hypogonadism.

Adrenal Medulla 5

Learning Objectives

- ❏ Answer questions about hormones of the adrenal medulla
- ❏ Demonstrate understanding of major metabolic actions of epinephrine
- ❏ Interpret scenarios on pheochromocytomas

HORMONES OF THE ADRENAL MEDULLA

- Secretion of the adrenal medulla is 20% norepinephrine and 80% epinephrine.
- Phenylethanolamine-N-methyltransferase (PMNT) converts norepinephrine into epinephrine.
- Half-life of the catecholamines is only about 2 minutes. Metabolic end-products include metanephrines and vanillylmandelic acid (VMA) both of which can be measured in plasma and urine
- Removal of the adrenal medulla reduces plasma epinephrine to very low levels but does not alter plasma norepinephrine. Most circulating norepinephrine arises from postganglionic sympathetic neurons.
- Because many of the actions of epinephrine are also mediated by norepinephrine, the adrenal medulla is not essential for life.
- The vasoconstrictive action of norepinephrine is essential for the maintenance of normal blood pressure, especially when an individual is standing. Plasma norepinephrine levels double when one goes from a lying to a standing position. People with inadequate production of norepinephrine suffer from orthostatic hypotension.
- Epinephrine is a stress hormone and rapidly increases in response to exercise, exposure to cold, emergencies, and hypoglycemia.

MAJOR METABOLIC ACTIONS OF EPINEPHRINE

- Liver: Epinephrine increases the activity of liver and muscle phosphorylase, promoting glycogenolysis. This increases glucose output by the liver.
- Skeletal muscle: Epinephrine promotes glycogenolysis but because muscle lacks glucose-6-phosphatase, glucose cannot be released by skeletal muscle; instead, it must be metabolized at least to lactate before being released into the circulation.
- Adipose tissue: Epinephrine increases lipolysis in adipose tissue by increasing the activity of hormone-sensitive lipase. Glycerol from TG breakdown is a minor substrate for gluconeogenesis.
- Epinephrine increases the metabolic rate. This will not occur without thyroid hormones or the adrenal cortex.

Metabolic Actions of Epinephrine on CHO and Fat

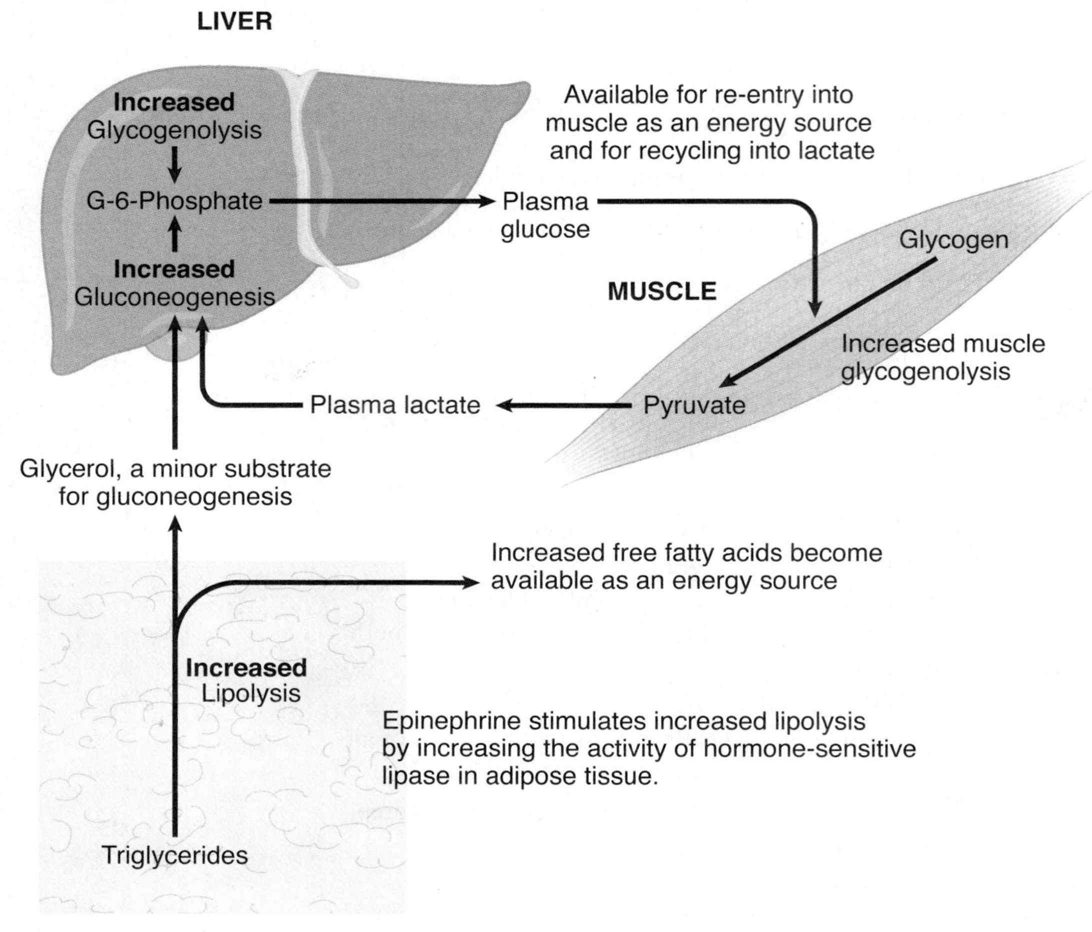

Figure X-5-1. Actions of Catecholamines

PHEOCHROMOCYTOMAS

- Adrenal tumors that secrete epinephrine and norepinephrine in various ratios
- Usually unilateral benign tumors
- Characteristic of MEN 2A and MEN 2B
- Paragangliomas are extra-adrenal pheochromocytomas of sympathetic ganglia located primarily within the abdomen and that secrete norepinephrine.
- Most consistent feature is hypertension. Symptoms include headache, diaphoresis, palpitations, and anxiety. Increased metabolic rate and hyperglycemia also occur.
- Pheochromocytomas are highly vascular and encapsulated.
- Episodic release of hormone, particularly when it is mainly norepinephrine, can abruptly cause a hypertensive crisis. Can be induced by physical stimuli that displaces abdominal contents.
- Most reliable initial test is plasma metanephrines or 24-hour urine catecholamines or metanephines.
- Usually curable but can be fatal if undiagnosed
- Treat with alpha blocker followed by surgical removal.

Chapter Summary

- Circulating epinephrine originates mainly from the adrenals, whereas circulating norepinephrine originates mainly from sympathetic nerve endings.
- Epinephrine is a stress hormone secreted in response to exercise, exposure to cold, emergencies, and hypoglycemia.
- Epinephrine increases blood glucose via liver glycogenolysis. It also stimulates muscle glycogenolysis, but muscle does not release glucose.
- Epinephrine increases the release of fatty acids from adipose tissue by increasing the activity of hormone-sensitive lipase.
- Pheochromocytomas secrete epinephrine and norepinephrine and are most consistently associated with hypertension.
- Episodic release, particularly of norepinephrine, can induce a hypertensive crisis.
- The most reliable test is urine metanephrines.

Endocrine Pancreas 6

Learning Objectives

- ❑ Use knowledge of hormones of the islets of Langerhans
- ❑ Use knowledge of actions of insulin
- ❑ Use knowledge of control of insulin secretion
- ❑ Explain information related to actions of glucagon
- ❑ Answer questions about control of glucagon secretion
- ❑ Use knowledge of diabetes mellitus
- ❑ Answer questions about pancreatic endocrine-secreting tumors

HORMONES OF THE ISLETS OF LANGERHANS

The location and proportion of each major hormone-secreting cell type of the islets of Langerhans are shown in Figure X-6-1. The local inhibitory paracrine action of each islet hormone is shown by dashed arrows. The diameter of each circle approximately represents the proportion of that cell type present in the islets.

Clinical Correlate

For many years, C-peptide was considered to have no biological function, but more recently this has been called into question. Studies suggest that C-peptide receptors exist on cells. In addition, C-peptide may serve a protective role, helping to prevent the renal, neural, and microvascular pathologies seen when it is absent, i.e., type I diabetes mellitus.

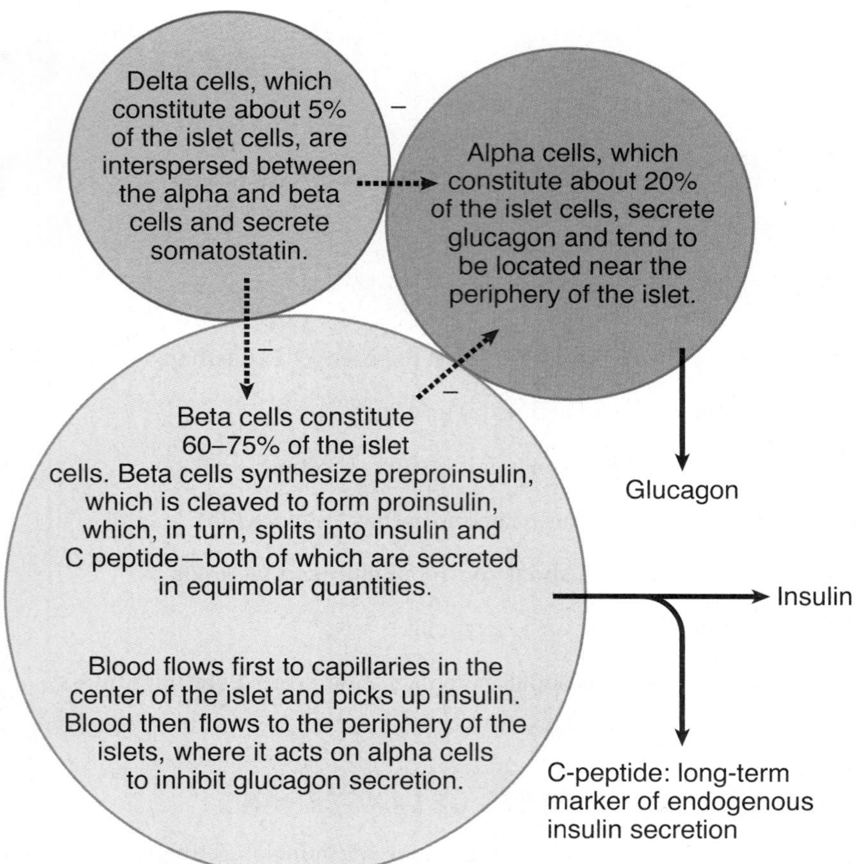

Delta cells, which constitute about 5% of the islet cells, are interspersed between the alpha and beta cells and secrete somatostatin.
Alpha cells, which constitute about 20% of the islet cells, secrete glucagon and tend to be located near the periphery of the islet.
–
–
–
Beta cells constitute 60–75% of the islet cells. Beta cells synthesize preproinsulin, which is cleaved to form proinsulin, which, in turn, splits into insulin and C peptide—both of which are secreted in equimolar quantities.
Blood flows first to capillaries in the center of the islet and picks up insulin. Blood then flows to the periphery of the islets, where it acts on alpha cells to inhibit glucagon secretion.
Glucagon
Insulin
C-peptide: long-term marker of endogenous insulin secretion

Figure X-6-1. Hormones of the Pancreatic Islets

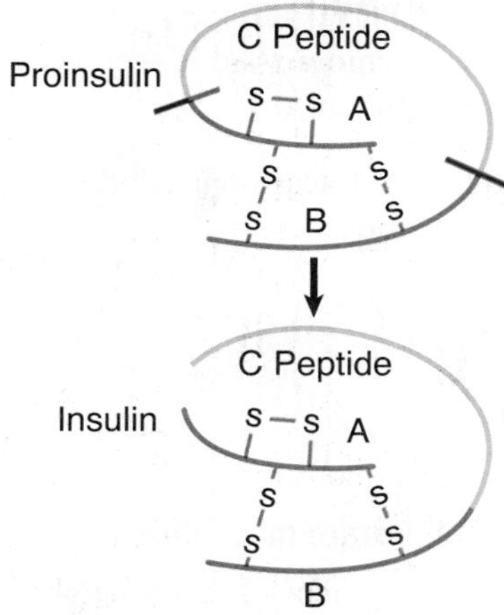

Figure X-6-2. Insulin

ACTIONS OF INSULIN

Insulin Receptor

- The portion of the insulin receptor that faces externally has the hormone-binding domain.
- The portion of the insulin receptor that faces the cytosol has tyrosine kinase activity.
- When occupied by insulin, the receptor phosphorylates itself and other proteins. (See Step 1 Biochemistry Lecture Notes for additional details.)

Peripheral Uptake of Glucose

Glucose is taken up by peripheral tissues by facilitated diffusion. Insulin facilitates this uptake in some tissues. Typically the insulin receptor causes the insertion of glucose transporters in the membrane.

Tissues that require insulin for effective uptake of glucose are:

- Adipose tissue
- Resting skeletal muscle (although glucose can enter working muscle without the aid of insulin)
- Liver because of glucokinase stimulation

Tissues in which glucose uptake is not affected by insulin are:

- Nervous tissue
- Kidney tubules
- Intestinal mucosa
- Red blood cells
- β-cells of pancreas

Metabolic Actions of Insulin

Insulin is a major anabolic hormone, and it secreted in response to a carbohydrate- and/or protein-containing meal.

Anabolic hormones tend to promote protein synthesis (increase lean body mass). Other anabolic hormones include:

- Thyroid hormones
- Growth hormone/IGF I
- Sex steroids (androgens)

Effects of insulin on carbohydrate metabolism

Insulin increases the uptake of glucose and its metabolism in muscle and fat. By increasing glucose uptake in muscle, its metabolism increases, i.e., its conversion to carbon dioxide and water is increased.

Insulin increases glycogen synthesis in liver and muscle. The activity of enzymes that promote glycogen synthesis (glucokinase and glycogen synthetase) is increased. The activity of those enzymes that promote glycogen breakdown (phosphorylase and glucose-6-phosphatase) is decreased.

- Glucokinase and glucose-6-phosphatase are expressed by the liver but not by muscle.

Effects of insulin on protein metabolism

- Insulin increases amino acid uptake by muscle cells.
- Insulin increases protein synthesis.
- Insulin decreases protein breakdown (deficiency of insulin results in a breakdown of protein).

Effects of insulin on fat metabolism

Insulin increases (Figure X-6-3):

- Glucose uptake by fat cells (increases membrane transporters). By increasing glucose uptake, insulin also makes triose phosphates available for triglyceride synthesis in adipose tissue.
- Triglyceride uptake by fat cells. It increases the activity of lipoprotein lipase. Lipoprotein lipase is located on the endothelium of capillaries, and it catalyzes the release of free fatty acids from triglycerides.
- Triglyceride synthesis (lipogenesis) in adipose tissue and liver by stimulating the rate-limiting step, namely the carboxylation of acetyl CoA to malonyl CoA. In other words, insulin stimulates the conversion of carbohydrate into fat.

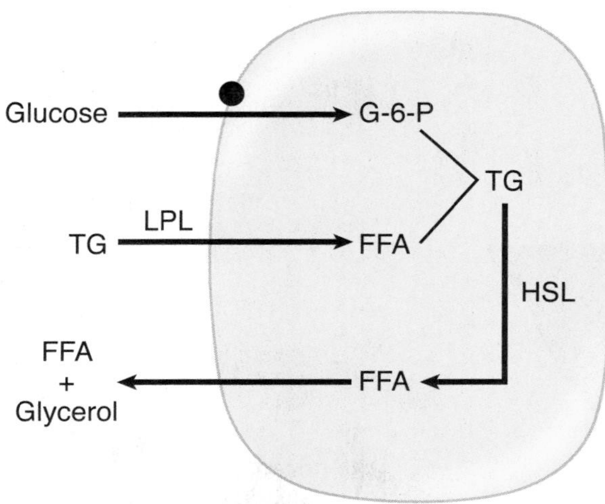

Figure X-6-3. The Adipose Cell

LPL = Lipoprotein lipase
HSL = Hormone-sensitive lipase

Insulin decreases:

- Triglyceride breakdown (lipolysis) in adipose tissue by decreasing the activity of hormone-sensitive lipase. This enzyme is activated by stress hormones (i.e., cortisol, growth hormone, epinephrine [glucagon]).
- Formation of ketone bodies by the liver.

Insulin Effects on Potassium

Insulin promotes K^+ movement into cells. Although the overall process is not well understood, insulin increases the activity of Na/K-ATPase in most body tissues.

This K^+-lowering action of insulin is used to treat acute, life-threatening hyperkalemia. For example, sometimes the hyperkalemia of renal failure is successfully lowered by the simultaneous administration of insulin and glucose. (The glucose is given to prevent severe insulin-induced hypoglycemia from developing.)

It does not work as quickly as calcium chloride, which is instantaneous, in protecting the heart from arrhythmias. Insulin and glucose administration is faster than Na^+/K^+ cation exchange resins such as kayexalate. Kayexalate is taken into the GI tract orally but needs 6–12 hours to be effective in lowering potassium levels.

Summary

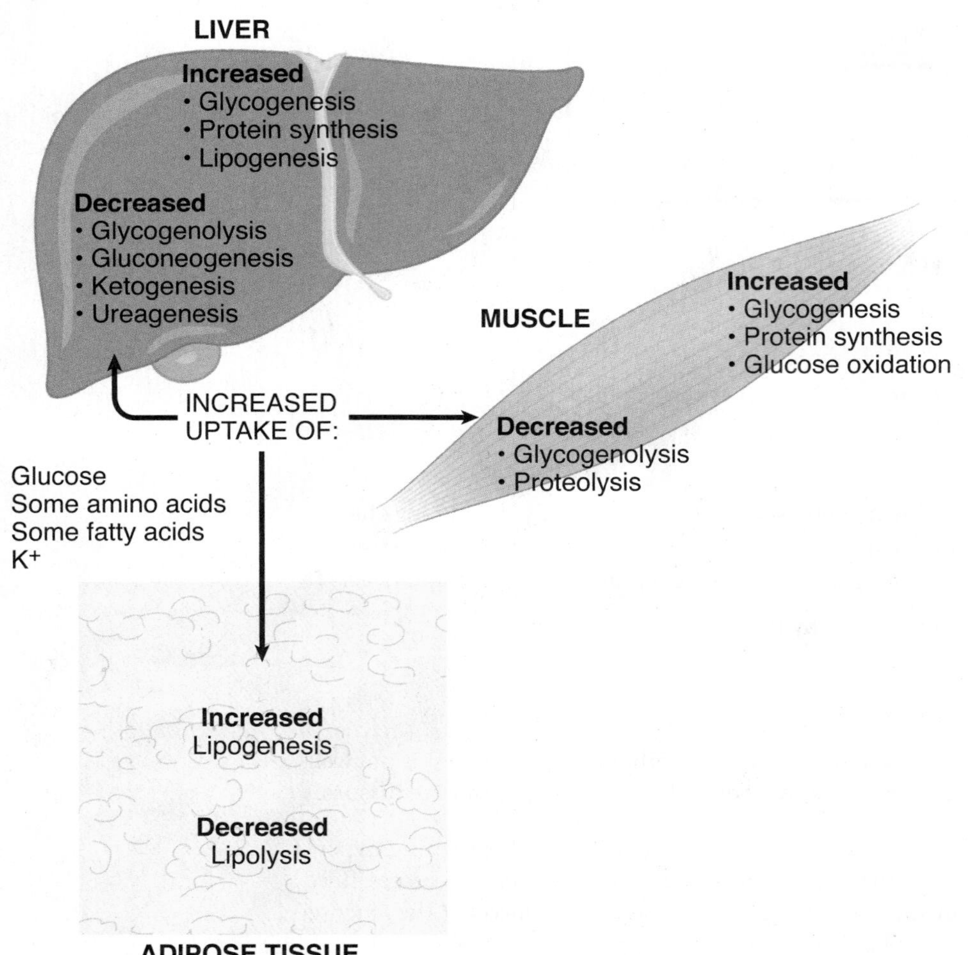

Figure X-6-4. Major Actions of Insulin

CONTROL OF INSULIN SECRETION

The most important controller of insulin secretion is plasma glucose. Above a threshold of 100 mg%, insulin secretion is directly proportional to plasma glucose.

Glucose enters the cell, causing a rise in intracellular ATP that closes ATP-sensitive K+ channels.

Closure of the ATP-sensitive K^+ channels results in depolarization, causing voltage-gated Ca^{2+} channels to open.

The rise in cytosolic Ca^{2+} causes exocytosis of the vesicles, which then secrete insulin and C-peptide into the blood.

All of the hormones or neurotransmitters named in Figure X-6-5 attach to membrane receptors (R). In contrast, the metabolic substrates, glucose and amino acids, enter the β-cell.

Bridge to Pharmacology

Sulfonylurea derivatives block the ATP-sensitive K^+ channels and thus increase insulin secretion.

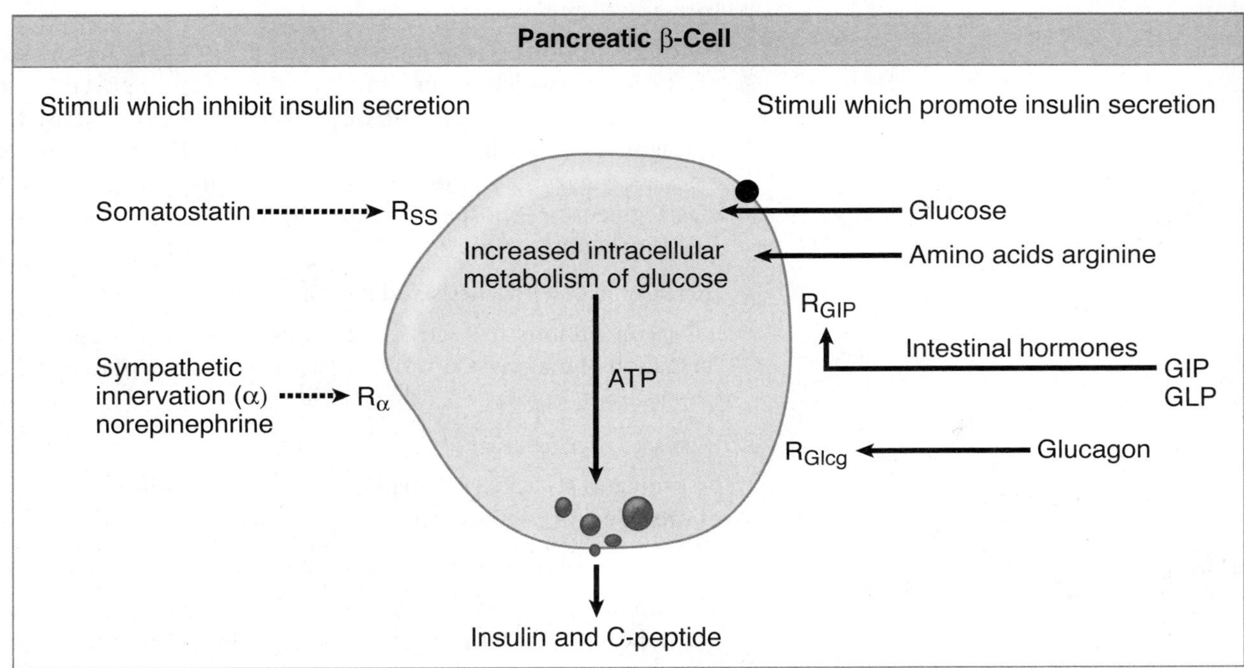

Figure X-6-5. Control of Insulin Secretion

Incretin
GIP = Gastric inhibitory peptide or glucose insulinotropic peptide

GLP = Glucagon-like peptide

ACTIONS OF GLUCAGON

Glucagon is a peptide hormone. It is secreted by the α-cells of the pancreatic islets.

The primary target for glucagon action is the liver hepatocyte, where its action is mediated by an increase in the concentration of cAMP. The cAMP activates protein kinase A, which, by catalyzing phosphorylation, alters the activity of enzymes mediating the actions given below.

Note: Skeletal muscle is not a target tissue for glucagon.

Specific Actions of Glucagon on the Liver

1. Increases liver glycogenolysis.

   Glucagon activates glycogen phosphorylase, breaking down glycogen to glucose-1-phosphate. Glucagon inactivates glycogen synthetase, preventing the glucose-1-phosphate from being recycled back into glycogen.

2. Increases liver gluconeogenesis.

   Glucagon inhibits phosphofructokinase-2 (PFK-2), thereby reducing 2,6 bisphosphate, which in turn inhibits PFK-1 (an important enzyme driving glycolysis). Inhibition of PFK-1 aids gluconeogenesis. In addition, glucagon, along with cortisol, enhances phosphoenolpyruvate carboxykinase, a key enzyme in the gluconeogenic pathway. Finally, glucagon stimulates glucose-6-phosphatase, thereby releasing glucose into the blood (see Biochemistry notes).

3. Increases liver ketogenesis and decreases lipogenesis.

   Glucagon inhibits the activity of acetyl CoA carboxylase, decreasing the formation of malonyl CoA. When the concentration of malonyl CoA is low, ketogenesis is favored over lipogenesis.

4. Increases ureagenesis.

   It stimulates N-acetylglutamate synthesis, which stimulates the production of urea (see Biochemistry notes).

5. Increases insulin secretion.

   The amino acid sequence of glucagon is similar to that of the duodenal hormone, secretin. Like secretin (and most other gut hormones), glucagon stimulates insulin secretion.

6. Increases lipolysis in the liver.

   Glucagon activates hormone-sensitive lipase in the liver, but because the action is on the liver and not the adipocyte, glucagon is not considered a major fat-mobilizing hormone.

CONTROL OF GLUCAGON SECRETION

Major factors that control glucagon secretion are summarized in Figure X-6-6. Stimuli that promote glucagon secretion are depicted on the right, and those that inhibit on the left. R designates a surface receptor for the particular hormone or neurotransmitter.

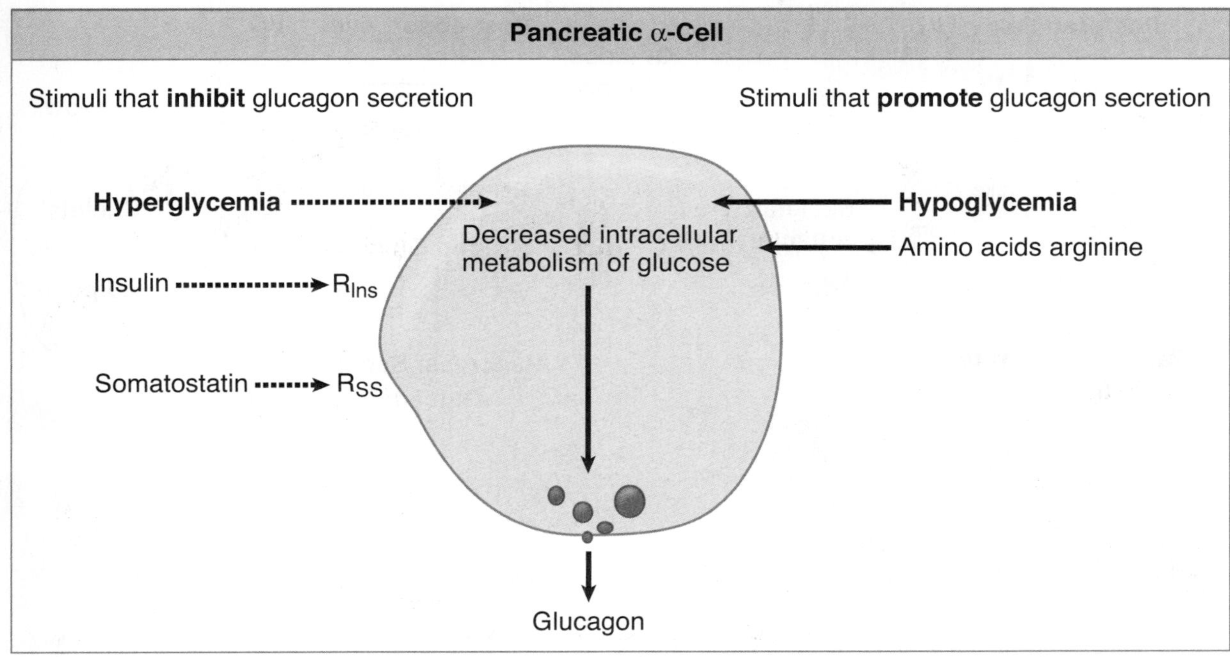

Figure X-6-6. Control of Glucagon Secretion

Low plasma glucose (hypoglycemia) is the most important physiologic promoter for glucagon secretion, and elevated plasma glucose (hyperglycemia) the most important inhibitor.

Amino acids, especially dibasic amino acids (arginine, lysine), also promote the secretion of glucagon. Thus, glucagon is secreted in response to the ingestion of a meal rich in proteins.

Overall View of Glucose Counterregulation

Glucose counterregulation is the concept that plasma glucose concentration is regulated by insulin and by hormones that oppose, or counter, its actions. Figure X-6-7 displays a diagram showing glucose regulation in the postprandial and post-absorptive states.

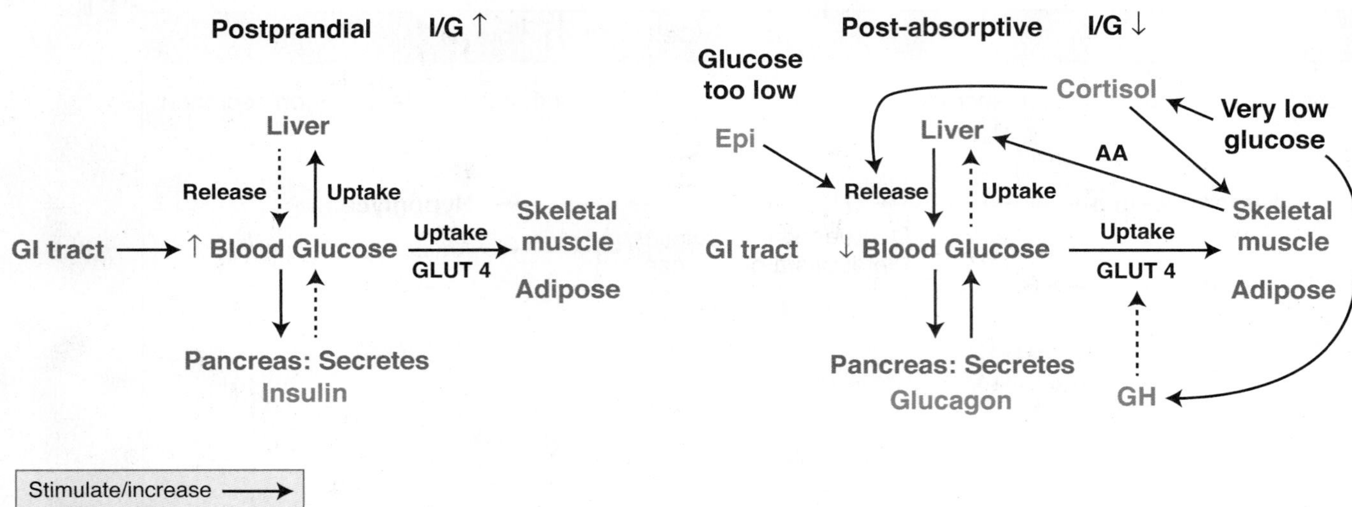

Figure X-6-7. Insulin Actions in Liver

Insulin : Glucagon Ratio

- Insulin and glucagon: move substrates in opposite directions. The direction of substrate fluxes is very sensitive to this ratio.
- Normal postabsorptive ratio: 2.0
- States requiring mobilization of substrates ratio: 0.5 or less
- Carbohydrate meal, ratio 10 or more
- Protein meal or fat meal produces little change in the ratio.

DIABETES MELLITUS

In both types of diabetes mellitus, there is hyperglycemia, polyuria, increased thirst and fluid intake, hyperosmolar state, recurrent blurred vision, mental confusion, lethargy, weakness, and abnormal peripheral sensation. Coma, if it does occur, is due to the hyperosmotic environment, not the acidosis.

Type 2

- Accounts for about 90% of all the cases of diabetes
- Strong genetic component
- Body build is usually obese (particularly central or visceral).
- Usually, but not always, middle-aged or older
- The number of younger individuals in this category is increasing.
- Characterized by variable degrees of insulin resistance, impaired insulin secretion, and increased hepatic output of glucose. Insulin resistance precedes secretory defects and in the early stages hyperinsulinemia is able to overcome tissue resistance. Ultimately beta cell failure can occur.
- Insulin levels may be high, normal, or low.
- Resistance to insulin is not well understood. It is thought to be due to postreceptor defects in signaling, which ultimately lead to a decrease in the number of glucose transporters. Reducing plasma glucose and thus plasma insulin can increase receptor sensitivity toward normal.
- Plasma glucose good screening for type 2. Elevated glucose due to elevated hepatic output.
- With a controlled diet and exercise, the symptoms of type 2 diabetes often disappear without the necessity for pharmacologic therapy.
- Individuals tend to be ketosis resistant. The presence of some endogenous insulin secretion appears to protect from development of a ketoacidosis. If it does develop, it is usually the result of severe stress or infection (increased counterregulatory homones, suppressed insulin).
- In nonobese patients, a deficient insulin release by the pancreas is often the problem, but varying degrees of insulin resistance can also occur.

Metabolic Syndrome (Syndrome X)

A group of metabolic derangements that includes atherogenic dyslipidemia (low HDL) and high triglycerides, elevated blood glucose, hypertension, central obesity, prothrombotic state, and a proinflammatory state. The clustering of these risk factors increases the probability of developing cardiovascular disease and type 2 diabetes.

Type 1

- Genetic association less marked than in type 2
- Genetically predisposed individuals whose immune system destroys pancreatic beta cells
- Symptoms do not become evident until 80% of the beta cells are destroyed.
- Body build usually lean
- Usually, but not always, early age of onset
- Due to an absence of insulin production
- Increased glucagon secretion also generally occurs
- Three target tissues for insulin—liver, skeletal muscle, and adipose tissue—fail to take up absorbed nutrients (glucose, amino acids, and fatty acids), thus increasing their levels in the blood.

Metabolic effects in insulin-deficient individuals

CHO

- Increased blood glucose concentration
- Increased glycogen breakdown
- Decreased peripheral glucose use

Protein

- Increased protein breakdown
- Increased catabolism of amino acids
- Increased gluconeogenesis
- Increased ureagenesis
- Decreased protein synthesis

Fat

- Increased triglyceride breakdown
- Increased level of circulating free fatty acids
- Increased ketosis, resulting in ketoacidosis (metabolic acidosis)
- Decreased fatty acid synthesis
- Decreased triglyceride synthesis

Renal System

The failure to reabsorb all the filtered glucose in the proximal tube also prevents normal water and electrolyte reabsorption in this segment, resulting in an osmotic diuresis (polyuria). This causes loss of glucose, water, and electrolytes from the body. Thus, even though the electrolyte concentration of the urine is low, body stores of electrolytes, particularly Na^+ and K^+, are lost.

Potassium Ion

- Hydrogen ions move intracellularly to be buffered, and potassium ions leave the cell, reducing the intracellular concentration.
- There is a lack of the normal insulin effect of pumping potassium ion into cells.
- Consequently, hyperkalemia is typical, but plasma K^+ may be normal or low because of renal loss. Regardless, the body stores of K^+ are reduced because of the renal loss.
- Insulin replacement can produce severe hypokalemia, and potassium replacement is a normal part of therapy.

Sodium Ion

- Polyuria decreases total body sodium but dehydration may keep sodium within or close to the normal range.
- Hyperosmolar state due to the hyperglycemia. Thus, 2 times the sodium concentration is not a good index of osmolarity.

$$\text{Effective osmolarity} = 2\ (\text{Na})\ \text{mEq/L} + \frac{\text{glucose mg/dL}}{18}$$

Hyperosmolar Coma

- Severe hyperglycemia shifts fluid from the intracellular to the extracellular space.
- Polyuria decreases volume of the extracellular space and leads to a decreased renal plasma flow and a reduced glucose excretion. Combined with the rise in counterregulatory hormones, the plasma glucose rises further.
- The severe loss of intracellular fluid from the brain causes the coma.
- Type 2 diabetics often present with the highest plasma glucose and greater states of dehydration. Thus these patients have a higher incidence of coma.

Diabetic Ketoacidosis (DKA)

- Without any insulin, excessive lipolysis provides fatty acids to the liver, where they preferentially converted to ketone bodies because of the unopposed action of glucagon.
- Blood pH and bicarbonate decrease due to the metabolic acidosis.
- Increased alveolar ventilation is the respiratory compensation for the metabolic acidosis. When the arterial pH decreases to about 7.20, ventilation becomes deep and rapid (Kussmaul breathing).
- An acidic urine results as the kidneys attempt to compensate for the acidosis.
- The severe acidosis is in addition to the dehydration and net decrease in total body sodium and potassium.
- Treatment is replacement of fluid and electrolytes and administration of insulin
- DKA treatment is first 2–3 liters of normal saline and IV insulin. Subcutaneous insulin may not be fully absorbed because of decreased skin perfusion. Hyponatremia is common because of hyperglycemia. For each 100 point increase in glucose above normal, there is a 1.6 decrease in sodium.

  100 mg ELEVATION glucose = 1.6 mEq DECREASE sodium

- When hyponatremia is present with hyperglycemia, management is correction of the elevated glucose level. When glucose comes to normal, the sodium corrects.

Hypoglycemia

- In the diabetic, overdosing with insulin causes hypoglycemia.
- Type 1 diabetics are particularly prone to hypoglycemia. In these individuals the glucagon response to hypoglycemia is absent.
- Initial symptoms due to catecholamine release followed by the direct effects of hypoglycemia include slowed mental processes and confusion.

PANCREATIC ENDOCRINE-SECRETING TUMORS

Insulinomas

- Most common islet cell tumor
- Found almost exclusively within the pancreas and hypersecrete insulin
- Most common symptoms due to the hypoglycemia (confusion, disorientation, headache)
- Association with MEN 1
- Insulin measured to determine insulin-mediated versus noninsulin-mediated hypoglycemia
- Insulin-secreting tumor: insulin and C-peptide both elevated
- Factitious hypoglycemia: C-peptide below normal
- Treat with removal

Other Endocrine-Secreting Tumors

- Gastrinomas
- Glucagonomas
- Somostatinomas
- VIPomas

Management of all neuroendocrine tumors is localization with CT, then surgical resection.

Glucagonoma

- Alpha cell oversecretion
- Hyperglycemia/diabetes
- Localize with CT scan
- Surgically remove

Summary

Table X-6-1. Summary of Insulin-Related Pathophysiologic States

	Glucose	Insulin	C-peptide	Ketoacidosis
Type 2 diabetes	↑	↑, ↔	↑, ↔	–
Type 1 diabetes	↑	↓	↓	+
Insulinoma	↓	↑	↑	–
Factitious hypoglycemia (self-injection of insulin)	↓	↑	↓	–

OTHER HORMONES INVOLVED IN ENERGY BALANCE AND APPETITE

Leptin

- Leptin is produced in adipose tissue and is thought to be a "long-term" regulator of appetite and energy balance.
- Secretion is circadian, with the highest levels occurring at night and the nadir in the morning. Individual meals do not stimulate the release of leptin.
- The leptin receptor is a member of the cytokine family of receptors, which activate gene transcription factors.
- Leptin decreases hypothalamic neuropeptide Y (NPY), which is a potent activator of feeding (orexigenic). By inhibiting NPY synthesis, leptin promotes satiety (anorexigenic).
- Leptin increases energy expenditure, in part by increasing fatty acid oxidation, and it decreases fat stores. Lack of and/or resistance to leptin causes obesity.

Adiponectin

- Adiponectin is produced in adipose tissue, and it increases insulin sensitivity and tissue fat oxidation.
- Dysregulation of adiponectin, along with production of cytokines by adipocytes, may play a role in obesity, insulin resistance, and cachexia. Plasma levels of adiponectin are low in Type II diabetics, and infusion of this hormone decreases plasma glucose in experimental animal models of diabetes mellitus.
  - The mechanism of action and regulation of secretion are not well understood, but it does appear to inhibit liver output of glucose.

Bridge to Pharmacology

Administration of the thiazolidinedione (TZD) class of compounds to diabetics increases the circulating levels of adiponectin, which may be part of the mechanism by which these drugs reduce plasma glucose.

Ghrelin

- Ghrelin is produced by cells of the stomach.
- Circulating levels of ghrelin are reduced in response to a meal and highest in the fasting state.
- Ghrelin activates hypothalamic NYP neurons (see leptin discussion above) and is thus a potent orexigenic hormone. It also stimulates the release of growth hormone (GH), although its physiologic significance/role is not well understood. Because of ghrelin's effects on GH and appetite, however, it may prove beneficial for restoring GH levels in the elderly and anorexic conditions, such as cancer.
- Ghrelin levels are decreased in obese individuals and elevated by low calorie diets, strenuous exercise, and patients with Prader-Willi syndrome.
- Ghrelin is a peptide hormone that works via Gq and Gs. Its mechanism of action and regulation of secretion are not well understood.

Bridge to Pathology

Prader-Willi syndrome is a genetic condition affecting many parts of the body. In infancy, this condition is characterized by hypotonia, feeding difficulties, poor growth, and delayed development. Beginning in childhood, affected individuals develop an insatiable appetite, which leads to chronic hyperphagia and obesity.

Chapter Summary

- C-peptide secreted in conjunction with insulin is an index of endogenous insulin secretion.
- The peripheral uptake of glucose is via facilitated transport. In some tissues, such as adipose and resting skeletal muscle, the number of functioning transporters is regulated by insulin.
- Insulin facilitates the metabolism of glucose to carbon dioxide and water and also its conversion to glycogen in liver and muscle.
- Insulin promotes protein synthesis and decreases protein breakdown.
- Insulin promotes lipogenesis. It inhibits lipolysis by decreasing the activity of hormone-sensitive lipase. Hyperglycemia is the major promoter of insulin secretion.
- The major target tissue for glucagon is the liver, where its primary action is glycogenolysis and increased glucose output.
- Hypoglycemia is the main promoter and hyperglycemia the main inhibitor of glucagon secretion.

Type 2 Diabetes

- Strong genetic component and accounts for at least 90% of all cases
- Body build exhibits central obesity
- Insulin resistance, impaired insulin secretion, and increased hepatic output of glucose
- Fasting plasma glucose provides good screening.
- Individuals can have extremely high plasma glucose levels without ketoacidosis.

Type 1 Diabetes

- Generally autoimmune origin
- Absence of insulin secretion but elevated glucagon
- High circulating glucose (glycogen, gluconeogenesis), amino acids (protein), fatty acids (triglyceride)
- Polyuria, dehydration, and electrolyte depletion
- Ketoacidosis, Kussmaul breathing
- Insulinomas: increased insulin, increased C-peptide, decreased plasma glucose

Hormonal Control of Calcium and Phosphate

7

Learning Objectives

- ❑ Solve problems concerning overview of calcium and phosphate
- ❑ Solve problems concerning bone remodeling
- ❑ Solve problems concerning parathyroid hormone
- ❑ Solve problems concerning calcitonin
- ❑ Demonstrate understanding of role of vitamin D (calcitriol) in calcium homeostasis
- ❑ Solve problems concerning disorders in calcium and phosphate
- ❑ Answer questions about metabolic bone disorders

OVERVIEW OF CALCIUM AND PHOSPHATE

- The percentage of dietary calcium absorbed from the gut is inversely related to intake.
- The dietary intake of and the percentage of calcium absorbed is diminished in the elderly.
- Ingested phosphate is also absorbed by the gut.
- Both calcium and phosphate absorption in the GI tract are stimulated by the active form of vitamin D (calcitriol).

The approximate percentage of the body's total calcium is given for each of the compartments in Figure X-7-1. In addition, the fraction of calcium is indicated. The calcium concentration in the interstitial fluid is 103 to 104 times higher than the intracellular calcium concentration. The initiation of many cellular processes (secretion, movement of intracellular organelles, cell division) is linked to a sudden brief increase in intracellular (cytosolic) calcium.

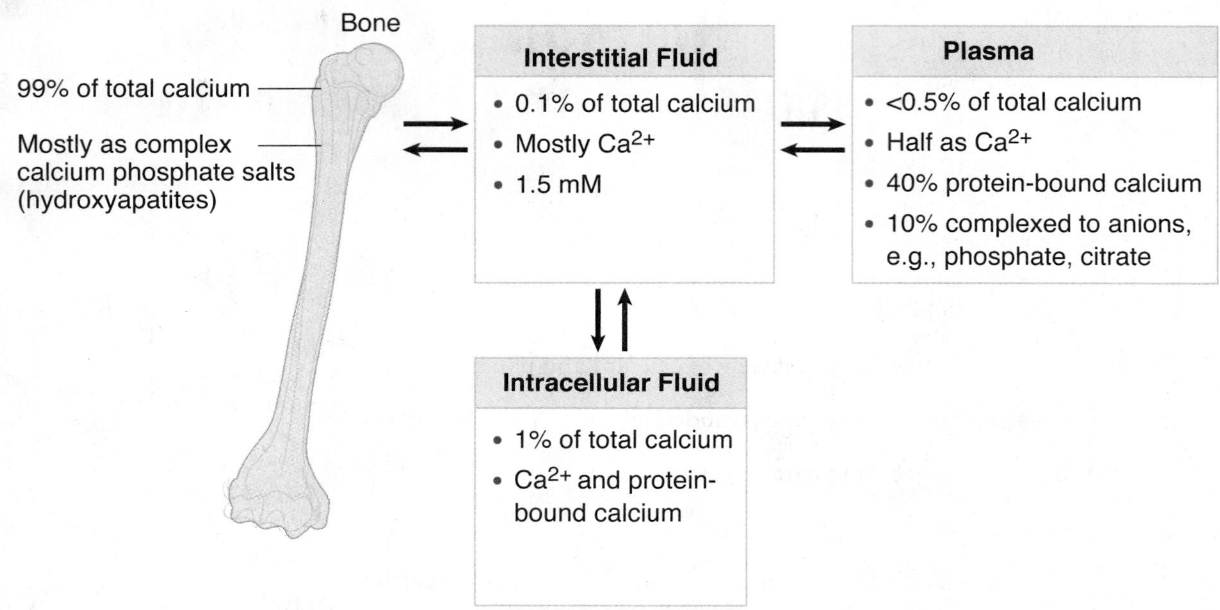

Figure X-7-1. Calcium Distribution in the Body

Plasma Calcium

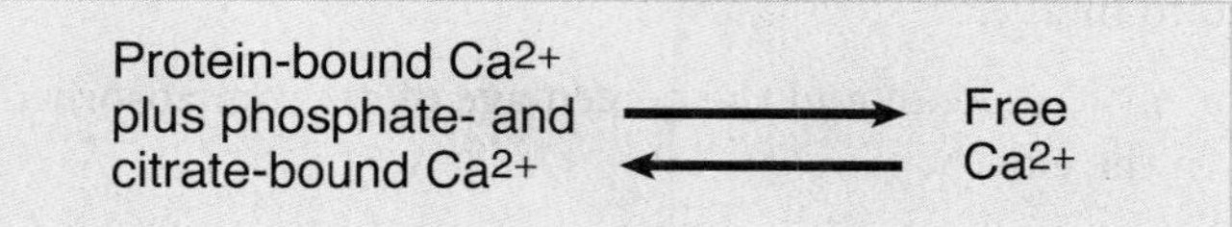

Figure X-7-2. Relationship of Bound and Free Calcium

- Plasma calcium represents 50% ionized free, 40% attached to protein, 10% associated with anions such as phosphate and citrate.
- The free calcium is the physiologically active and precisely regulated form.
- Alkalosis (hyperventilation) decreases and acidosis increases free plasma calcium by varying the amount bound to protein.
- Alkalosis lowers free calcium by increasing protein-binding, while acidosis raises free calcium by decreasing protein-binding.

Relationship Between Calcium and Phosphate

Bone is a complex precipitate of calcium and phosphate to which hydroxide and bicarbonate ions are added to make up the mature hydroxyapatite crystals, which are laid down in a protein (osteoid) matrix. Whether calcium and phosphate are laid down in bone (precipitate from solution) or are resorbed from bone (go into solution) depends on the product of their concentrations rather than on their individual concentrations.

When the product exceeds a certain number (solubility product or ion product), bone is laid down:

$$[Ca^{2+}] \times [PO^{-}_{4}] > \text{solubility product} = \text{bone deposition}$$

- Under normal conditions the ECF product of calcium times phosphate is close to the solubility product.
- Thus, an increase in the interstitial fluid concentration of either Ca^{2+} or phosphate increases bone mineralization.
- For example, an increase in plasma phosphate would increase the product of their concentrations, promote precipitation, and lower free calcium in the interstitial fluid.
- A malignant increase in the concentration of calcium or phosphate due to chronic renal disease or rhabdomyolysis can cause the precipitation of calcium phosphate within tissues.

When the product is below the solubility product, bone is resorbed:

$$[Ca^{2+}] \times [PO^{-}_{4}] < \text{solubility product} = \text{bone resorption}$$

- Thus, a decrease in the interstitial concentration of either Ca^{2+} or phosphate promotes the resorption of these salts from bone (demineralization).
- For example, a decrease in plasma phosphate alone would promote bone demineralization. Increasing renal excretion of phosphate would promote bone demineralization and a rise in interstitial free calcium.

It is the free Ca^{2+}, not the phosphate, that is regulated so precisely. Hormonal control of free Ca^{2+} levels is via a dual hormonal system; parathyroid hormone and vitamin D.

BONE REMODELING

- Bone is undergoing continual remodeling throughout life, although the turnover is faster in younger individuals. As many as 300,000 bone-remodeling sites are active in a normal person.
- Bone remodeling involves the interplay between bone-building cells (osteoblasts) and cells that break down bone (osteoclasts), as illustrated in Figure X-7-3.
- Osteoblasts cause bone deposition and they secrete two proteins (Figure X-7-3):
  - RANK-L (Receptor Activator of Nuclear KappaB Ligand): This protein binds to the RANK receptor, which is expressed on precursor cells resulting in their differentiation into active osteoclasts. Active osteoclasts also express the RANK receptor, which, when stimulated, activates osteoclastic activity.
  - OPG (osteoprotegerin): This protein binds RANK-L, thereby preventing it from binding onto precursor or osteoclast cells. This reduces differentiation and overall osteoclastic activity. Thus, OPG acts as a "decoy" for RANK-L.

- Bone remodeling is influenced by parathyroid hormone (PTH), and the active form of vitamin D, both of which are covered below. Estrogen is well known for conserving bone integrity and it does so by at least two mechanisms. First, it induces the synthesis of OPG. Second, it reduces the secretion of cytokines by T-lymphocytes. These cytokines stimulate differentiation of precursor cells into active osteoclasts and they stimulate activity of mature osteocytes. By inhibiting these cytokines and increasing OPG, estrogen reduces the activity of osteoclasts.
- Glucocorticoids increase bone breakdown by inducing the synthesis and release of RANK-L and by inhibiting the synthesis of OPG.

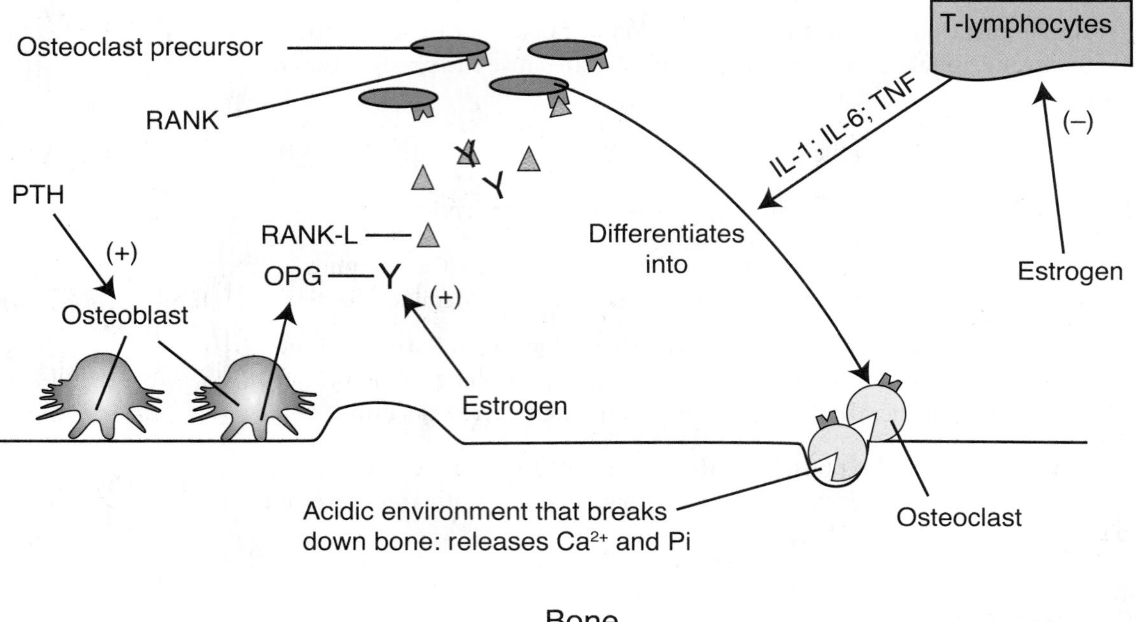

RANK = receptor activator of nuclear factor kappaB

RANK-L = receptor activator of nuclear factor kappaB ligand

OPG = osteoprotegerin (endogenous blocker of RANK-L)

Pi = phosphate

Figure X-7-3. Relationship between Osteoblasts and Osteoclasts

Weight-Bearing Stress

Weight-bearing mechanical stress increases the mineralization of bone.

The absence of weight-bearing stress (being sedentary, bedridden, or weightless) promotes the demineralization of bone. Under these conditions, the following occurs:

- Plasma Ca^{2+} tends to be in the upper region of normal.
- Plasma PTH decreases.
- Urinary calcium increases.

Indices

Indices can be utilized to detect excess bone demineralization and remodeling:

- Increased serum osteocalcin and alkaline phosphatase are associated with osteoblastic activity.
- Increased urinary excretion of hydroxyproline is a breakdown product of collagen

PARATHYROID HORMONE (PTH)

Actions of PTH

A decrease in the free calcium is the signal to increase PTH secretion and the function of PTH is to raise free calcium, which it does by several mechanisms.

- Increases Ca^{2+} reabsorption in distal tubule of the kidney (chapter 4, section VIII)
- Inhibits phosphate (Pi) reabsorption in proximal tubule of the kidney.
- Stimulates the 1-alpha-hydroxylase enzyme in kidney, converting inactive vitamin D to its active form.
- Causes bone resorption, releasing Ca^{2+} and Pi into the blood.

Bone resorption

The mechanisms of PTH-induced bone resorption are complex and not fully understood. However, the following generalizations do apply.

- Osteoblasts express receptors for PTH. Binding of PTH stimulates the osteoblast to release RANK-L. This in turn, increases osteoclastic activity resulting in bone resorption and the release of calcium and phosphate into the blood, as shown in Figure X-7-3.
- Although counterintuitive, intermittent spikes in PTH, e.g., intravenous or subcutaneous injection, stimulates osteoblastic activity resulting in bone deposition. Thus, PTH can be useful in treating osteoporosis in the clinical setting.

Parathyroid Hormone-Related Peptide

- PTHrP is a paracrine factor secreted by many tissues; e.g., lung, mammary tissue, placenta.
- It may have a role in fetal development. In postnatal life, its role is unclear.
- The majority of humoral hypercalcemias of malignancy are due to overexpression of PTHrP.
- PTHrP has a strong structural homology to PTH and binds with equal affinity to the PTH receptor.

Regulation of PTH Secretion

- PTH is a peptide hormone released from the parathyroid glands in response to lowered plasma free Ca^{2+} (Figure X-7-4).
- Free Ca^{2+} in the plasma is the primary regulator of PTH.

- The negative feedback relationship between plasma calcium and PTH secretion is highly sigmoidal, with the steep portion of the curve representing the normal range of plasma free calcium.
- To sense the free calcium, the parathyroid cell depends upon high levels of expression of the calcium-sensing receptor (CaSR).
- In most cells, exocytosis depends on a rise in intracellular free calcium. In the parathyroid gland, a fall in intracellular free calcium causes release.
- Depletion of magnesium stores can create a reversible hypoparathyroidism.

Normal range = region between dashed lines

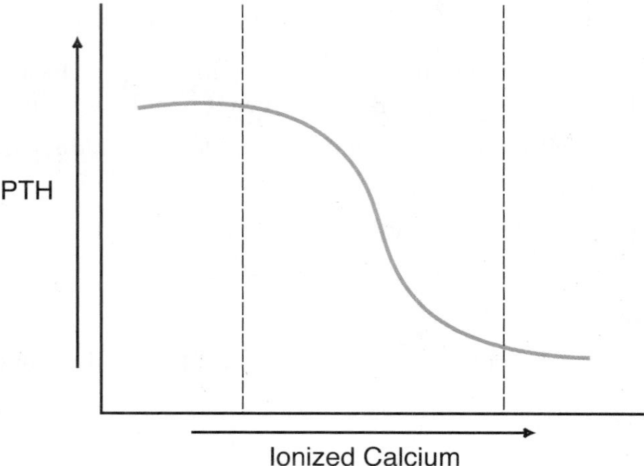

Figure X-7-4. Relationship between Plasma Calcium and PTH

CALCITONIN

- Calcitonin (CT) is a peptide hormone secreted by the parafollicular cells (C cells) of the thyroid gland. It is released in response to elevated free calcium.
- Calcitonin lowers plasma calcium by decreasing the activity of osteoclasts, thus decreasing bone resorption. Calcitonin is useful in the treatment of Paget's disease, severe hypercalcemia, and osteoporosis.
- Calcitonin is not a major controller of Ca^{2+} in humans. Removing the thyroid (with the C cells) or excess of calcitonin via a C cell tumor (medullary carcinoma of the thyroid) has little impact on plasma calcium.
- No deficiency or excess disease has been described.

ROLE OF VITAMIN D (CALCITRIOL) IN CALCIUM HOMEOSTASIS

Sources and Synthesis

Vitamin D_2 (ergocalciferol) is a vitamin but can functionally be considered a prohormone. It is a normal dietary component. A slightly different form, vitamin D_3 (cholecalciferol), is synthesized in the skin. The synthesis of active 1,25 di-OH vitamin D (calcitriol) is outlined in Figure X-7-5.

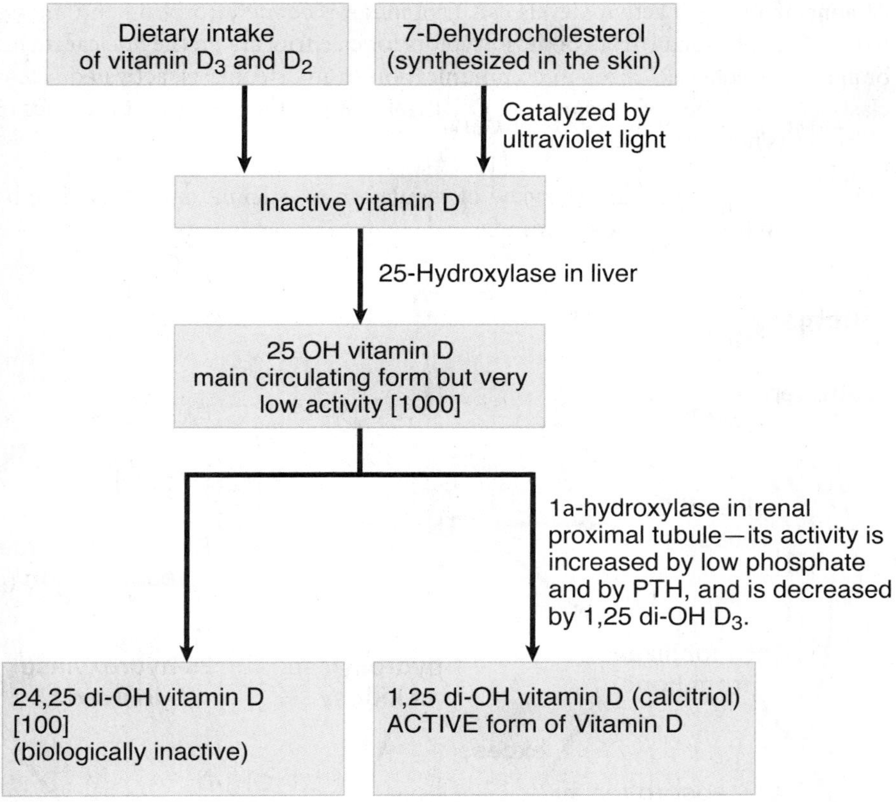

Figure X-7-5. Vitamin D Metabolism

The synthesis of calcitriol occurs sequentially in the skin → liver → kidney. The relative numbers of molecules of each of the hydroxylated forms of D present in the blood of a normal person are given in brackets. After its conversion to the 25 OH form in the liver, it can be stored in fat tissue. The serum levels of 25 OH vitamin D represent the best measure of the body stores of vitamin D when a deficiency is suspected. Most of the 25 OH form, which is the immediate precursor of 1,25 di-OH D, is converted to the inactive metabolite, 24,25 di-OH D. Ultraviolet (UV) light also evokes skin tanning, decreasing the penetration of UV light, and thus decreases the subsequent formation of D_3. This mechanism may prevent overproduction of D_3 in individuals exposed to large amounts of sunlight.

Actions of Calcitriol

Under normal conditions, vitamin D acts to raise plasma Ca^{2+} and phosphate. Thus, vitamin D promotes bone deposition. This is accomplished by:

- Calcitriol increases the absorption of Ca^{2+} and phosphate by the intestinal mucosa by increasing the production of the Ca^{2+}-binding protein calbindin. The details of this process are poorly understood.
- The resulting high concentrations of Ca^{2+} and phosphate in the extracellular fluid exceed the solubility product, and precipitation of bone salts into bone matrix occurs.
- Calcitriol enhances PTH's action at the renal distal tubule.

At abnormally high activity levels calcitriol increases bone resorption and release of Ca^{2+} and phosphate from bone. Receptors for calcitriol are on the nuclear membranes of osteoblasts. Through communication from osteoblasts, activated osteoclasts carry out the bone resorption. Calcitriol requires the concurrent presence of PTH for its bone-resorbing action.

Figure X-7-6 provides an overview of regulation of calcium and phosphate by parathyroid hormone and vitamin D.

Summary

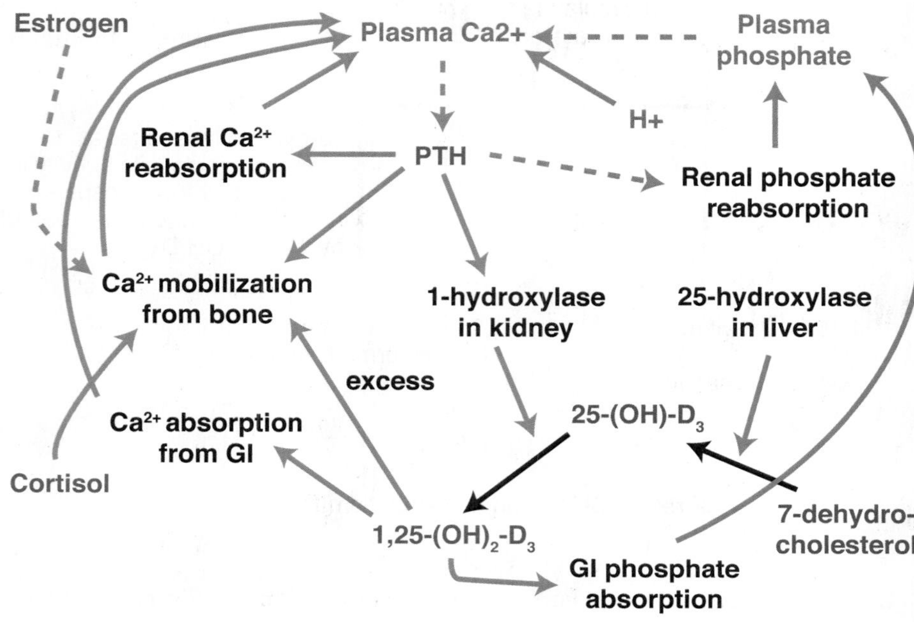

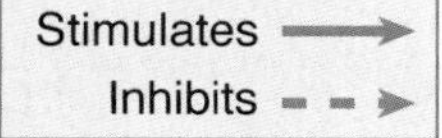

Figure X-7-6. Regulation of Calcium and Phosphate

DISORDERS IN CALCIUM AND PHOSPHATE

Hypercalcemia

Hypercalcemia of primary hyperparathyroidism

- Initiating factor is primary hypersecretion of PTH
- Consequences include increased plasma calcium, decreased plasma phosphate, polyuria, hypercalciuria, and decreased bone mass
- 80% due to a single parathyroid adenoma
- High calcium can lead to nephrogenic diabetes insipidus. This is why there is massive volume deficit in hypercalcemia.
- High calcium makes it harder to depolarize neural tissue. This is why hypercalcemia causes lethargy, confusion, and constipation.
- 15% due to primary hyperplasia as in MEN 1 or MEN 2A
- Parathyroid carcinoma rare

- Ectopic hormonal hypercalcemia usually PTHrP
- Most patients asymptomatic
- Symptoms include lethargy, fatigue, depression, neuromuscular weakness, and difficulty in concentrating
- Increased plasma alkaline phosphatase, osteocalcin and increased excretion of cAMP (second messenger for PTH in the kidney), and hydroxyproline
- Severe dehydration
- Bone manifestation is osteitis fibrosa cystica in which there are increased osteoclasts in scalloped areas of the surface bone and replacement of marrow elements with fibrous tissue. Increased alkaline phosphatase is due to high bone turnover.
- Hypercalcemia decreases QT interval and in some cases causes cardiac arrhythmias.

Related causes of hypercalcemia

- Lithium shifts the sigmoid Ca/PTH curve to the right. Higher calcium levels are thus needed to suppress PTH. Similarly, the CaSR is mutated in patients with familial hypocalciuric hypercalcemia (FHH; see Renal Physiology section, chapter 4), resulting in more PTH for any given calcium concentration in the plasma.
- Sarcoidosis and other granulomatous disorders (10%) due to increased activity of 1-alpha hydroxylase activity in granulomas.
- Thyrotoxicosis, milk-alkali syndrome
- Thiazide diuretics increase renal calcium absorption.

Differential diagnosis and treatment

- Elevated plasma calcium and PTH normal or elevated; conclusion is primary hyperparathyroidism
- Elevated plasma calcium and decreased PTH; conclusion is something other than primary hyperparathyroidism
- Treatment is usually surgery; i.e., removing the adenoma or with hyperplasia removing most of the parathyroid tissue
- Treat with high volume fluid replacement
- Bisphosphonates need 2–3 days to be fully effective
- Calcitonin rapidly inhibits osteoclastic activity

Hypocalcemia

Hypocalcemia of primary hypoparathyroidism

- Can be hereditary or autoimmune
- Caused by thyroid surgery or surgery to correct hyperparathyroidism
- The initiating factor is inadequate secretion of PTH by the parathyroid glands.
- The decrease in plasma calcium is accompanied by an increased plasma phosphate. Even though less phosphate is resorbed from bone, plasma

phosphate increases because the normal action of PTH is to inhibit phosphate reabsorption and increase excretion by the kidney. Therefore, without PTH, more of the filtered load is reabsorbed.

- Symptoms focus on the hypocalcemic induced increased excitability of motor neurons creating muscular spasms and tetany
- Chvostek's sign is induced by tapping the facial nerve just anterior to the ear lobe.
- Trousseau's sign is elicited by inflating a pressure cuff on the upper arm. A positive response is carpal spasm.
- Hypomagnesemia prevents PTH secretion and induces hypocalcemia. This condition responds immediately to an infusion of magnesium.

Pseudohypoparathyroidism

- This is a rare familial disorder characterized by target tissue resistance to parathyroid hormone.
- Exhibits same signs and symptoms as primary hypoparathyroidism except PTH elevated
- It is usually accompanied by developmental defects: mental retardation, short and stocky stature, one or more metacarpal or metatarsal bones missing (short 4th or 5th finger).

Additional causes of hypocalcemia

- Acute hypocalcemia can occur even with intact homeostatic mechanisms. Included would be alkalosis via hyperventilation, transfusions of citrated blood, rhabdomyolysis or tumor lysis, and the subsequent hyperphosphatemia
- Hyperphosphatemia of chronic renal failure
- Failures with vitamin D system
- Congenital absence of parathyroids rare (DiGeorge's syndrome)
- Damaged muscle binds calcium. Rhabdomyolysis binds free calcium.

Predictive indices for a primary disorder

When plasma calcium and phosphate levels are changing in opposite directions, the cause is usually a primary disorder. An exception may be chronic renal failure. This state is not a primary disorder but is usually associated with hypocalcemia and hyperphosphatemia (hypocalcemic-induced secondary hyperparathyroidism).

Renal Failure and Secondary Hyperparathyroidism

- Most common cause of secondary hyperparathyroidism
- Loss of nephrons prevents kidneys from excreting phosphate (Pi)
- Elevated Pi lowers free Ca^{2+}, which in turn increases PTH

Vitamin D Deficiency and Secondary Hyperparathyroidism

- Causes include a diet deficient in vitamin D, inadequate sunlight exposure, malabsorption of vitamin D, enzyme deficiencies in the pathway to activation of vitamin D
- In all cases there is a decrease in plasma calcium, which elicits an increase in PTH secretion and a secondary hyperparathyroidism.
- A similar consequence is the increased demand for calcium as in pregnancy.
- Characterized by increased PTH, decreased plasma calcium, and decreased plasma phosphate. Even though the elevated PTH increases phosphate resorption from bone, PTH also inhibits phosphate reabsorption by the kidney, thereby promoting phosphate excretion and a drop in plasma phosphate.
- Bone mass is lost to maintain plasma calcium.
- Diagnostic test is a low plasma 25(OH) vitamin D.

Excess Vitamin D and Secondary Hypoparathyroidism

- An excessive intake of vitamin D raises plasma calcium, which elicits a decrease in PTH
- Characterized by decreased PTH, increased plasma calcium, and increased plasma phosphate but normal or decreased phosphate excretion. Because PTH increases the excretion of phosphate by inhibiting reabsorption in the proximal tubule, decreased PTH causes increased reabsorption of phosphate and elevated plasma levels.
- Excessive vitamin D promotes bone resorption and bone mass decreases.

Predictive indices for a secondary disorder

When the plasma calcium and phosphate are changing in the same direction, the origin is usually a secondary disorder.

- Secondary hyperparathyroidism: both decrease
- Secondary hypoparathyroidism: both increase

Note also that in either a deficiency or an excess of vitamin D, there is a decrease in bone mass but mechanism differs (high PTH in deficiency; direct effect of vitamin D with excess).

METABOLIC BONE DISORDERS

Osteoporosis

- Osteoporosis is a loss of bone mass (both mineralization and matrix) with fractures, due to normal age-related changes in bone remodeling as well as additional factors that exaggerate this process.
- If bone mineral density is 2.5 standard deviations below the average, then this equals osteoporosis.
- If bone mineral density is 1 to 2.5 standard deviations below the average, then this equals osteopenia.

- Bone mass reaches a peak subsequent to puberty. Heredity accounts for most of the variation but physical activity, nutrition, and reproductive hormones play a significant role, especially estrogens even in men.
- Secondary osteoporosis can occur in thyrotoxicosis and particularly with elevations in glucocorticoids.
- A mainstay of treatment involves the use of bisphosphonates that are rapidly incorporated into bone and reduce the activity of osteoclasts.
- Calcitonin inhibits bone resorption.

Osteoporosis can also be treated with:

- **Denosumab:** inhibitor of RANKL. RANKL is a TNF family of cytokine that activates osteoclasts; denosumab therefore, inhibits osteoclasts.
- **Teriparatide:** synthetic PTH. When used intermittently, teriparatide has a stimulatory effect on osteoblastic bone formation.
- Calcitonin
- Raloxifene: selective estrogen receptor modifier

Rickets and Osteomalacia

- Origin is the abnormal mineralization of bone and cartilage
- Rickets is before plate closure, osteomalacia is after plate closure.
- In rickets there is expansion of the epiphyseal plates and the most striking abnormalities are the bowing of the legs and protuberant abdomen.
- In osteomalacia, symptoms are more subtle.
- Most common cause in adults is a malabsorption disorder, e.g., celiac disease; a vitamin D deficiency can also cause
- Rarely caused by enzyme deficiencies when substrate availability is normal.

Chapter Summary

- Only a percentage of the ingested calcium is absorbed from the small intestine and this percentage is decreased in the elderly.
- It is the ECF free calcium that is the biological active, precisely regulated form.
- Alkalosis decreases the ECF free calcium.
- Bone deposition and resorption depend upon the product of the calcium and phosphate concentrations.
- ECF free calcium is regulated by parathyroid hormone (PTH) and vitamin D.
- At the kidney, PTH (1) increases distal tubule calcium reabsorption, (2) inhibits proximal tubule phosphate reabsorption, and (3) stimulates the 1-alphahydroxylase enzyme.
- Bone is constantly being remodeled and mechanical stress increases, while bed rest decreases overall bone mass.
- The main circulating form of vitamin D is the 25-OH form, but the active physiologic form is the 1,25 di-OH form.
- The most common cause of hypercalcemia is primary hyperparathyroidism (↑ calcium, ↓ phosphate).
- Hypercalcemia is usually associated with bone loss.
- The most common cause of primary hypoparathyroidism is surgery (↓ calcium, ↑ phosphate).
- Hypocalcemia induces muscular tetany.
- Vitamin D deficiency induces a secondary hyperparathyroidism (↓ calcium, ↓ phosphate) and a decrease in bone mass (rickets, osteomalacia).
- Vitamin D excess induces a secondary hypoparathyroidism (↑ calcium, ↑ phosphate) and the increased activity of vitamin D directly decreases bone mass.
- Chronic renal failure often induces a hyperphosphatemia and a secondary hyperparathyroidism (↓ calcium, ↑ phosphate).
- Osteoporosis is mainly an age-related process in which the bone matrix and mineralization decrease.
- In rickets and osteomalacia there is mainly a decrease in the mineralization of bone.

Thyroid Hormones 8

Learning Objectives

- ❏ Solve problems concerning overview of the thyroid gland
- ❏ Use knowledge of biosynthesis and transport of thyroid hormones
- ❏ Interpret scenarios on physiologic actions of thyroid hormones
- ❏ Answer questions about control of thyroid hormone secretion
- ❏ Answer questions about pathologic changes in thyroid hormone secretion

OVERVIEW OF THE THYROID GLAND

In mammals, thyroid hormones are essential for normal growth and maturation. Therefore, thyroid hormones are major anabolic hormones.

Dietary intake of about 500 µg per day is typical, mainly in the form of iodide (I^-) or iodine (I). To maintain normal thyroid hormone secretion, 150 µg is the minimal intake necessary. I^- is the form absorbed from the small intestine.

- The functional unit of the thyroid gland is the follicle.
- The lumen is filled with thyroglobulin, which contain large numbers of thyroid hormone molecules.
- Surrounding the lumen are the follicle cells, which function to both synthesize and release thyroid hormones.
- These relationships are schematically represented in Figure X-8-1.

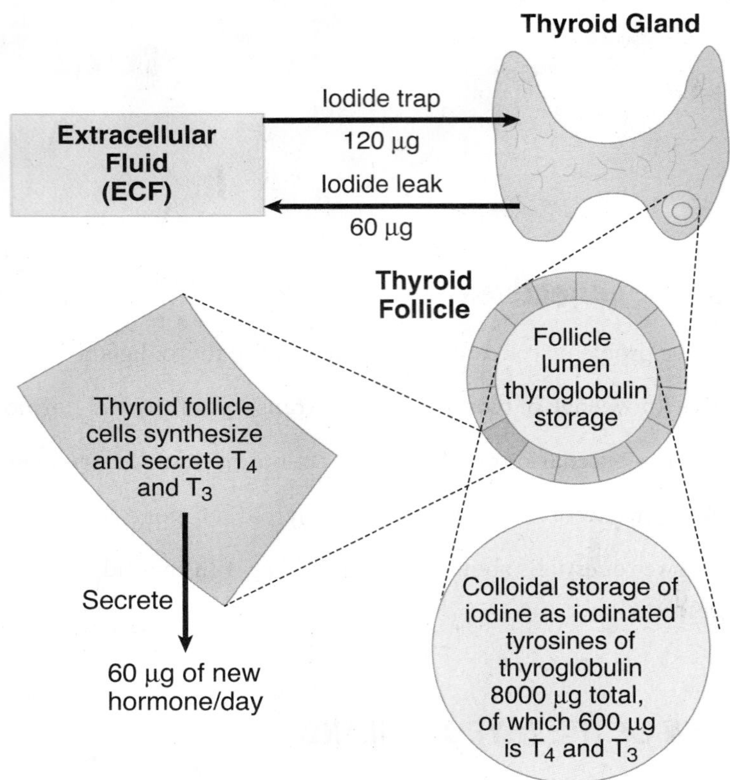
Thyroid Gland
Iodide trap
120 µg
Iodide leak
60 µg
Extracellular Fluid (ECF)
Thyroid Follicle
Follicle lumen thyroglobulin storage
Thyroid follicle cells synthesize and secrete T_4 and T_3
Secrete
60 µg of new hormone/day
Colloidal storage of iodine as iodinated tyrosines of thyroglobulin 8000 µg total, of which 600 µg is T_4 and T_3

Figure X-8-1. The Thyroid Follicle

BIOSYNTHESIS AND TRANSPORT OF THYROID HORMONES

Synthesis of Thyroid Hormones

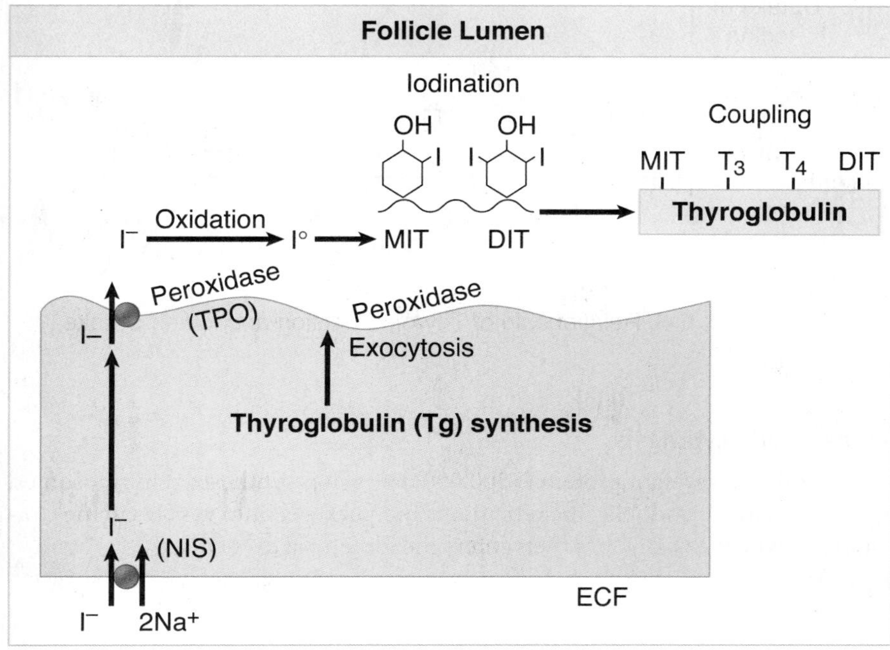

Figure X-8-2. Steps in Thyroid Synthesis

Iodide transport

Iodine uptake is via a sodium/potassium pump powered sodium/iodide symporter on the basal membrane (NIS). This pump can raise the concentration of I^- within the cell to as much as 250 times that of plasma. The pump can be blocked by anions like perchlorate and thiocyanate, which compete with I.

Along the apical membrane, the I^- is transported into the lumen by an anion-exchanger called pendrin.

The 24-hour iodine uptake by the thyroid is directly proportional to thyroid function. This is shown in Figure X-8-3.

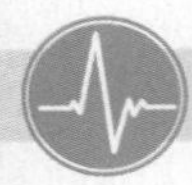

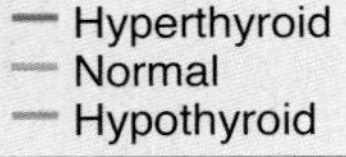

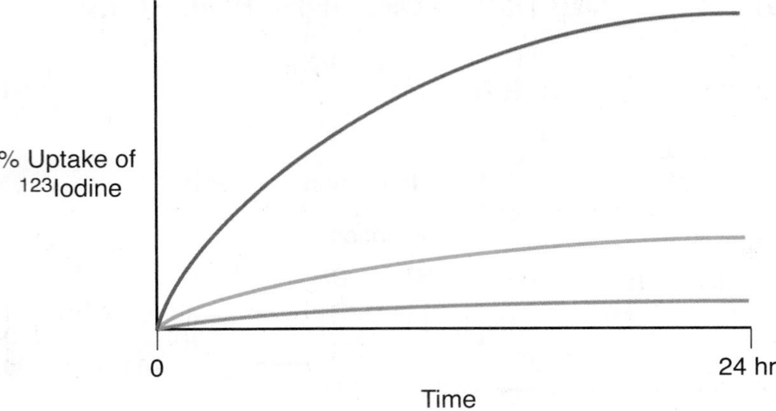

Figure X-8-3. Relationship of Thyroid Function and Iodine Uptake

Thyroglobulin synthesis

A high molecular weight protein (>300,000 daltons) is synthesized in ribosomes, glycosylated in the endoplasmic reticulum, and packaged into vesicles in the Golgi apparatus. The thyroglobin then enters the lumen via exocytosis.

Oxidation of I^- to I^o

The enzyme thyroperoxidase (TPO), which is located at the apical border of the follicle cell, catalyzes oxidation. Peroxidase also catalyzes iodination and coupling.

Iodination

As thyroglobulin is extruded into the follicular lumen, a portion (<20%) of its tyrosine residues are iodinated. The catalyst for this reaction is peroxidase. The initial products of iodination are mono- and diiodotyrosine (MIT and DIT), respectively, with the latter form predominating, except when iodine is scarce.

Coupling

Peroxidase also promotes the coupling of iodinated tyrosine in the thyroglobulin molecule. When two DITs couple, tetraiodothyronine (T4) is formed. When one DIT and one MIT combine, triiodothyronine (T3) is formed. When iodine is abundant, mainly T4 is formed. But when iodine becomes scarce, the production of T3 increases.

Storage of thyroid hormones

Enough hormone is stored as iodinated thyroglobulin in the follicular colloid to last the body for 2–3 months.

Structure of Thyroid Hormones

The chemical structures of T4, T3, and reverse T3 (rT3) are shown in Figure X-8-4. Do not memorize structure; note the number and location of iodines, instead, attached to the tyrosine residues.

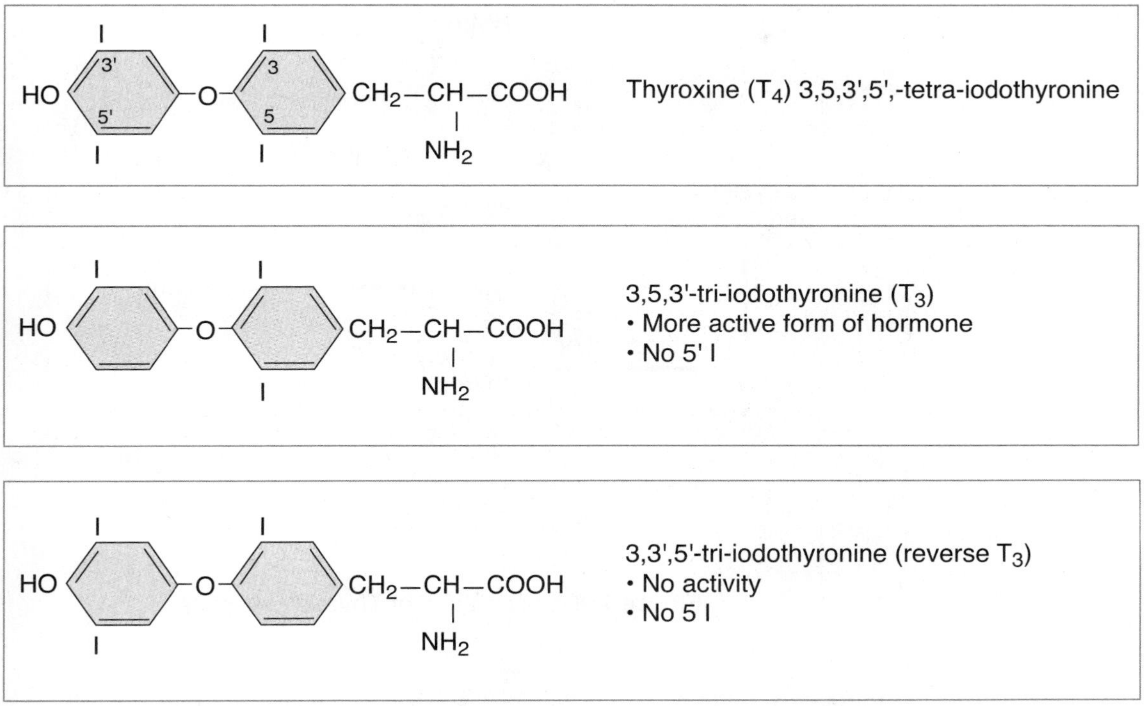

I I
3' 3
HO —O— CH_2—CH—COOH
5' 5
I I
NH_2

Thyroxine (T_4) 3,5,3',5',-tetra-iodothyronine

I I
HO —O— CH_2—CH—COOH
I
NH_2

3,5,3'-tri-iodothyronine (T_3)
- More active form of hormone
- No 5' I

I I
HO —O— CH_2—CH—COOH
I
NH_2

3,3',5'-tri-iodothyronine (reverse T_3)
- No activity
- No 5 I

Figure X-8-4. Active and Inactive Forms of Thyroid Hormones

Secretion of Thyroid Hormone

Figure X-8-5 illustrates the main steps in thyroglobulin degradation and the release of thyroid hormones.

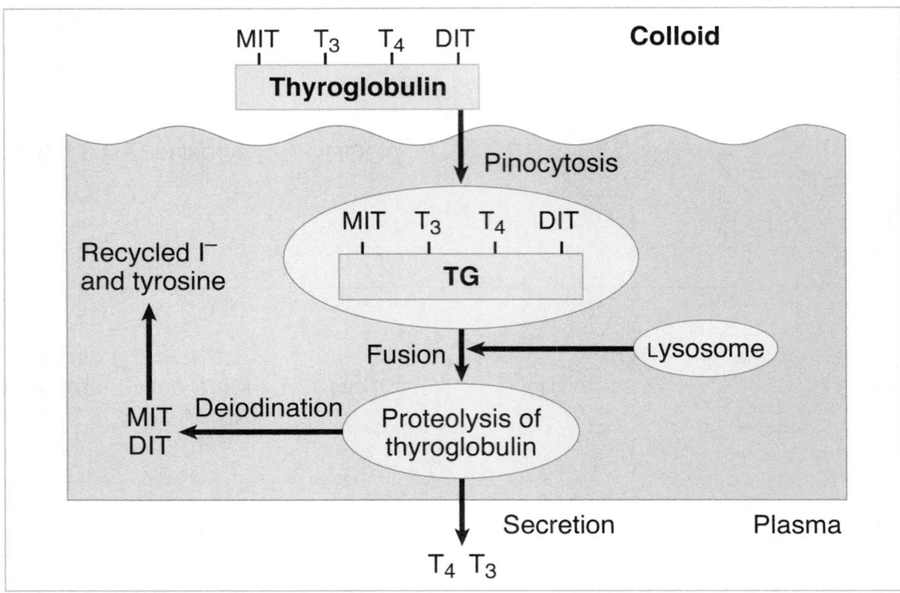

Figure X-8-5. Secretion of Thyroid Hormone

Pinocytosis: Pieces of the follicular colloid are taken back into the follicle by endocytosis.

Fusion: The endocytosed material fuses with lysosomes, which transport it toward the basal surface of the cell.

Proteolysis of thyroglobulin: Within the lysosomes, the thyroglobulin is broken into free amino acids, some of which are T4, T3, DIT, and MIT.

Secretion: T4 and T3 are secreted into the blood, with the T4:T3 ratio being as high as 20:1. The thyroid has the same 5'-mono-deiodinase found in many peripheral tissues and in an iodine- deficient state more of the hormone can be released as T3.

Along with thyroid hormones a small amount of thyroglobulin is also released into the circulation. Its release is increased in a number of states including thyroiditis, nodular goiter, and by cancerous thyroid tissue. After the surgical removal of cancerous thyroid tissue, any residual thyroglobulin in the circulation indicates cancerous cells are still present.

Deiodination: A microsomal deiodinase removes the iodine from iodinated tyrosines (DIT and MIT) but not from the iodinated thyronines (T3 and T4). The iodine is then available for resynthesis of hormone. (Individuals with a deficiency of this enzyme are more likely to develop symptoms of iodine deficiency.)

Transport of Thyroid Hormones in Blood

There is an equilibrium between bound and free circulating thyroid hormone in the bloodstream. Figure X-8-6 illustrates this equilibrium.

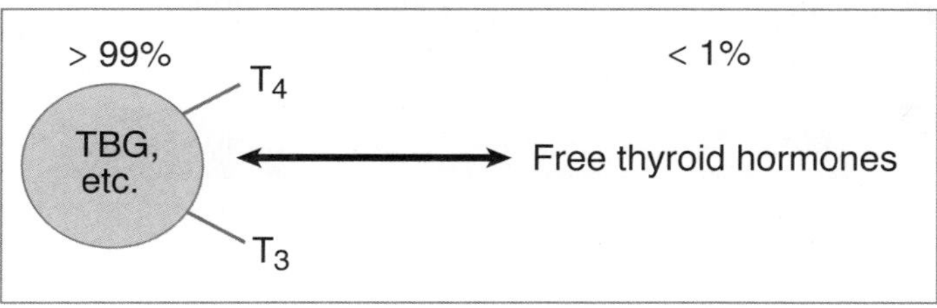

Figure X-8-6. Plasma Transport of Thyroid Hormone

TBG = thyroid-binding globulin

About 70% of the circulating thyroid is bound to thyroid-binding globulin (TBG). The remainder of the bound protein is attached to thyroxine-binding prealbumin (transthyretin) and albumin. Large variations in TBG do not normally affect the free form. A rare congenital deficiency or excess of TBG drastically alters the bound fraction but because the free fraction is normal, the individuals are all euthyroid.

Also, T4 has the higher affinity for binding proteins; therefore, it binds more tightly to protein than does T3, and consequently has a greater half-life than T3. Most circulating thyroid hormone is T4. Normally, there is 50 times more T4 than T3.

- T4 half-life = 6 days
- T3 half-life = 1 day

The amount of circulating thyroid hormone is about 3 times the amount normally secreted by the thyroid gland each day. Thus, circulating protein-bound thyroid hormones act as a significant reserve.

Activation and Degradation of Thyroid Hormones

- T3 and T4 bind to the same nuclear receptor but T3 binds with 10 times more affinity than T4.
- Thus, because it has greater affinity for the receptor, T3 is the more active form of thyroid hormone.
- Many target tissues can regulate the conversion of T4 to either T3 or rT3, thereby locally controlling hormone activity.
- Most of the circulating T3 is derived from the peripheral conversion of T4 into T3 and its release again into the circulation (e.g., liver, kidney, and skeletal muscle).
- This peripheral conversion of thyroid hormone is represented in Figure X-8-7.

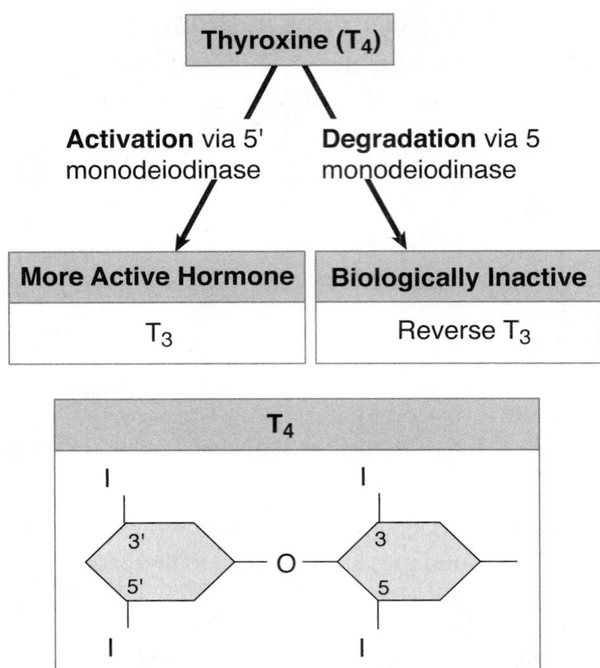

Figure X-8-7. Peripheral Conversion of Thyroid Hormone

Certain clinical states are associated with a reduction in the conversion of T4 into T3, often with an enhanced conversion of T4 into rT3 (low T3 syndrome). Such states would include fasting, medical and surgical stresses, catabolic diseases, and even excess secretion of cortisol could be included here. The result is a reduction in metabolic rate and a conservation of energy resources. In the early stages, the circulating T4 is normal but in many cases as the metabolic problem or stress becomes more severe, T4 can fall as well.

PHYSIOLOGIC ACTIONS OF THYROID HORMONES

In many tissues, thyroid hormones are not the prime indicators or the major inhibitors of specific cellular processes. Rather, a multitude of processes function properly only when optimal amounts of thyroid hormones are present. This underscores the permissive nature of thyroid hormones.

Metabolic Rate

- Thyroid hormones increase metabolic rate, as evidenced by increased O_2 consumption and heat production.
- Thyroid hormones increase the activity of the membrane-bound Na/K^- ATPase in many tissues, and it can be argued that it is the increased pumping of Na^+ that accounts for most of the increase in metabolic rate.
- The increase in metabolic rate produced by a single dose of T4 occurs only after a latency of several hours but may last 6 days or more.
- Thyroid hormones are absolutely necessary for normal brain maturation and essential for normal menstrual cycles. Hypothyroidism leads to menstrual irregularities (menorrhagia) and infertility (anovulatory cycles).

Growth and Maturation (T4 and T3 Anabolic Hormones)

Fetal growth rates appear normal in the absence of thyroid hormone production (i.e., if the fetus is hypothyroid). However, without adequate thyroid hormones during the perinatal period, abnormalities rapidly develop in nervous system maturation.

- Synapses develop abnormally and there is decreased dendritic branching and myelination. These abnormalities lead to mental retardation.
- These neural changes are irreversible and lead to cretinism unless replacement therapy is started soon after birth.

Lipid Metabolism

- Thyroid hormone accelerates cholesterol clearance from the plasma.
- Thyroid hormones are required for conversion of carotene to vitamin A, and, as a consequence, hypothyroid individuals can suffer from night blindness and yellowing of the skin.

CHO Metabolism

- Thyroid hormone increases the rate of glucose absorption from the small intestine.

Cardiovascular Effects

- Thyroid hormones have positive inotropic and chronotropic effects on the heart.
- The increased contractility is partly direct and partly indirect: they increase the number and affinity of β-adrenergic receptors in the heart, thereby increasing the sensitivity to catecholamines.
- Acting on the SA node, they directly increase heart rate.
- Cardiac output is increased, and both heart rate and stroke volume are elevated.
- Systolic pressure increases are due to increased stroke volume, and diastolic pressure decreases are due to decreased peripheral resistance.
- Thyroid hormones in the normal range are required for optimum cardiac performance.

Additional Effects

- Thyroid hormones maintain the ventilatory response to hypoxia, increase erythropoietin, and increase gut motility and bone turnover.
- Hypothyroidism is associated with an increased prolactin. TRH in excess amounts will stimulate prolactin.

CONTROL OF THYROID HORMONE SECRETION

Feedback Relationships

Figure X-8-8 shows the overall control of thyroid function.

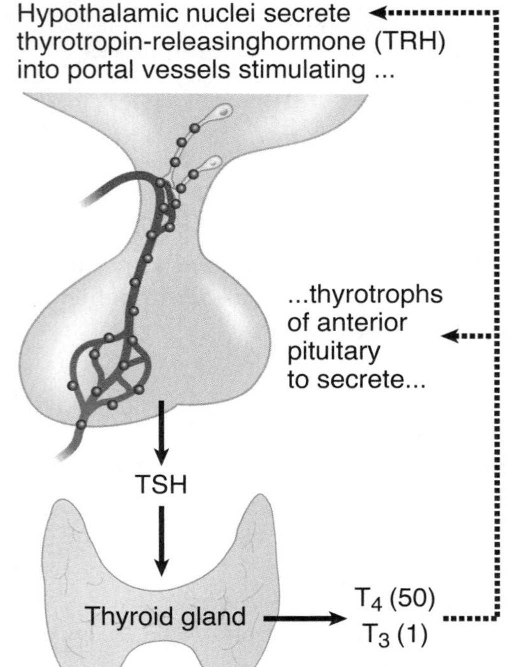
Hypothalamic nuclei secrete
thyrotropin-releasinghormone (TRH)
into portal vessels stimulating ...
...thyrotrophs
of anterior
pituitary
to secrete...
TSH
Within the thyrotroph, thyroid hormones decrease the sensitivity of the thyrotroph to TRH, thereby decreasing TSH secretion.
Thyroid gland
T_4 (50)
T_3 (1)

Figure X-8-8. Hypothalamic–Pituitary Control of Thyroid-Hormone Secretion

- TRH provides a constant and necessary stimulus for TSH secretion. In the absence of TRH, the secretion of TSH (and T4) decreases to very low levels. The target tissue for TSH is the thyroid, where it increases the secretion of thyroid hormone, T4 being the predominant form.
- Negative feedback of thyroid hormones is exerted mainly at the level of the anterior pituitary gland.
- Because the main circulating form is T4, it is T4 that is responsible for most of the negative feedback.
- However, within the thyrotrophs the T4 is converted to T3 before it acts to reduce the sensitivity of the thyrotroph to TRH.
- As long as circulating free T4 remains normal, changes in circulating T3 have minimal effects on TSH secretion. However, TSH secretion increases if there is a significant drop in circulating free T4, even in the presence of an increase in circulating T3.

Overall Effects of Thyrotropin (TSH) on the Thyroid

Rapidly induced TSH effects

TSH tends to rapidly increase (within minutes or an hour) all steps in the synthesis and degradation of thyroid hormones, including:

- Iodide trapping
- Thyroglobulin synthesis and exocytosis into the follicular lumen
- Pinocytotic reuptake of iodinated thyroglobulin back into the thyroid follicular cell
- Secretion of T4 into the blood

Slowly induced TSH effects

Changes that occur more slowly (hours or days) in response to TSH include:

- Increased blood flow to the thyroid gland
- Increased hypertrophy or hyperplasia of the thyroid cells, which initially leads to increased size of the gland or goiter

Tests of Thyroid Function

- Determining the serum TSH is the first step in evaluating thyroid function.
- Secondly, free T4 (FT4) measurements are now readily available and would confirm an initial conclusion based on the TSH measurement. An alternative test would be an index of the free T4 via resin uptake.
- Autoimmune thyroid disease is sometimes detected by measuring circulating antibodies. Most notably are the TPO antibodies, which are elevated in Hashimoto's thyroiditis (hypothyroidism) and Graves' disease (hyperthyroidism).
- Additional antibodies are those against thyroglobulin and the TSI antibodies that stimulate the TSH receptor in Graves' disease.
- Uptake of iodine isotopes by the thyroid allows thyroid imaging and quantitation of tracer uptake.
- Subacute thyroiditis: overall a below-normal uptake of isotope
- Graves' disease: increased tracer uptake that is distributed evenly throughout the enlarged gland
- Toxic adenomas: local areas of increased uptake with below-normal uptake in the remainder of the gland
- Toxic multinodular goiter: enlarged gland that often has an abnormal architecture and with multiple areas of high and low uptake.

PATHOLOGIC CHANGES IN THYROID HORMONE SECRETION

Table X-8-1. Changes in Feedback Relationships in Several Disorders

	T4	TSH	TRH
Primary hypothyroidism	↓	↑	↑
Pituitary hypothyroidism (secondary)	↓	↓	↑
Pituitary hyperthyroidism (secondary)	↑	↑	↓
Graves' disease (autoimmune)	↑	↓	↓

A goiter can develop in all of the disorders shown in the preceding table except secondary and tertiary hypothyroidism.

Thyroidal Response to Low Intake of Iodine

In most cases, if iodine is deficient in the diet but not absent, the individual will remain euthyroid but will develop a goiter. The changes are shown in Figure X-8-9. The adaptive sequence occurs when dietary intake of iodine is deficient. The sequence of events begins with 1 (decreased secretion of T4) and proceeds through 4, the development of a goiter.

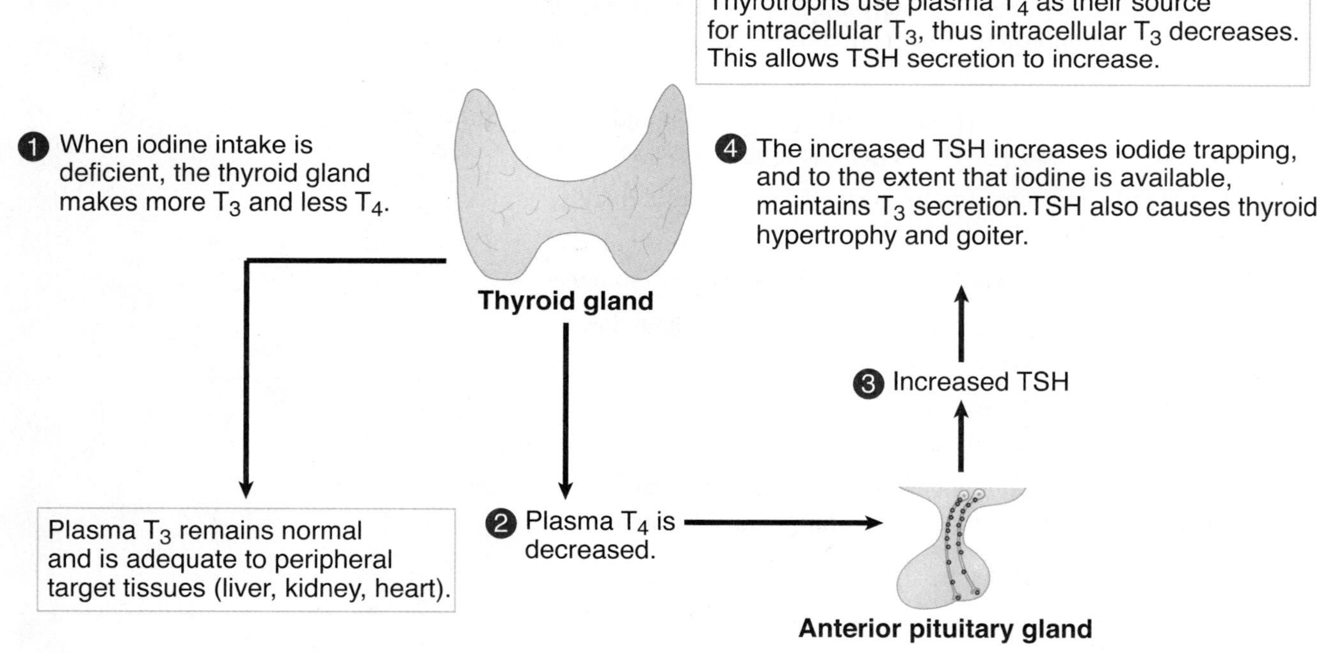
Thyrotrophs use plasma T_4 as their source for intracellular T_3, thus intracellular T_3 decreases. This allows TSH secretion to increase.
1 When iodine intake is deficient, the thyroid gland makes more T_3 and less T_4.
Thyroid gland
4 The increased TSH increases iodide trapping, and to the extent that iodine is available, maintains T_3 secretion. TSH also causes thyroid hypertrophy and goiter.
3 Increased TSH
Plasma T_3 remains normal and is adequate to peripheral target tissues (liver, kidney, heart).
2 Plasma T_4 is decreased.
Anterior pituitary gland

Figure X-8-9. Iodine Deficiency

Primary Hypothyroidism

Primary changes and clinical presentation

- Most common cause is Hashimoto's thyroiditis, an autoimmune destruction of the thyroid with lymphocytic infiltration; ↑ TPO antibodies; early stages have a diffusely enlarged thyroid progressing in the later stages to a smaller atrophic and fibrotic gland.
- ↑ TSH, ↓ FT4; in subclinical hypothyroidism the TSH is on the high side of normal and the FT4 is on the low side of normal.
- Decreased basal metabolic rate and oxygen consumption
- Plasma cholesterol and other blood lipids tend to be elevated.
- Increased TRH drives a hyperprolactinemia. In women it may result in amenorrhea with galactorrhea; more often anovulatory cycles with menorrhagia. In men infertility and gynecomastia.
- Decreased GFR and an inability to excrete a water load, which may lead to hyponatremia.
- Inability to convert carotene to vitamin A may cause yellowing of the skin and night blindness.
- Slow thinking and lethargy; some patients have severe mental symptoms, dementia, or psychosis ("myxedema madness")
- Decreased food intake but individuals tend to be overweight
- Deep tendon reflexes with slow relaxation phase
- In the early stages, a decreased cardiac performance due to diminished contractility. In the later stages, cardiac features suggestive of cardiomyopathy
- Anemia, constipation, hoarseness in speech, and the skin is dry and cool
- A decreased ventilatory drive to hypercapnia and hypoxia
- Accumulation of subcutaneous mucopolysaccharides that give rise to a nonpitting edema (myxedema)
- Myxedema coma is the end stage of untreated hypothyroidism. The major features are hypoventilation, fluid and electrolyte imbalances, and hypothermia and ultimately shock and death.

Cretinism

- Untreated postnatal hypothyroidism results in cretinism, a form of dwarfism with mental retardation.
- Individuals often appear normal following delivery but may display some respiratory difficulty, jaundice, feeding problems, and hypotonia.
- Abnormalities rapidly develop in nervous system maturation, which are irreversible and result in mental retardation.
- Prepubertal growth, including bone ossification, is retarded in the absence of thyroid hormones. A stippled epiphysis is a sign of hypothyroidism in children.
- There is no evidence that thyroid hormones act directly on growth or bone formation. Rather, thyroid hormone appears to be permissive or act synergistically with growth hormone or growth factors acting directly on bone. Thyroid hormone is required for normal synthesis and secretion of growth hormone.

- Acquired hypothyroidism during childhood results in dwarfism but there is no mental retardation.
- At puberty, increased androgen secretion drives an increased growth hormone secretion. This will not occur with depressed levels of thyroid hormones.

Additional causes of hypothyroidism

- Secondary generally associated with panhypopituitarism
- Secondary or tertiary characterized by ↓ FT4 and inappropriately normal TSH.
- Severe iodine deficiency (not in the United States)
- Drug induced, e.g., lithium
- Failure to escape from the Wolff-Chaikoff effect following excessive iodine intake
- Rarely there can be resistance to thyroid hormone

Treatment

- Replacement doses of T4. The goal is to give enough T4 to normalize serum TSH.
- Because metabolism of T4 decreases and the plasma half-life increases with age, higher doses of T4 are required in younger individuals.
- Overall levels of TSH must be checked on occasion to make sure of the proper dosage of T4.
- In women beyond menopause, overprescribing T4 can contribute to the development of osteoporosis.

Primary Hyperthyroidism (Graves' Disease)

- Thyrotoxicosis by definition is the clinical syndrome whereby tissues are exposed to high levels of thyroid hormone (= hyperthyroidism)
- The most common cause of thyrotoxicosis is Graves' disease, a primary hyperthyroidism.
- Graves' disease is an autoimmune problem in which one antibody is directed against the thyroid receptor. It is referred to as the thyroid stimulating antibody (TSI or TSH-R).
- In addition TPO antibodies and those against thyroglobulin are also found in Graves' disease.
- ↑ FT4, ↓ TSH; it is the TSI stimulating the TSH receptor on the thyroid that is driving the hyperthyroidism.
- In Graves' disease the thyroid is symmetrically enlarged.
- Increased radioiodine uptake by the thyroid and decreased serum cholesterol.
- Only Graves' disease has thyroid-stimulating antibodies. The only types of hyperthyroidism with increased radioactive iodine uptake are Graves' disease and toxic nodular goiter.
  - Subacute thyroiditis and "silent" or "painless" thyroiditis do not have increased radioactive iodine uptake; they are "leaking" of thyroid hormone out of a gland damaged by antibodies.

- Increased metabolic rate and heat production. Individuals tend to seek a cool environment.
- Cardiac output, contractility, and heart rate are increased with possibly palpitations and arrhythmias (increased β-adrenergic stimulation)
- Many symptoms suggest a state of excess catecholamines but circulating catecholamines are usually normal.
- Weight loss with increased food intake, protein wasting, and muscle weakness.
- Tremor, nervousness, and excessive sweating.
- The wide-eyed stare (exophthalmos) in patients with Graves' is caused by an infiltration of orbital soft tissues and extraocular muscles and the resulting edema, and this process is caused by the antibodies.
- Untreated hyperthyroidism may decompensate into a condition called "thyroid storm."
- The end-stage of Graves' disease is often a hypothyroidism.

Acute treatment

- Beta blockers are the most rapid in effect
- Methimazole or propylthiouracil stops the production of hormone
- Iodine in high dose stops incorporation of iodine into the gland
- Steroids such as dexamethasone stop conversion of T4 to T3
- Long-term permanent cure is ablation of the gland with radioactive iodine

Additional origins of hyperthyroidism (thyrotoxicosis)

- Autonomously functioning thyroid adenoma
- Toxic multinodular goiter
- Subacute and silent thyroiditis
- TSH-secreting pituitary adenoma (secondary hyperthyroidism) (very rare)

Goiter

- A goiter is simply an enlarged thyroid and does not designate functional status. A goiter can be present in hypo-, hyper-, and euthyroid states. There is no correlation between thyroid size and function.
- A generalized enlargement of the thyroid is considered a "diffuse goiter."
- Diffuse enlargement often results from prolonged stimulation by TSH or TSH-like factor; e.g., Hashimoto's thyroiditis, Graves' disease, diet deficient in iodine
- An irregular or lumpy enlargement of the thyroid is considered a "nodular goiter."
- With time, excessive stimulation by TSH can result in a multinodular goiter e.g. iodine deficiency initially produces a diffuse nontoxic goiter. Long term however, focal hyperplasia with necrosis and hemorrhage results in the formation of nodules. Nodules vary from "hot nodules" that can trap iodine to "cold nodules " that cannot trap iodine.

Chapter Summary

- Thyroid hormones are anabolic and are required for normal growth and maturation.
- Thyroid follicles store several months supply of thyroid hormone.
- The thyroid synthesizes and releases mainly T4 but on an iodine-deficient diet, the production and release of T3, a more active form of the hormone, increases.
- Most of the activity of T4 is due to the peripheral conversion to T3.
- Thyroid hormones increase metabolic rate, conversion of carotene to vitamin A and increase cardiac performance.
- Thyroid hormone is required for postnatal brain maturation. Cretinism is a form of dwarfism with mental retardation.
- Circulating T4 creates most of the negative feedback to the anterior pituitary but the T4 entering the thyrotropes must be converted into T3 before it creates negative feedback.
- Tests of thyroid function focus on the circulating TSH and FT4.
- Primary hypothyroidism is mainly due to Hashimoto's thyroiditis and results in decreased FT4 and increased TSH.
- Primary hyperthyroidism is mainly due to Graves' disease. The autoimmune factor stimulating the thyroid increases FT4 and decreases TSH.
- A goiter, which can be described as diffuse or nodular, is simply an enlarged thyroid and does not designate functional status.
- Individuals on an iodine-deficient diet develop large goiters but they are usually euthyroid.

Growth, Growth Hormone, and Puberty

9

Learning Objectives

- ❏ Explain information related to in-utero and prepubertal growth
- ❏ Explain information related to physiologic actions of growth hormone
- ❏ Use knowledge of control of growth hormone secretion
- ❏ Answer questions about puberty
- ❏ Use knowledge of acromegaly

IN-UTERO AND PREPUBERTAL GROWTH

Intrauterine Growth

- Important roles for growth hormone, IGF-II (early in gestation), IGF-I (later in gestation) and insulin
- Infants of diabetic mothers have increased insulin levels and are large.
- Smoking decreases vascularity of the placenta and decreases birth weight.
- Poor maternal nutrition leading cause of low birth weight worldwide.

Postnatal Growth

- Although fetal hypothyroidism does not decrease birth weight, hypothyroidism following delivery causes irreversible abnormalities in nervous system maturation, which in turn lead to mental retardation (cretinism).
- Growth hormone, insulin, and thyroid hormone play major roles. Acquired hypothyroidism later in childhood will slow growth and reduce bone advancement more than growth hormone deficiency, but will not cause mental retardation.
- Replacement of hormone deficiencies creates a period of catch-up growth, but it is soon replaced with a normal growth rate.
- There is no major role for gonadal sex steroids on prepubertal growth or for glucocorticoids but glucocorticoid excess will slow growth.
- Hypersecretion of growth hormone pre-puberty (pituitary adenoma) results in giantism. It also delays pubertal changes, and the subsequent hypogonadism contributes to the giantism.

Prepubertal Growth Hormone Deficiency

- Deficiencies can be congenital (decreased birth length), idiopathic (low GHRH), or acquired (hypothalamic-pituitary tumor).
- A deficiency causes dwarfism, which is characterized by: short stature, chubby, immature facial appearance, delayed skeletal maturation, and tendency to episodes of hypoglycemia.
- Tissue resistance to growth hormone (↑ growth hormone, ↓ IGF-I) results in Laron syndrome (Laron dwarfism).
- Stimulation test is with an arginine infusion.
- Growth hormone deficiency following puberty decreases lean body mass, and replacement therapy is now considered an acceptable treatment.
- Treatment of GH deficiency is simple replacement of GH.
- Treatment of Laron dwarfism (lack of GH receptor) is synthetic IGF. Mecasermin is the name of recombinant IGF.

PHYSIOLOGIC ACTIONS OF GROWTH HORMONE

Growth hormone is a major anabolic growth-promoting hormone and a stress hormone. All anabolic hormones (i.e., growth hormone, insulin, thyroid hormones, and androgens) are required for normal growth. The major stress and anabolic actions of growth hormone are shown in Figure X-9-1. This figure shows that most of the direct actions of growth hormone are consistent with its actions as a stress hormone. A direct anabolic action is the promotion of amino acid entry into cells, thus making them more available for protein synthesis. However, most of the anabolic actions of growth hormone are indirect via the production of growth factors.

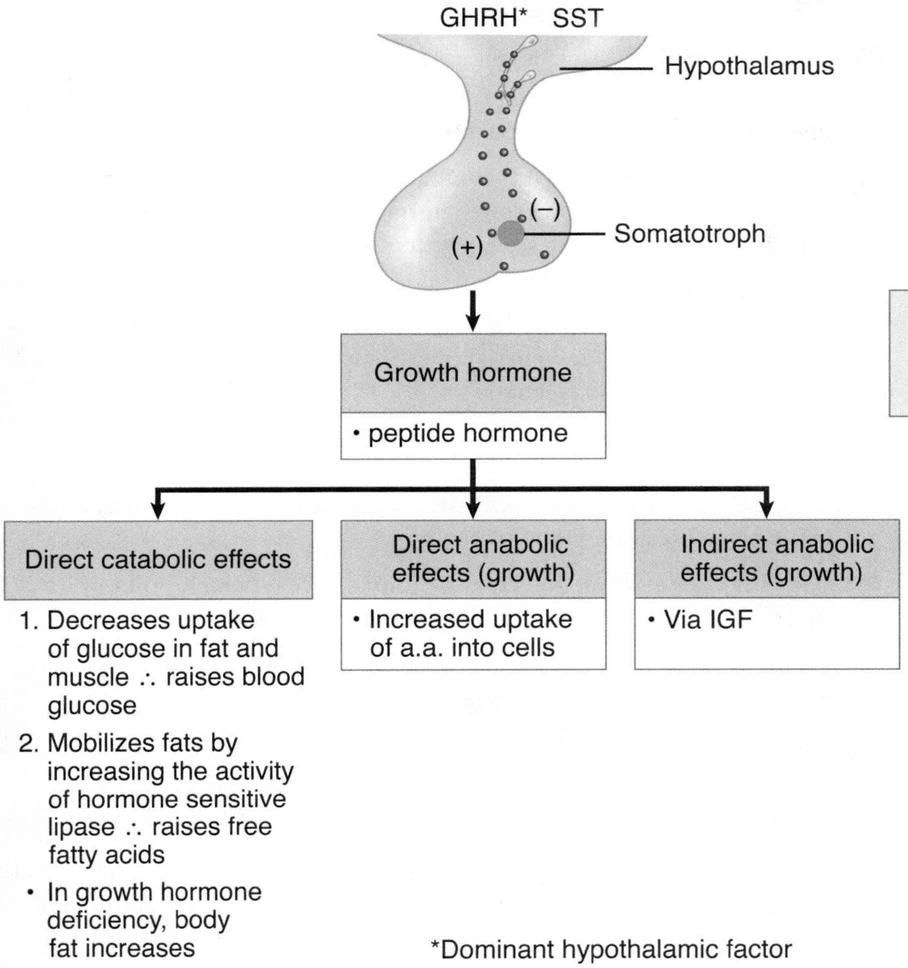

GHRH* SST
Hypothalamus
(–)
(+)
Somatotroph
Growth hormone
• peptide hormone
Direct catabolic effects
1. Decreases uptake of glucose in fat and muscle ∴ raises blood glucose
2. Mobilizes fats by increasing the activity of hormone sensitive lipase ∴ raises free fatty acids
• In growth hormone deficiency, body fat increases
Direct anabolic effects (growth)
• Increased uptake of a.a. into cells
Indirect anabolic effects (growth)
• Via IGF
*Dominant hypothalamic factor

Figure X-9-1. Overview of Growth Hormone

GHRH = growth hormone-releasing hormone

SST = somatostatin

Indirect Anabolic Actions of Growth Hormone

Most of the anabolic actions of growth hormone are an indirect result of increased production of insulin-like growth factors (IGFs). A major growth factor is IGF-I.

The steps in the production and release of IGF-I are shown in Figure X-9-2.

GH
acts on
Liver and other tissues (e.g., skeletal muscle)
Increased production and release of
Growth factors (especially IGF-I)

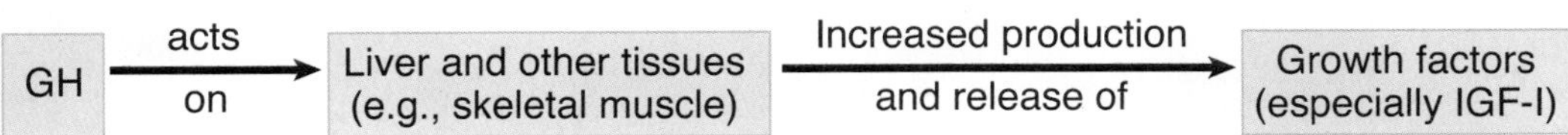

Figure X-9-2. IGF-Mediated Effects of Growth Hormone

Specific Properties of the IGFs

IGF-I is a major anabolic growth factor. It has the following characteristics:

- A circulating peptide growth factor similar in structure to proinsulin and has some insulin-like activity
- Circulates in the blood tightly bound to a large protein, whose production is also dependent on growth hormone. Protein binding increases the half-life and thus serves as a better 24-hour marker of GH (half-life 15–20 minutes).
- The major known anabolic effect of IGF-I is that it increases the synthesis of cartilage (chondrogenesis) in the epiphyseal platès of long bones, thereby increasing bone length.
- It is also hypothesized that circulating IGFs increase lean body mass. The decreased lean body mass of aging may, in part, be due to the concomitant decrease in IGFs. IGFs also decrease in catabolic states, especially protein-calorie malnutrition.
- IGF-II is another growth factor, the importance of which is not well understood but may have a role in fetal development.

CONTROL OF GROWTH HORMONE (GH) SECRETION

- GH secretion is pulsatile. The secretory pulses are much more likely to occur during the night in stages III and IV (non-REM) of sleep than during the day.
- Secretion of GH requires the presence of normal plasma levels of thyroid hormones. GH secretion is markedly reduced in hypothyroid individuals.
- During the sixth decade of life and later, GH secretion diminishes considerably in both men and women. What initiates this decrease is unknown.

Each of the promoters could act by increasing GHRH secretion, decreasing SST secretion, or both.

Notice that most of the factors that regulate GH secretion are identical to those that regulate glucagon (except for those boxed). These factors are consistent with their shared role as stress hormones.

The inhibitory effect of IGF-I represents a negative feedback loop to the hypothalamus.

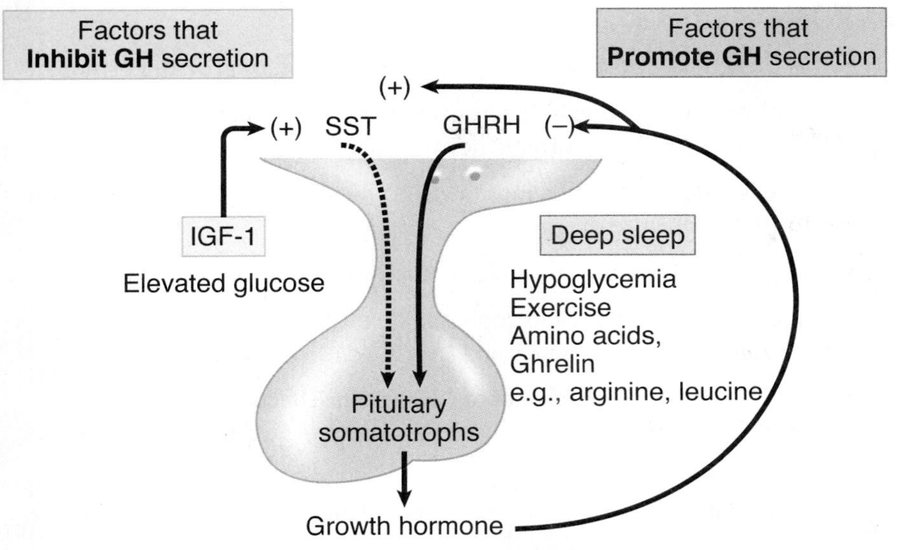

Figure X-9-3. Control of Growth Hormone Secretion

SST = somatostatin

PUBERTY

Reproductive Changes

- Hypothalamic pulse generator increases activity just before physical changes at puberty.
- First noted sign in a female is breast development; first by estrogen (promotes duct growth) then progesterone (promotes development of milk-producing alveolar cells). First noted sign in a male is enlargement of the testes (mainly FSH stimulating seminiferous tubules).
- Pubic hair development in males and females is dependent on androgen.

Growth Changes

- During puberty, androgens promote the secretion in the following anabolic sequence:

At puberty, if T4 is normal, ↑ androgens drive ↑ growth hormone, which drives ↑ IGF-I.

- IGF-I is the major stimulus for cell division of the cartilage-synthesizing cells located in the epiphyseal plates of long bones.
- In males, the increased androgen arises from the testes (testosterone); in females, from the adrenals (adrenarche).
- Near the end of puberty, androgens promote the mineralization (fusion or closure) of the epiphyseal plates of long bones. Estrogen can also cause plate closure, even in men.
- In females, the growth spurt begins early in puberty and is near completion by menarche. In males, the growth spurt develops near the end of puberty.

ACROMEGALY

- It is caused by a post pubertal excessive secretion of growth hormone.
- It is almost always due to macroadenoma (> 1 cm dia) of the anterior pituitary and second in frequency to prolactinomas.
- There is a slow onset of symptoms, and the disease is usually present for 5 to 10 years before diagnosis.
- Ectopic GHRH secretion has been documented but is rare.
- Some tumors contain lactotrophs, and elevated prolactin can cause hypogonadism and galactorrhea.
- Increased IGF-I causes most of the deleterious effects of acromegaly but growth hormone excess directly causes the hyperglycemia and insulin resistance.
- There is characteristic proliferation of cartilage, bone and soft tissue, visceral, and cardiomegaly.
- Observable changes include enlargement of the hands and feet (acral parts) and coarsening of the facial features, including downward and forward growth of the mandible. Also, increased hat size.
- Measurement of IGF-I is a useful screening measure and confirms diagnosis with the lack of growth hormone suppression by oral glucose.
- Diagnosis: Treatment should only be done when 3 steps are completed:
  - Elevated IGF level
  - Failure of suppression of GH/IGF after giving glucose
  - MRI shows lesion in brain in pituitary
- Never start with a scan in endocrinology. Benign pituitary "incidentaloma" is common in 2–10% of the population. Always confirm the presence of an overproduction of a hormone before doing a scan. This is true for adrenal lesions as well.
- Treatment:
  - Surgical removal by trans-sphenoidal approach is first. Removal of an over-producing adenoma is the first treatment in most of endocrinology with the exception of prolactinoma.
  - If surgical removal fails, use the growth hormone receptor antagonist, pegvisomant, or octreotide. Octreotide is synthetic somatostatin. Cabergoline is a dopamine agonist used when other medications have failed.
  - Radiation is used last, only after surgery, pegvisomant, octreotide and cabergoline have failed.

Chapter Summary

- Anabolic hormones except thyroid hormone are required for intrauterine growth.
- Thyroid hormone is required in the perinatal period to prevent mental retardation.
- Sex steroids have no major role prepuberty.
- Excess glucocorticoids slow growth.
- Excess growth hormone accelerates growth, delays pubertal changes, and creates gigantism.
- Prepubertal growth hormone deficiency or tissue resistance to growth hormone (Laron syndrome) leads to dwarfism.
- Most of the direct actions of growth hormone are consistent with its actions as a stress hormone; i.e., it decreases the peripheral uptake of glucose and promotes lipolysis.
- Most of the anabolic actions of growth hormone are indirect via growth factors.
- The most important growth factor is IGF-I, which increases the synthesis of cartilage in the epiphyseal plates of long bones.
- Growth hormone secretion is pulsatile and a great deal is released during the night.
- Plasma IGF-I is usually a good index of overall growth hormone secretion.
- The first noted female change at puberty is breast development; in the male it is testes enlargement.
- The increased secretion of growth hormone during puberty is driven by a concurrent increase in androgen secretion.
- The acute factors regulating growth hormone secretion are similar to those regulating glucagon and are consistent with their role as stress hormones.
- Acromegaly is almost always due to pituitary adenoma and most of the deleterious effects due to IGF-I. Noted changes include acral enlargement and coarse facial features. Measurement of IGF-I is useful screening, lack of growth hormone suppression by oral glucose diagnostic.

Male Reproductive System 10

Learning Objectives

- ❑ Solve problems concerning hypothalamic-pituitary-gonadal axis in males
- ❑ Solve problems concerning age-related hormonal changes in males
- ❑ Demonstrate understanding of erection, emission, and ejaculation
- ❑ Use knowledge of gonadal dysfunction in the male

HYPOTHALAMIC-PITUITARY-GONADAL (HPG) AXIS IN MALES

The factors involved in the overall control of adult male hormone secretion are summarized in Figure X-10-1.

Note

LH, FSH, TSH, and human chorionic gonadotropin (hCG) are glycoproteins with identical alpha subunits. The beta subunits differ and thus confer specificity.

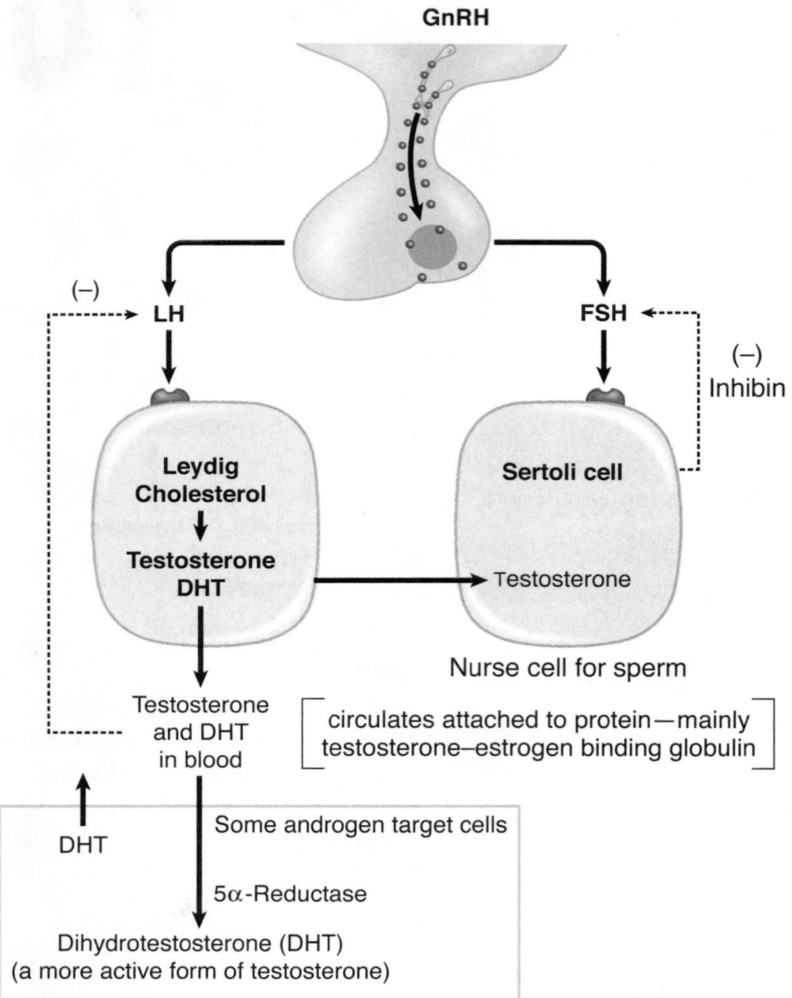

GnRH—synthesized in preoptic region of hypothalamus and secreted in pulses into hypophyseal portal vessels

- produces pulsatile release of LH and FSH
- pulsatile release of GnRH prevents downregulation of its receptors in anterior pituitary

LH and **FSH**—produced and secreted by gonadotrophs of anterior pituitary

- LH stimulates Leydig cells to produce testosterone.
- FSH stimulates Sertoli cells (see below).

Leydig cell testosterone—some diffuses directly to Sertoli cells, where it is required for Sertoli cell function.

- produces negative feedback for LH

Sertoli cell inhibin B—produces negative feedback for FSH

Figure X-10-1. Control of Testes

LH/Leydig Cells

- Leydig cells express receptors for LH
- LH is a peptide hormone that activates Gs--cAMP, which in turn initiates testosterone production by activating steroidogenic acute regulatory protein (StAR).
- Testosterone diffuses into Sertoli cells (high concentration) and into the blood.
- Circulating testosterone provides negative feedback to regulate LH secretion at the level of the hypothalamus and anterior pituitary.
- Leydig cells aromatize some of this testosterone into estradiol (see Figure X-10-2).

5α-reductase

Some target tissue express this enzyme, which converts testosterone into the more potent dihydrotestosterone. Some important physiologic effects primarily mediated by dihydrotestosterone are as follows:

- Sexual differentiation: differentiation to form male external genitalia
- Growth of the prostate
- Male-pattern baldness
- Increased activity of sebaceous glands
- Synthesis of NO synthase in penile tissue

FSH/Sertoli Cells

- FSH binds to Sertoli cells and activates a Gs--cAMP pathway.
- Sertoli cells release inhibin B, which has negative feedback on FSH secretion.

Hormonal Control of Testicular Function

Figure X-10-2 illustrates the source and nature of the hormones controlling testicular function.

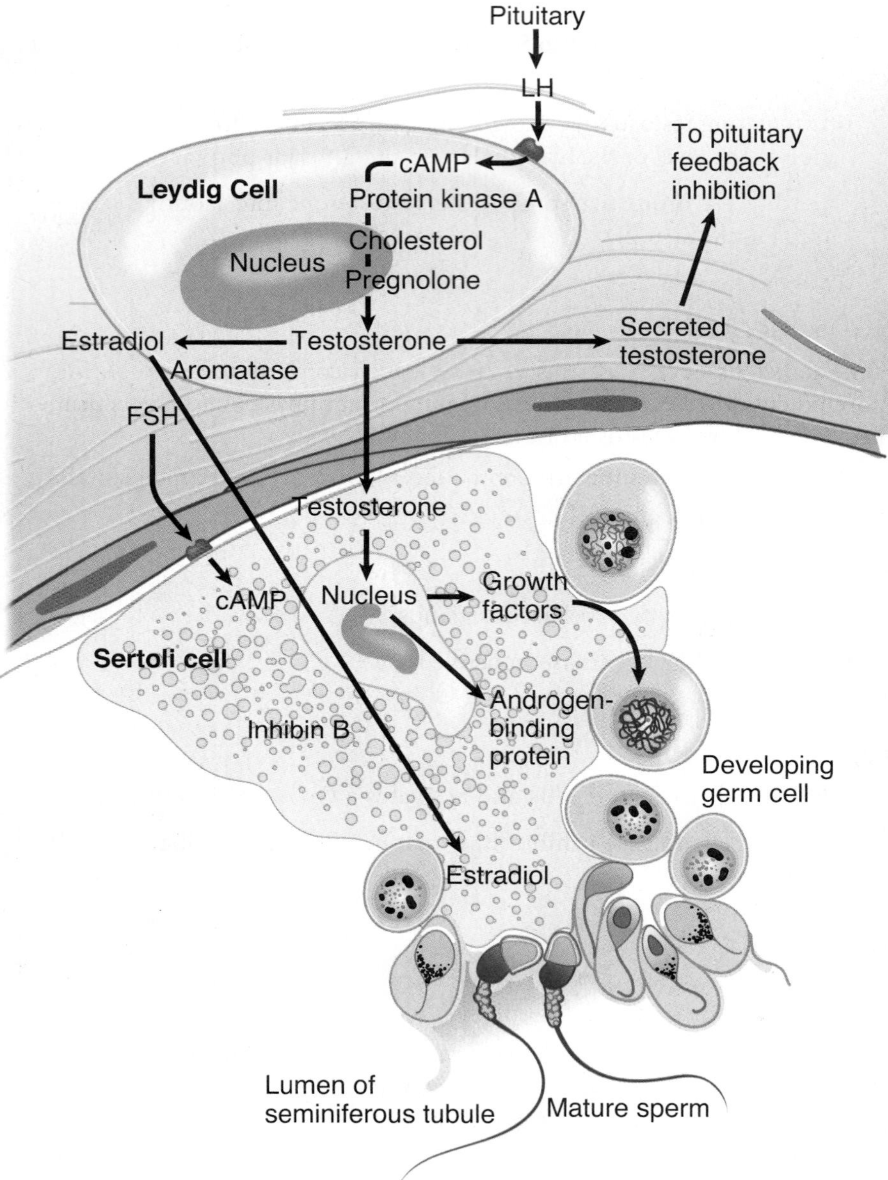

Figure X-10-2. Endocrine Function of Testes

Note

Sertoli cells provide the nourishment that is required for normal spermatogenesis.

- FSH, along with a very high level of testosterone from the neighboring Leydig cells, produces growth factors necessary for growth and maturation of the sperm.
- FSH and testosterone induce the synthesis of androgen binding protein, which helps maintain high local levels of testosterone.
- Leydig cells express aromatase, which aromatizes testosterone into estradiol, an important hormone for growth and maturation of the sperm.
- Sertoli cells secrete inhibin B, which produces feedback regulation on FSH.

Definitions

Androgen: any steroid that controls the development and maintenance of masculine characteristics

Testosterone: a natural male androgen of testicular origin, controlled by the luteinizing hormone (LH)

Dihydrotestosterone: a more active form of testosterone made by 5-alpha-reductase. Dihydrotestosterone makes the penis, prostate, and scrotum on an embryo.

Methyl testosterone: a synthetic androgen, which is an anabolic steroid sometimes used by athletes

Adrenal androgens: natural weak androgens (male and female) of adrenal origin, controlled by ACTH. These are DHEA and androstenedione.

Inhibins: peptide hormones secreted into the blood. They inhibit the secretion of FSH by pituitary gonadotrophs.

Aromatase: an enzyme that stimulates the aromatization of the A-ring of testosterone, converting it into estradiol. The physiologic importance of this conversion is not understood; however, approximately a third of the estradiol in the blood of men arises from Sertoli cells, and the remainder arises from peripheral conversion of testosterone to estradiol by an aromatase present in adipose tissue. One sign of a Sertoli cell tumor is excessive estradiol in the blood of the affected man.

AGE-RELATED HORMONAL CHANGES IN MALES

Figure X-10-3 depicts the relative plasma LH and testosterone concentrations throughout the life of the normal human male. The numbers refer to the descriptions that follow the figure.

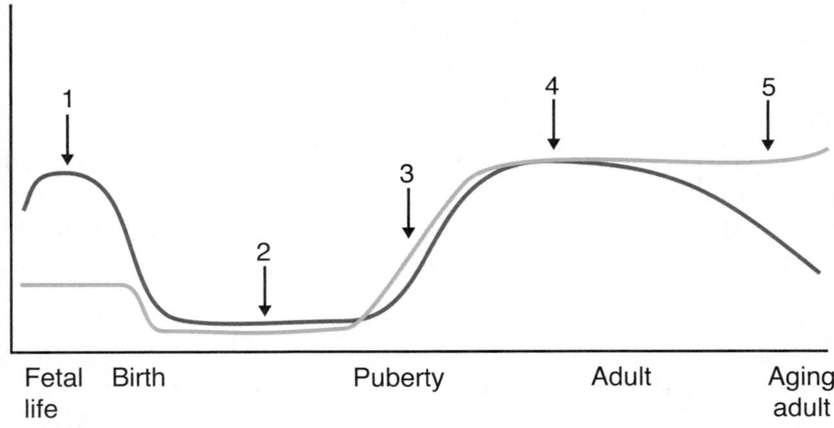

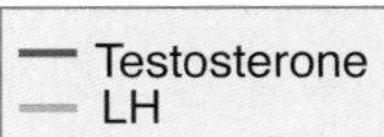

Figure X-10-3. Development and Aging in Male Reproduction

1. Fetal life

The development of male and female internal and external structures depends on the fetal hormonal environment. The Wolffian and Müllerian ducts are initially present in both male and female fetuses. If there is no hormonal input (the situation in the normal female fetus), female internal and female external structures develop (Müllerian ducts develop, Wolffian ducts regress).

Normal male development requires the presence of 3 hormones: testosterone, dihydrotestosterone, and the Müllerian inhibiting factor (MIF).

1. (hCG) + LH → Leydig cells → testosterone → Wolffian ducts
2. testosterone $\xrightarrow{5\text{-}\alpha\text{-reductase}}$ dihydrotestosterone → urogenital sinus & genital organs
3. Sertoli cells → MIF → absence of female internal structures

MIF prevents the development of the Müllerian ducts, which would otherwise differentiate into female internal structures. In the absence of MIF, the Müllerian ducts develop. Thus, in addition to normal male structures, a uterus will be present.

- Wolffian ducts differentiate into the majority of male internal structures; namely, epididymis, vas deferens, and seminal vesicles.
  - In the absence of testosterone, the Wolffian ducts regress.
- Dihydrotestosterone induces the urogenital sinus and genital tubercle to differentiate into the external scrotum, penis, and prostate gland.
  - In the absence of dihydrotestosterone, female external structures develop.

2. Childhood

Within a few months after birth, LH and testosterone drop to low levels and remain low until puberty. The cause of this prolonged quiescence of reproductive hormone secretion during childhood is not known. Interestingly, LH secretion remains low in spite of low testosterone.

3. Puberty

Near the onset of puberty, the amplitude of the LH pulses becomes greater, driving the mean level of LH higher. Early in puberty, this potentiation of the LH pulses is especially pronounced during sleep. This increased LH stimulates the Leydig cells to again secrete testosterone.

4. Adult

During adulthood, LH secretion drives testosterone secretion. Thus, it is not surprising that the relative levels of the two hormones parallel one another.

5. Aging adult

Testosterone and inhibin secretions decrease with age. Men in their seventies generally secrete only 60–70% as much testosterone as do men in their twenties. Nevertheless, there is no abrupt decrease in testosterone secretion in men that parallels the relatively abrupt decrease in estrogen secretion that women experience at menopause. The loss of feedback will cause an increase in LH and FSH secretion.

Effect on Muscle Mass

The capacity of androgens to stimulate protein synthesis and decrease protein breakdown, especially in muscle, is responsible for the larger muscle mass in men as compared with women. Exogenous androgens (anabolic steroids) are sometimes taken by men and women in an attempt to increase muscle mass.

Spermatogenesis Is Temperature Dependent

Effect on fertility

For unknown reasons, spermatogenesis ceases at temperatures typical of the abdominal cavity. Thus, when the testes fail to descend before or shortly after birth, and the condition (cryptorchidism) is not surgically corrected, infertility results.

Cooling mechanisms

Normally, the scrotum provides an environment that is 4°C cooler than the abdominal cavity. The cooling is accomplished by a countercurrent heat exchanger located in the spermatic cord. Also, the temperature of the scrotum and the testes is regulated by relative degree of contraction or relaxation of the cremasteric muscles and scrotal skin rugae that surround and suspend the testes.

Effect on FSH and LH

Sertoli cells, and therefore germ cell maturation, are adversely affected by the elevated temperatures of cryptorchid testes. In adults with bilaterally undescended testes, FSH secretion is elevated, probably as a result of decreased Sertoli cell production of inhibins. Testosterone secretion by the Leydig cells of cryptorchid testes also tends to be low, and as a result, LH secretion of adults with bilateral cryptorchidism is elevated.

ERECTION, EMISSION, AND EJACULATION

Erection

- Erection is caused by dilation of the blood vessels (a parasympathetic response) in the erectile tissue of the penis (the corpora- and ischiocavernous sinuses).
- This dilation increases the inflow of blood so much that the penile veins get compressed between the engorged cavernous spaces and the Buck's and dartos fasciae.
- Nitric oxide (NO), working through cGMP, mediates the vasodilation.

Emission

- Emission is the movement of semen from the epididymis, vas deferens, seminal vesicles, and prostate to the ejaculatory ducts.
- The movement is mediated by sympathetic (thoracolumbar) adrenergic transmitters.

- Simultaneously with emission, there is also a sympathetic adrenergic-mediated contraction of the internal sphincter of the bladder, which prevents retrograde ejaculation of semen into the bladder. Destruction of this sphincter by prostatectomy often results in retrograde ejaculation.
- Emission normally precedes ejaculation but also continues during ejaculation.

Ejaculation

- Ejaculation is caused by the rhythmic contraction of the bulbospongiosus and the ischiocavernous muscles, which surround the base of the penis.
- Contraction of these striated muscles that are innervated by somatic motor nerves causes the semen to exit rapidly in the direction of least resistance, i.e., outwardly through the urethra.

GONADAL DYSFUNCTION IN THE MALE

The consequences of deficient testosterone production depend upon the age of onset:

- Testosterone deficiency in the second to third month of gestation results in varying degrees of ambiguity in the male genitalia and male pseudohermaphrodism.
- Testosterone deficiency in the third trimester leads to problems in testicular descent (cryptorchidism) along with micropenis.
- Pubertal testosterone deficiency leads to poor secondary sexual development and overall eunuchoid features.
- Postpubertal testosterone deficiency leads to decreased libido, erectile dysfunction, decrease in facial and body hair growth, low energy, and infertility.

Causes of Hypogonadism

- Noonan syndrome
- Klinefelter's syndrome
- Hypothalamic-pituitary disorders (Kallman's syndrome, panhypopituitarism)
- Gonadal failure/sex steroid synthesis failure

Definitions

- Pseudohermaphrodite: an individual with the genetic constitution and gonads of one sex and the genitalia of the other.
- Female pseudohermaphroditism: female fetus exposed to androgens during the 8th to 13th week of development, e.g., congenital virilizing adrenal hyperplasia.
- Male pseudohermaphroditism: lack of androgen activity in male fetus, e.g., defective testes, androgen resistance
- When the loss of receptor function is complete, testicular feminizing syndrome results. Here MIF is present and testosterone is secreted, usually at elevated levels. The external structures are female, but the vagina ends blindly because there are no female internal structures.

Table X-10-1. Hormonal Changes in Specific Altered States

	Sex Steroids	LH	FSH
Primary hypogonadism	↓	↑	↑
Pituitary hypogonadism	↓	↓	↓
Kallman's (↓ GnRH)	↓	↓	↓
Postmenopausal women	↓	↑	↑
Anabolic steroid therapy (male)*	↑	↓	(↓)
Inhibin infusion (male)†	–	–	↓
GnRH infusion (constant rate)‡	↓	↓	↓
GnRH infusion (pulsatile)	↑	↑	↑

*LH suppression causes Leydig cell atrophy in an adult male and therefore reduced testicular androgen production. Because Leydig cell testosterone is required for spermatogenesis, anabolic steroids suppress spermatogenesis.

Although testosterone is not the normal feedback regulating FSH, high circulating testosterone activity will suppress the release of FSH.

†Because FSH is required for spermatogenesis, giving inhibin suppresses spermatogenesis.

‡A constant rate of infusion of the gonadotropin-releasing hormone (GnRH) will cause a transient increase in LH and FSH secretion, followed by a decrease caused by the downregulation of gonadotroph receptors.

Chapter Summary

- GnRH regulates the secretion of both FSH and LH. A pulsatile input of GnRH to the gonadotrophs is required to prevent downregulation of its receptors.
- LH stimulates Leydig cell testosterone, and testosterone is the negative feedback loop for LH. Sertoli cells possess FSH receptors, and inhibin B is the normal feedback loop for FSH.
- The testes secrete testosterone and some dihydrotestosterone (DHT). Most of the circulating DHT is due to the peripheral conversion of testosterone.
- Both FSH and Leydig cell testosterone are required for normal spermatogenesis.
- The fetal ovary does not secrete hormones. Regardless of genetics (i.e., XX or XY), without input of the male developmental hormones, the fetus will develop female internal and external structures.
- Normal male development requires testosterone (internal structures), dihydrotestosterone (external structures), and MIF (suppresses female internal structures).
- Erection is mainly a parasympathetic response, whereas ejaculation requires sympathetic involvement.
- Hypogonadism can have many origins, including genetic, structural, environmental, and hormonal.

Female Reproductive System 11

Learning Objectives

- ❏ Interpret scenarios on menstrual cycle
- ❏ Explain information related to female sex steroid metabolism and excretion
- ❏ Answer questions about menstrual irregularities
- ❏ Explain information related to pregnancy
- ❏ Solve problems concerning lactation

MENSTRUAL CYCLE

The Phases

The menstrual cycle (approximately 28 days) can be divided into the following phases or events. By convention, the first day of bleeding (menses) is called day 1 of the menstrual cycle.

- Follicular phase (first 2 weeks) is also called the proliferative or preovulatory phase. This phase is dominated by the peripheral effects of estrogen, which include the replacement of the endometrial cells lost during menses.
- Ovulation (approximately day 14) is preceded by the LH surge, which induces ovulation.
- Luteal phase (approximately 2 weeks) is dominated by the elevated plasma levels of progesterone, and along with lower levels of secreted estrogen, creates a secretory quiescent endometrium that prepares the uterus for implantation.
- Menses. Withdrawal of the hormonal support of the endometrium at this time causes necrosis and menstruation.

Follicular phase (approximately days 1 to 14)

- By convention, the first day of bleeding (menses) is called day 1 of the menstrual cycle.
- During the follicular phase, FSH secretion is slightly elevated, causing proliferation of granulosa cells and increased estrogen secretion within a cohort of follicles.
- One follicle has greater cellular growth and secretes more estradiol (dominant follicle). Estradiol promotes growth and increased sensitivity to FSH; thus the follicle continues to develop. The remaining follicles, lacking sufficient FSH, synthesize only androgen and become atretic (die).

Figures X-11-1 through X-11-4 illustrate the hormonal regulation of the menstrual cycle. The graphs represent the plasma hormonal levels throughout the cycle. The length of the menstrual cycle varies, but an average length is 28 days. Each of the plasma hormone concentrations is plotted relative to the day on which its concentration is lowest, i.e., just prior to menses (day 28). The accompanying diagram illustrates specific aspects of the phase under consideration.

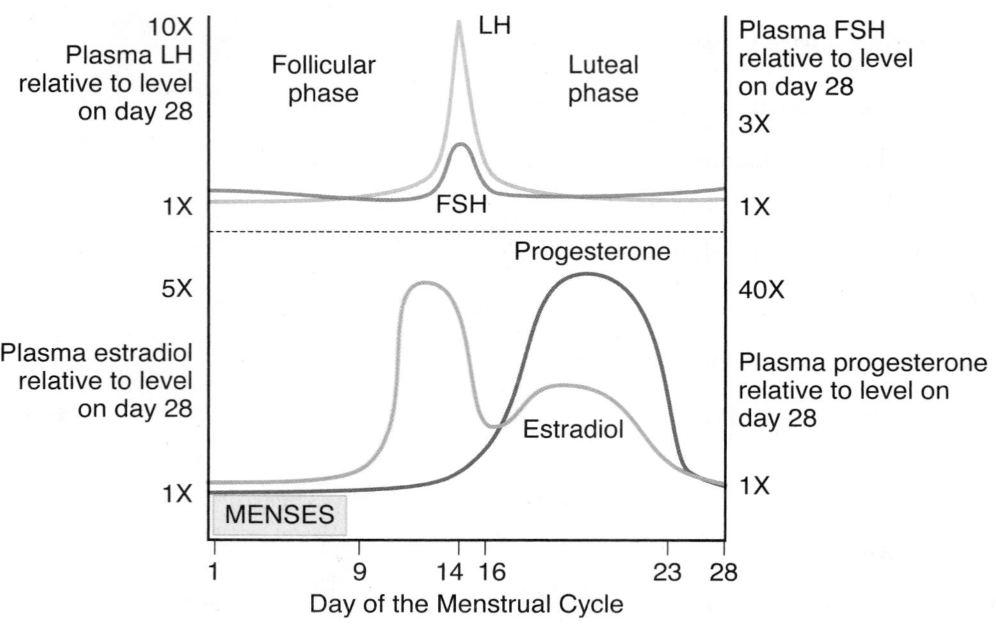

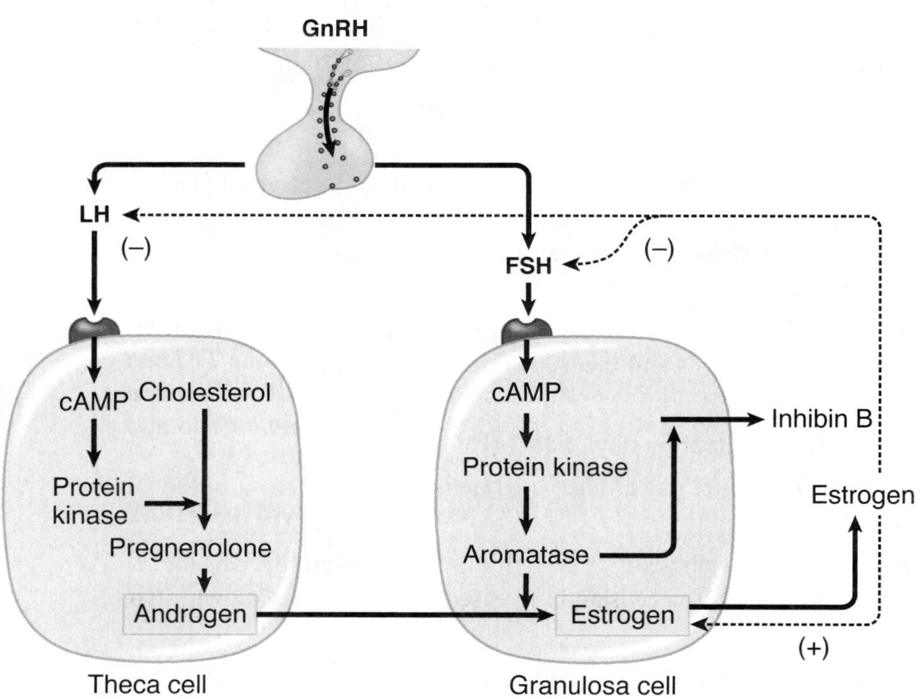

Figure X-11-1. Follicular Phase Relationships Approximately Days 1 to 14

Theca Cells: Under LH stimulation, which acts intracellularly via cAMP, cholesterol is transported into the mitochondria (StAR is activated). The pathway continues through intermediates to androgens. Little androgen is secreted into the blood; most of the androgen enters the adjacent granulosa cells.

Granulosa Cells: Possess the follicle's only FSH receptors. When coupled to FSH, these act via cAMP to increase the activity of aromatase; aromatase converts the androgens to estrogens (mainly estradiol).

Estrogen: Some of the estrogen produced by the granulosa cells is released into the blood and inhibits the release of LH and FSH from the anterior pituitary. However, another fraction of the estrogen acts locally on granulosa cells, increasing their proliferation and sensitivity to FSH.

- This local positive effect of estrogens causes a rising level of circulating estrogens during the follicular phase, but at the same time FSH is decreasing because of the inhibitory effect of estrogen on FSH release.
- Granulosa cells also release inhibin B.
- Inhibin B inhibits the secretion of FSH by the pituitary but their role in the menstral cycle is poorly understood.

Peripheral effects of estrogen produced by the granulosa cells during the follicular phase include:

- Circulating estrogens stimulate the female sex accessory organs and secondary sex characteristics.
- Rising levels of estrogens cause the endometrial cells of the uterine mucosal layers to increase their rate of mitotic division (proliferate).
- Circulating estrogens cause the cervical mucus to be thin and watery, making the cervix easy for sperm to traverse.

Ovulation

Ovulation takes place approximately on day 14. This is an approximation. Since ovulation is always 14 days before the end of the cycle, you can subtract 14 from the cycle length to find the day of ovulation.

Cycle length – 14 = ovulation day

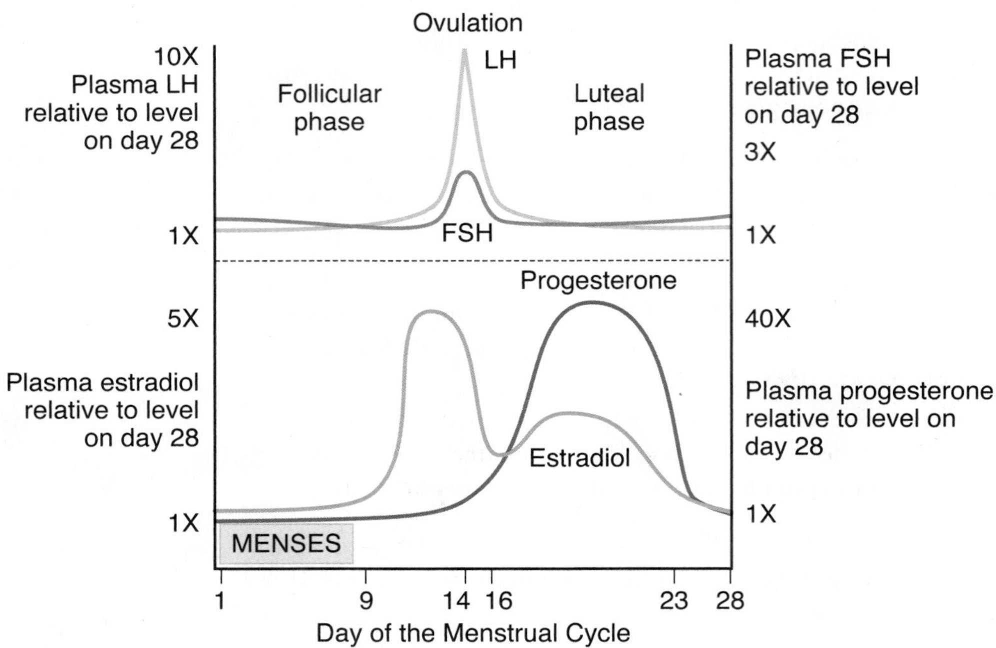

Ovulation occurs approximately day 14

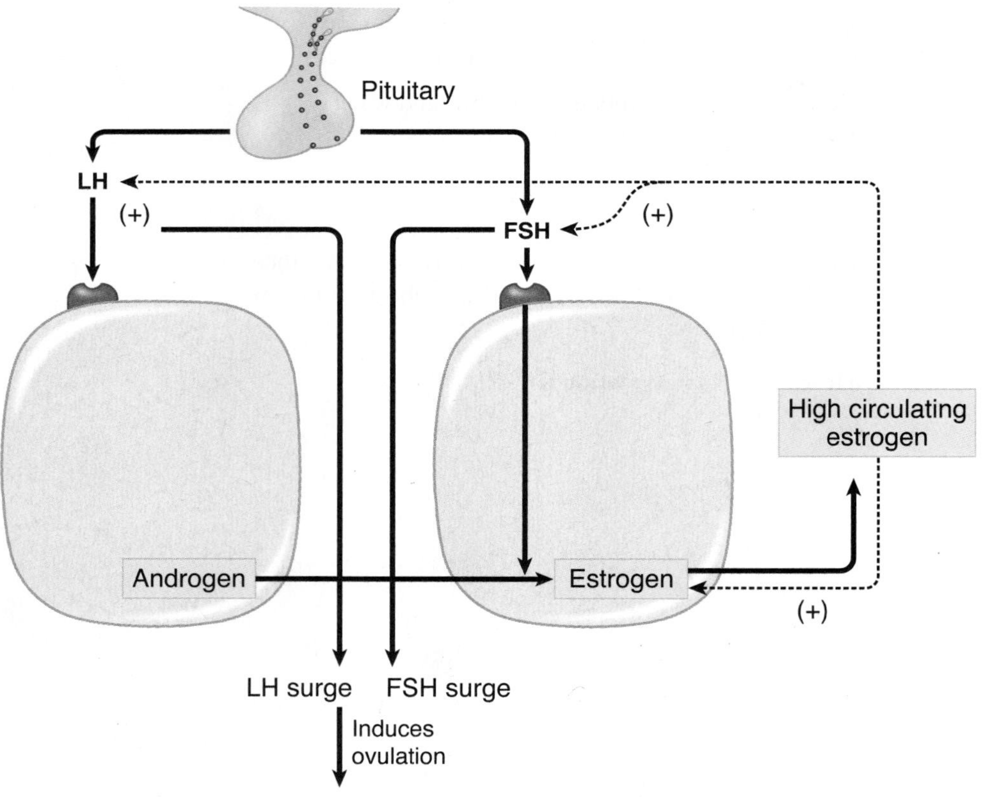

Figure X-11-2. Pituitary-Ovarian Relationships at Ovulation

Estrogen Levels

As shown in Figure X-11-2, near the end of the follicular phase, there is a dramatic rise in circulating estrogen. When estrogens rise above a certain level, they no longer inhibit the release of LH and FSH. Instead, they stimulate the release of LH and FSH (negative feedback loop to positive feedback loop).

This causes a surge in the release of LH and FSH. Only the LH surge is essential for the induction of ovulation and formation of the corpus luteum. Notice from the figure that the LH surge and ovulation occur after estrogen peaks. Therefore, if estrogens are still rising, ovulation has not occurred.

Follicular rupture occurs 24–36 hours after the onset of the LH surge. During this time interval, LH removes the restraint upon meiosis, which has been arrested in prophase for years. The first meiotic division is completed, and the first polar body is extruded.

Positive feedback loops are rare in the body. Only ovulation with estrogen and parturition with oxytocin represent positive feedback loops.

Luteal phase (approximately days 14 to 28)

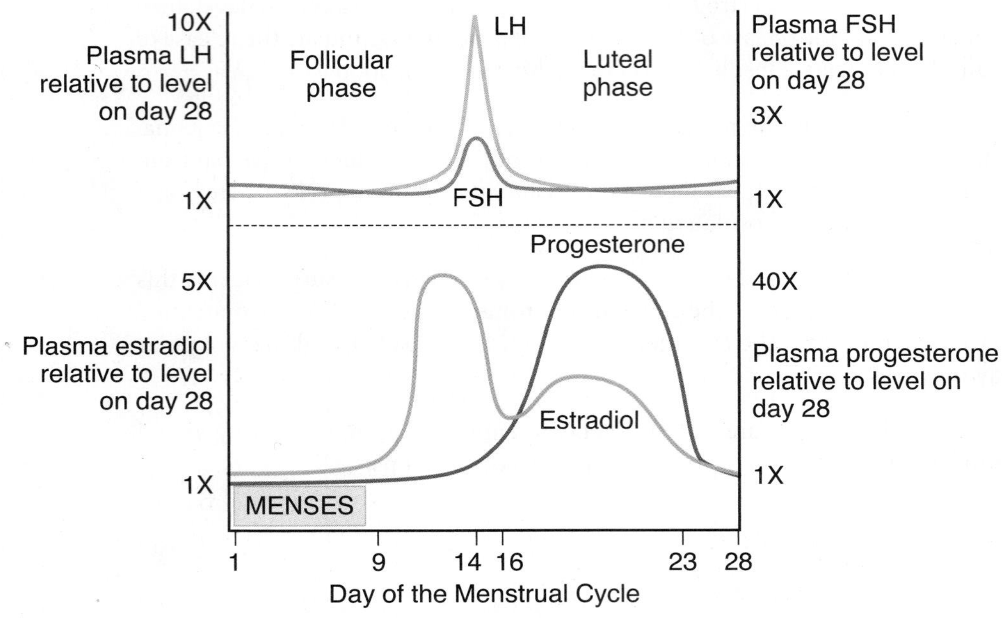

Luteinization of the preovulatory follicle

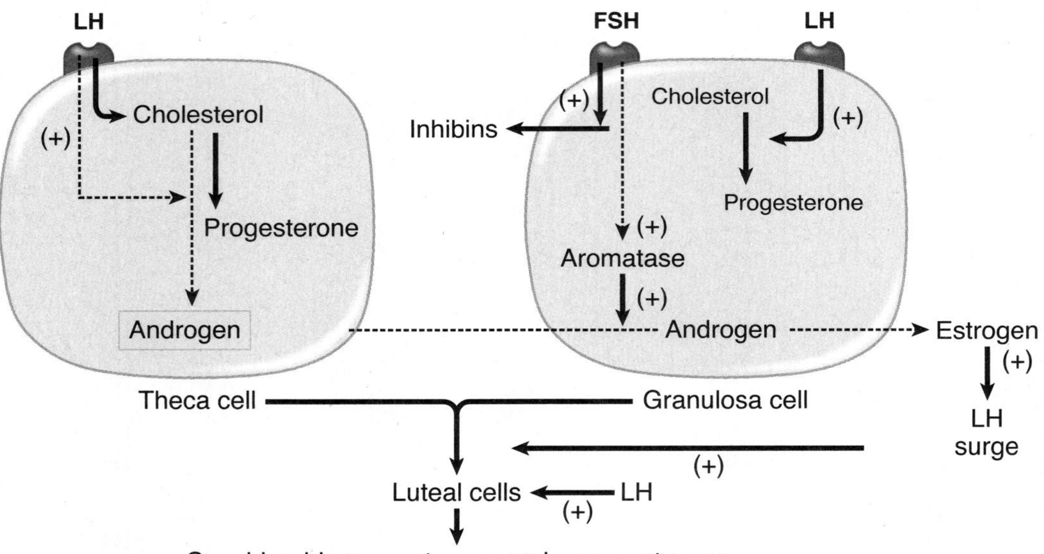

Figure X-11-3. The Luteal Phase Reactions

Preovulatory Follicle

In the latter stages of the follicular phase, intracellular changes within the granulosa and theca cells occur in preparation for their conversion into luteal cells.

- Estradiol, in conjunction with FSH, causes the granulosa cells to produce LH receptors.
- The metabolic pathways are then altered to favor the production of progesterone.
- This would include a decrease in the activity of aromatase and a drop in estrogen production.

LH Surge

Induced by the elevated estrogens, it causes the granulosa cells and theca cells to be transformed into luteal cells and increases the secretion of progesterone.

Corpus Luteum

The process of luteinization occurs following the exit of the oocyte from the follicle. The corpus luteum is made up of the remaining granulosa cells, thecal cells, and supportive tissue. Once formed, the luteal cells are stimulated by LH to secrete considerable progesterone and some estrogen. Progesterone inhibits LH secretion (negative feedback). The corpus luteum secretes inhibin A, which has negative feedback on FSH.

The increased plasma level of progesterone has several actions:

- It causes the uterine endometrium to become secretory, providing a source of nutrients for the blastocyst.
- It causes the cervical mucus to become thick, sealing off the uterus from further entry of sperm or bacteria.
- It has thermogenic properties, causing the basal body temperature to increase by 0.5–1.0° F.

Menses

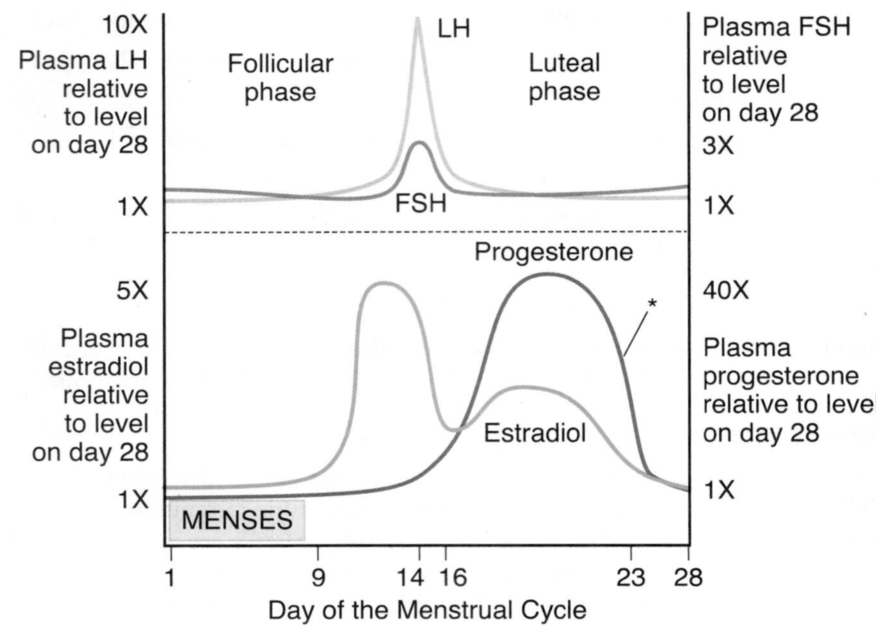

*The fall in sex steroids causes menses.

Figure X-11-4. Onset of Menses

- The life of the corpus luteum is finite, hence the luteal phase is only 14 days.
- Initially, the corpus luteum is very responsive to LH. Over time however, as the corpus luteum becomes less functional, it becomes less responsive to LH.
- Progesterone exerts negative feedback on LH, which contributes to the demise of the corpus luteum.
- With the demise of the corpus luteum, progesterone and estradiol fall to levels that are unable to support the endometrial changes, and menses begins.

Menstruation is due to a lack of gonadal sex steroids.

FEMALE SEX STEROID METABOLISM AND EXCRETION

Solubilization and Excretion

The female sex steroids undergo oxidation or reduction in the liver (and other target tissues), and a glucuronide or sulfate group is attached to the steroidal metabolite. This "conjugation" increases the solubility of the steroids in water, and they thus become excretable in urine.

Estradiol can be excreted as a conjugate of estradiol, but most is first converted to estrone or estriol.

Progesterone is converted in the liver to pregnanediol and is excreted as pregnanediol glucuronide.

Monitoring the Menstrual Cycle

The amount of sex steroids excreted in the urine can be used to monitor the menstrual cycle. For example:

- Low progesterone metabolites and low but slowly rising estrogen metabolites characterize the early follicular phase.
- Low progesterone metabolites and rapidly rising estrogen metabolites characterize the latter part of the follicular phase just before ovulation.
- Elevated levels of progesterone metabolites characterize the luteal phase and pregnancy. In the early luteal phase progesterone is rising, in the latter half it is falling.

Estrogens and Androgen Formation

- Estrogen: Generic term for any estrus-producing hormone, natural or synthetic
- 17 β-Estradiol: Major hormone secreted by the ovarian follicle
- Estrone: Some is secreted from the ovary but much is formed in peripheral tissues such as adipose tissue from androgens. These androgens originate from both the ovary and the adrenal glands. This is the main circulating estrogen following menopause. Fat cells have aromatase. Adipose tissue creates modest levels of estrogen.
- Estriol: Major estrogen synthesized from circulating androgens by the placenta
- Potency: Estradiol > estrone > estriol
- Androgens: The follicles also secrete androgen; DHEA, androstenedione, and testosterone. Additional testosterone production is from the peripheral conversion of adrenal and ovarian androgen. Some testosterone is also converted via 5 α-reductase to dihydrotestosterone in the skin.

New Cycle

During the 3 days prior to and during menses, plasma levels of progesterone and estradiol are at their low point; negative feedback restraint for gonadotropin secretion is removed. FSH secretion rises slightly and initiates the next cycle of follicular growth.

The length of the follicular phase of the menstrual cycle is more variable than the length of the luteal phase. Long cycles are usually due to a prolonged follicular phase and short cycles to a short follicular phase. Once ovulation has occurred, menses generally follows in about 14 days. The length of the menstrual cycle in days minus 14 gives the most likely day of ovulation.

MENSTRUAL IRREGULARITIES

Amenorrhea

- By definition, amenorrhea means the lack of menstral bleeding.
- Though in itself it does not cause harm, it may be a sign of genetic, endocrine, or anatomic abnormalities.

- In the absence of anatomic abnormalities (and pregnancy), it usually indicates a disruption of the hypothalamic–pituitary axis or an ovarian problem.
- A hypothalamic–pituitary origin would include Kallman's syndrome, functional hypothalamic amenorrhea, amenorrhea in female athletes, eating disorders, hypothyroidism (possibly because high TRH stimulates prolactin), and pituitary tumors such as prolactinomas.
- Ovarian causes could be premature ovarian failure (premature menopause), repetitive ovulation failure, or anovulation (intermittent bleeding), or a polycystic ovary.

Polycystic Ovarian Syndrome

- Characterized by elevated LH/FSH ratio.
- Clinical signs include: infertility, hirsutism, obesity, insulin resistance, and amenorrhea or oligomenorrhea
- The enlarged polycystic ovaries are known to be associated with increased androgen levels (DHEA).
- It originates in obese girls. The high extraglandular estrogens (mainly estrone) selectively suppress FSH. Ovarian follicles do have a suppressed aromatase activity and thus a diminished capacity to convert androgen into estrogen, but the adrenals may also contribute to the excess androgens as well.
- High androgens promote atresia in developing follicles and disrupt feedback relationships. Look for high LH and DHEA levels.
- The overall result is anovulation-induced amenorrhea with an estrogen-induced endometrial hyperplasia and breakthrough bleeding.
- Although poorly understood the hyperinsulinemia is believed to be a key etiologic factor.
- Treat amenorrhea in PCOS with metformin.
- Treat androgenization with spironolactone.

Hirsutism

- Defined as an excessive generally male pattern of hair growth.
- Virilization refers to accompanying additional alterations, such as deepening of the voice, clitoromegaly, increased muscle bulk, and breast atrophy.
- It is often associated with conditions of androgen excess such as congenital adrenal hyperplasia and polycystic ovarian syndrome.
- Axillary and pubic hair are sensitive to low levels of androgen.
- Hair on the upper chest, face (scalp region not involved), and back requires more androgen and represents the pattern seen in males.
- Circulating androgens involved are testosterone, DHEA, DHEAS, and androstenedione in response to LH and ACTH.
- Measurements of DHEAS as well as a dexamethasone suppression test helps in separating an adrenal from an ovarian source.
- Polycystic ovarian syndrome is the most common cause of ovarian androgen excess.

PREGNANCY

Ovum Pickup and Fertilization

In women, the ovum is released from the rupturing follicle into the abdominal cavity, where it is "picked up" by the fimbria of the oviduct. Failure of ovum pick-up may result in ectopic pregnancy, i.e., the implantation of the blastocyst at any site other than the interior of the uterus.

Fertilization occurs in the upper end of the oviduct within 8–25 hours after ovulation. After this, the ovum loses its ability to be fertilized. Sperm retain their capacity to fertilize an ovum for as long as 72 hours after ejaculation. For about 48 hours around the time of ovulation the cervical mucus is copious and slightly alkaline. This environment represent a good conduit for the sperm.

Weeks of gestation (gestational age) to estimate the delivery date are commonly taken from the first day of the last menstrual period.

Sperm are transported from the vagina to the upper ends of the oviduct by contraction of the female reproductive tract. The swimming motions of the sperm are important for penetration of the granulosa cell layer (cumulus oophorus) and membranes surrounding the ovum.

Low sperm counts (<20 million/mL of ejaculate) are associated with reduced fertility because sperm from ejaculates with low counts often contain many sperm with poor motility and an abnormal morphology. The first step in infertility evaluation is semen analysis.

Implantation

At the time of implantation, which occurs about 5-7 days after fertilization, the development is at the blastocyst stage. The trophoblastic cells of the fetus now begin to secrete a peptide hormone, human chorionic gonadotropin (hCG). HCG starts 10 days after fertilization.

Fetal hCG possesses a β subunit similar to that of LH, and therefore it has considerable LH activity.

The presence of the beta subunit of hCG in the urine can be detected by a variety of test kits for the detection of pregnancy.

Hormonal Maintenance of the Uterine Endometrium

Figure X-11-5 illustrates the production of estrogen and progesterone during pregnancy. The figure is divided into 3 phases:

- Part of the luteal phase before implantation
- Early pregnancy
- Late pregnancy

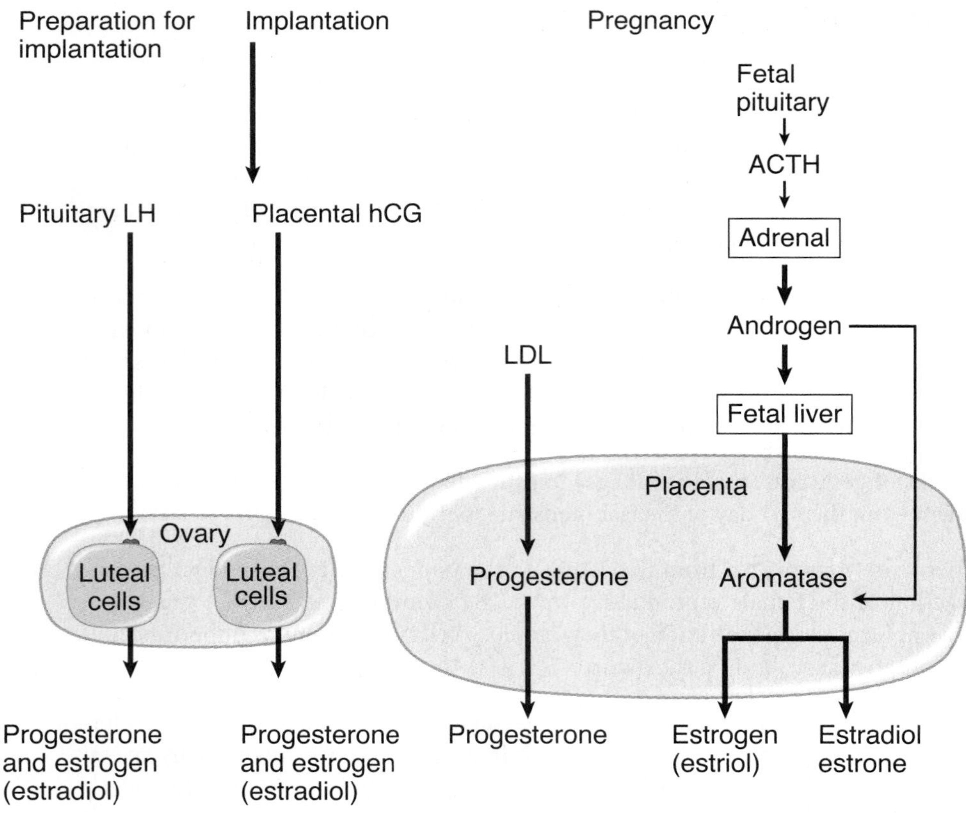

Figure X-11-5. Steroids During Pregnancy

Preparation for implantation (luteal phase)

Pituitary LH stimulates luteal cells to secrete progesterone and some estrogen. Because the ovaries are the source of the estrogen, it is mainly estradiol.

Implantation to second month

- Within a week or two of fertilization, trophoblastic cells of the placenta begin secreting hCG. In short, hCG prevents regression of the corpus luteum, thus allowing it to continue producing estrogens and progesterone.
- hCG doubles in the early weeks of pregnancy. Because it maintains secretion of progesterone from the corpus luteum, progesterone is a sensitive marker of early fetal well-being.
- Loss of the corpus luteum during this period terminates the pregnancy. However, in lieu of the corpus luteum, exogenous progesterone would be a functional substitute.

Third month to term

- Placenta secretes enough progesterone and estrogen to maintain the uterus. This is not controlled by hCG. At this time, the ovaries (corpus luteum) can be removed and pregnancy continues.

- Progesterone secretion of the placenta is limited only by the amount of precursor (cholesterol) delivered by low-density lipoproteins (LDL) to the placenta. Progesterone maintains uterine quiescence during pregnancy.
- The secretion of estrogen involve both the fetus and the placenta.
- The fetal adrenal gland secretes dehydroepiandrosterone (DHEA). The fetal liver then converts DHEA to androstenodione (A) and testosterone.
- The placenta expresses aromatase. This enzyme converts the A and testosterone from the fetus into estrogens, estriol being the primary one. Thus, estriol becomes a good marker for fetal well-being.

Peripheral Effects of Hormonal Changes

The large amount of estrogen and progesterone secreted by the placenta during pregnancy stimulates the following important changes within the mother:

- Massive growth of the uterus, especially the myometrium
- Increased growth of all components (glands, stroma, and fat) of the breasts

Additional hormonal changes

Increased prolactin secretion by the pituitary in response to elevated estrogens

Secretion of human placental lactogen (hPL), also called human chorionic somatomammotropin (hCS), by the placenta. This markedly increases during the latter half of the pregnancy.

- hPL (hCS) has considerable amino acid sequence homology with growth hormone but has very little growth-stimulating activity.
- hPL (hCS) has metabolic actions similar to growth hormone; that is, it increases maternal lipolysis and ketogenesis and decreases maternal glucose utilization, thereby making maternal energy stores more available for the fetus.
- During the second trimester pregnancy becomes a hyperinsulinemic state with peripheral resistance to the metabolic effects of insulin. This reserves glucose for fetal needs and the mother depends more heavily on fatty acids as a source of energy. Under these conditions even modest fasting can cause ketosis.
- These anti-insulin actions of hPL (hCS) may also account for the gestational diabetes that develops in some pregnant women.
- hPL (hCS) is secreted in proportion to the size of the placenta and is an index of placental well-being.

PRL = prolactin
Prog = progesterone

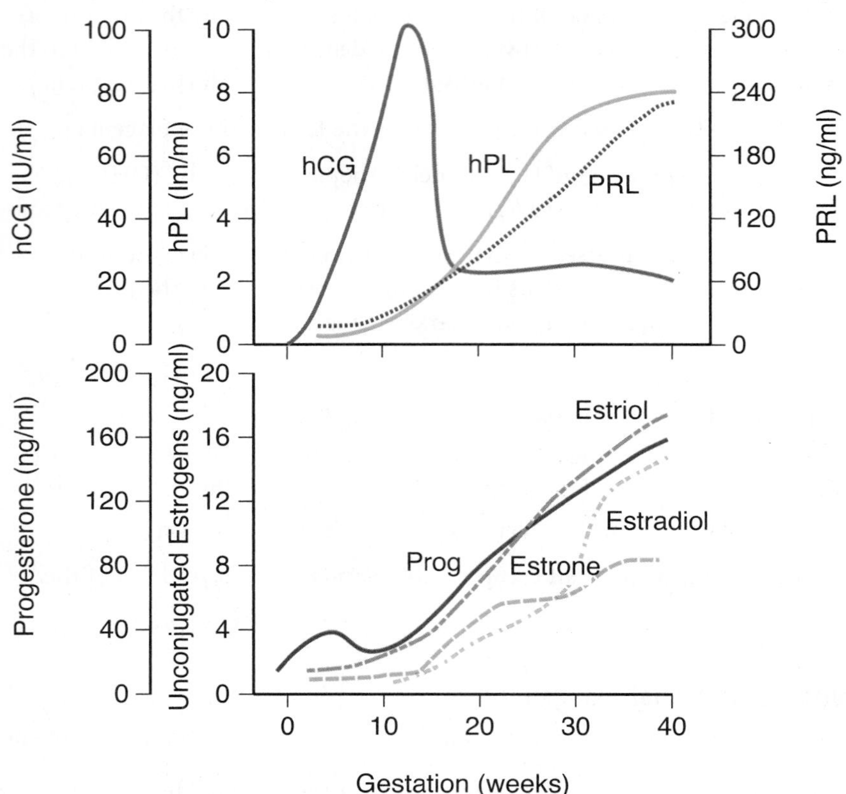

Figure X-11-6. Hormone Levels During Pregnancy

Maternal Compensatory Changes of Pregnancy

Cardiovascular/renal

Cardiac output increases but peripheral resistance decreases and as a result there is no hypertension associated with a normal pregnancy (parallel circuit of placenta). Blood pressure declines in the first trimester and gradually rises toward prepregnancy levels thereafter.

GFR increases and renal threshold decreases. Combined with the increased plasma glucose, glucose often appears in the urine.

Endocrine

The anterior pituitary enlarges by about one-third, due to a hyperplasia of the lactotrophs driven by the rise in estrogen. Postpartum pituitary necrosis (Sheehan syndrome) is preceded by obstetric hemorrhage. The posterior pituitary is usually spared. Failure to lactate is the most common clinical sign. Other manifestations would include the consequences of hypothyroidism and hypocortisolism.

Estrogen increases the circulating steroid-binding globulins and bound hormone increases but FT4 is normal. Hyperthyroidism increases the risk of preterm delivery. Hypothyroidism is unusual in pregnancy.

Estrogen increases renin secretion, and overall increased activity of the renin-angiotensin-aldosterone system causes fluid retention and hemodilution.

Changes induced near the end of pregnancy

The pubic symphysis, cervix, and vagina become more distensible. These changes make passage of the fetus through the birth canal easier. The peptide hormone relaxin, which is secreted by the placenta, also promotes these changes. Its action is not essential. Parturition in humans is normal in the absence of ovaries.

In response to elevated plasma estrogens, oxytocin receptors increase in the myometrium. Thus, the sensitivity of the uterine myometrium to the excitatory action of oxytocin is increased.

Parturition

The factors that initiate parturition are not well understood, but the following facts are known:

- As indicated above, estrogens and progesterone are high throughout pregnancy. Estrogens upregulate phospholipase A2 in the amnion as well as oxytocin receptors in the myometrium.
- Prostaglandins cause contraction of the uterus and are thought to initiate the labor process. Contraction of the myometrium pushes the fetus towards the cervix.
- Dilation of the cervix stimulates afferent neurons that cause the release of oxytocin from the posterior pituitary gland. Oxytocin contracts the myometrium and stimulates local production of prostaglandins. This contraction is thought to participate in parturition, and contraction of the uterus by oxytocin is thought to play an important role in limiting blood loss after the fetus is expelled.
- When a fetus dies, toxic products originating from the fetus increase prostaglandin release in the uterus, thus initiating contractions and a spontaneous abortion (miscarriage). Similarly, administration of prostaglandins induces abortion.

LACTATION

Mammary Gland Growth and Secretion

Growth of mammary tissue is stimulated by the female sex steroids estrogen and progesterone. However, for these steroids to stimulate maximum growth, prolactin, growth hormone, and cortisol also must be present.

During pregnancy, the high levels of plasma estrogen greatly increase prolactin secretion, but milk synthesis does not occur because the high level of estrogen (and progesterone) blocks milk synthesis. At parturition, plasma estrogen drops, withdrawing the block on milk synthesis. As a result, the number of prolactin receptors in mammary tissue increases several-fold, and milk synthesis begins.

Maintaining Lactation

Suckling is required to maintain lactation.

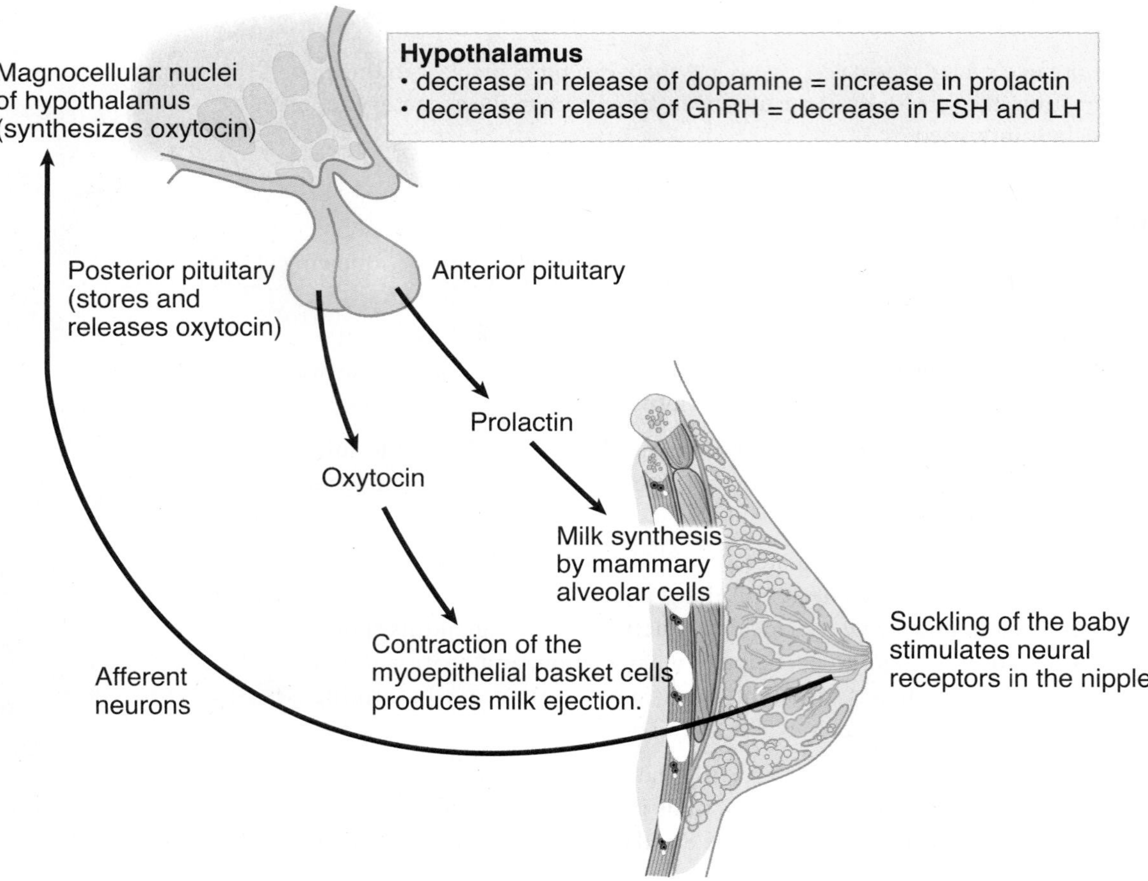

Figure X-11-7. Lactation and the Suckling Reflex

The suckling of the baby at the mother's breast stimulates receptors in the mother's nipples. Signals from these receptors are transmitted to the hypothalamus and have the following effects:

- Oxytocin synthesis and secretion are increased. Oxytocin causes the myoepithelial basket cells that surround the alveoli to contract. Preformed milk is ejected into the ducts and out the openings of the nipple; that is, milk ejection is initiated.
- The release of dopamine by the hypothalamus into the hypophyseal portal vessels is inhibited. This removes a chronic restraint on prolactin secretion. Prolactin secretion increases, and milk secretion is stimulated each time the baby suckles.
- The secretion of GnRH into the hypophyseal portal vessels is inhibited; secretion of FSH and LH decreases. Thus, follicular growth, estrogen secretion, ovulation, and menses cease. High prolactin levels also contribute to the amenorrhea.

For the suckling stimulus to inhibit GnRH secretion completely, the stimulus must be prolonged and frequent. Supplementation of the mother's milk with other fluids or sources of energy reduces the baby's suckling and allows gonadotropin secretion, follicular growth, and ovulation to occur.

Women who do not wish to breastfeed their children are sometimes administered large doses of estrogen. The estrogen inhibits lactation (by its inhibitory action of milk synthesis), even though estrogen promotes increased prolactin secretion.

Breastfeeding is a form of contraceptive because it should stop ovulation.

Chapter Summary

- Estrogen slowly rises during the early follicular stage. This is followed by a more rapid rise as ovulation approaches. This latter rise occurs because estrogen acts locally to enhance its own production.
- Once estrogen rises above a certain level, it no longer suppresses LH and FSH secretion but instead enhances their secretion. This induces a surge in the secretion of both LH and FSH. However, only the LH surge is required for ovulation.
- In the luteal phase, LH stimulates the luteal cells to secrete considerable progesterone as well as estrogen. Progesterone in this phase inhibits LH secretion.
- It is the drop in progesterone (and estrogen) that withdraws the hormonal support of the endometrium, causing menstruation.
- Variations in the length of the menstrual cycle are due to the follicular phase. Once ovulation has occurred, menstruation begins almost exactly 14 days later.
- Fertilization and biological pregnancy occur at the beginning of the luteal phase. Implantation occurs at about the middle of the luteal phase.
- In the first 2 to 3 months of pregnancy, fetal production of hCG is required for continued secretion of progesterone and estrogen by the ovary.
- In pregnancy, cardiac output increases, TPR decreases, and blood pressure is usually below prepregnancy levels.
- Pregnancy increases GFR and decreases the renal threshold for glucose.
- Pregnancy is a euthyroid state but there is activation of the renin-angiotensin-aldosterone system, which increases ECF volume.
- The ovaries are not required for the last 6 months of pregnancy because the placenta takes over the secretion of both progesterone and estrogen.
- hCG is an index of fetal well-being in early pregnancy. hPL is an index of placental function later in pregnancy. Estriol in an index of fetal well-being and placental function.
- Postpartum hemorrhaging can cause pituitary infarction (Sheehan's syndrome).
- Near the end of pregnancy, estrogen induces the appearance of oxytocin receptors in the myometrium. Once this occurs, oxytocin can be administered to induce labor. However, it is unlikely that a rise in oxytocin is the natural signal that begins delivery.
- During pregnancy, the rising estrogens drive an increase in prolactin secretion, but the estrogen blocks milk synthesis.
- At delivery, it is the drop in estrogen that initiates milk synthesis, but suckling is required to maintain lactation.

SECTION XI

Gastrointestinal Physiology

Gastrointestinal Physiology 1

Learning Objectives

- ❑ Answer questions about overview of the gastrointestinal tract
- ❑ Explain information related to motility
- ❑ Demonstrate understanding of secretions
- ❑ Demonstrate understanding of digestion
- ❑ Demonstrate understanding of absorption

OVERVIEW OF THE GASTROINTESTINAL TRACT

Structure

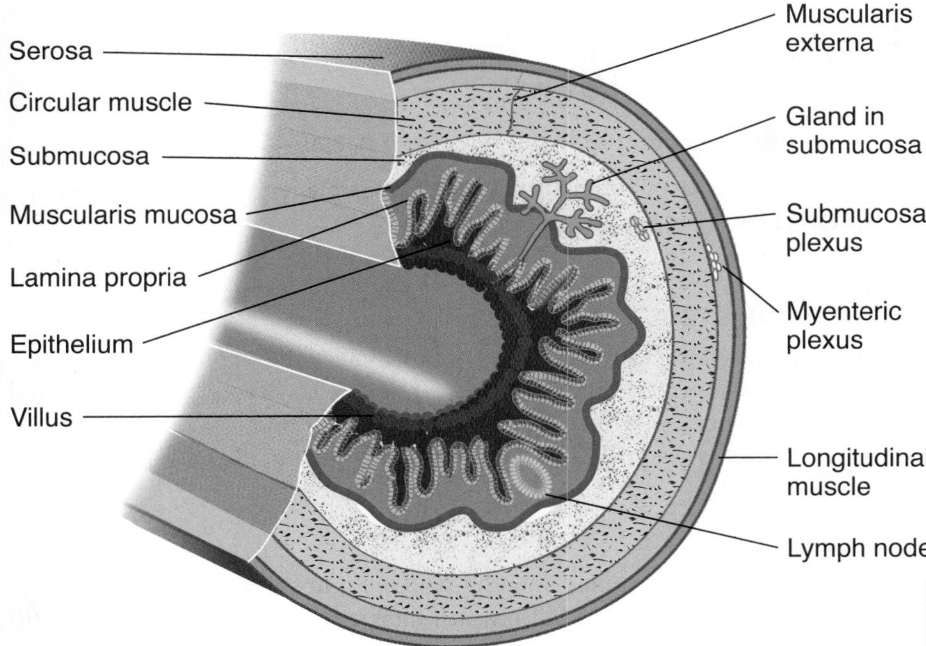

Figure XI-1-1. Gastrointestinal Tract

Mucosa

- Epithelium: consists of a single layer of specialized cells; some are involved in secretions and some release hormones
- Lamina propria: layer of connective tissue which contains glands, hormone-containing cells, lymph nodes, and capillaries
- Muscularis mucosa: a thin layer of muscle, the contraction of which causes folding and ridges in the mucosal layers

Submucosa

- A layer of connective tissue that contains glands, large blood vessels, and lymphatics.
- Outermost region has a nerve net called the submucosal (Meissner's) plexus.
- Meissner's plexus is part of the enteric nervous system and is involved in secretory activity.

Muscularis externa

- Inner layer of circular muscle
- Outer layer of longitudinal muscle
- Myenteric nerve plexus involved in motor activity is between the muscle layers.

Serosa

- Outermost layer of the GI tract
- Consists of connective tissue and a layer of epithelial cells
- Within this layer autonomic nerve fibers run and eventually synapse on target cells and the enteric nerve plexes

Note

Sympathetic regulation of the splanchnic circulation does not involve the enteric nervous system.

Nervous Control

Residing in the GI tract is a vast neural network called the enteric nervous system (Meissner's and myenteric plexi). Normal GI function is dependent on this neural network. The enteric nervous system is innervated by the autonomic nervous systems and serves as the final mediator for virtually all neurally mediated changes.

Sympathetic

The diagram below illustrates how the synaptic junction at the end of a nerve fiber secretes norepinephrine (NE), which then induces responses in the gastrointestinal (GI) system.

———————————< NE

↓ motility
↓ secretions
↑ constriction of sphincters

An increase in sympathetic activity slows processes.

Parasympathetic

———< ACh		↑ motility ↑ secretions
———< VIP		↓ constriction of sphincters
———< GRP	G cell	↑ gastrin

An increase in parasympathetic activity promotes digestive and absorptive processes.

VIP: vasoactive intestinal peptide, an inhibitory parasympathetic transmitter

GRP: gastrin-releasing peptide; stimulates the release of gastrin from G cells

Endocrine Control

Table XI-1-1. The Endocrine Control of the GI System

Hormone**	Source	Stimulus	Stomach Motility and Secretion	Pancreas	Gallbladder
Secretin	S cells lining duodenum	Acid entering duodenum	Inhibits	Stimulates fluid secretion (HCO_3^-)	
CCK	Cells lining duodenum	Fat and amino acids entering duodenum	Inhibits emptying	Stimulates enzyme secretion	1. Contraction 2. Relaxation sphincter (Oddi)
Gastrin	G cells of stomach	Stomach distension	Stimulates		
	Antrum	Parasym (GRP) Peptides			
	Duodenum	Stomach acid inhibits*			
GIP **GLP**	Duodenum	Fat, CHO, amino acids	Inhibits	Increases insulin Decreases glucagon	

CCK = cholecystokinin; GIP = gastric inhibitory peptide (glucose insulinotropic peptide), GLP = glucagon-like peptide

*Note: In a non–acid-producing stomach (e.g., chronic gastritis), the reduced negative feedback increases circulating gastrin.

**All four hormones stimulate insulin release.

MOTILITY

Characteristics of Smooth Muscle

Electrical activity

- Resting membrane potential –40 to –65 mV. Close to depolarization.
- Oscillation of membrane potential is generated by interstitial cells (interstitial cells of Cajal) that act as pacemakers. This is referred to as slow waves or basic electrical rhythm, and if threshold is reached it generates action potentials.

Note

Anticholinergic medications such as atropine or tricyclic antidepressants slow GI motility.

- Action potentials are generated by the opening of slow channels that allow the entry of both sodium and calcium.
- The duodenum contracts the most often.

Note

Nerve gas increases GI and bronchial secretions.

Motor activity

- Stretch produces a contractile response.
- Gap junctions create an electrical syncytium within the smooth muscle.
- Slow waves create low level contractions, and action potentials strengthen the contractions.
- Pacemaker activity from the interstitial cells creates the intrinsic motor activity.
- Tonic contraction at sphincters act as valves.

Swallowing

Swallowing is a reflex controlled from the brain stem.

Efferent input is via the vagus nerve for all events, and these are summarized in Figure XI-1-2.

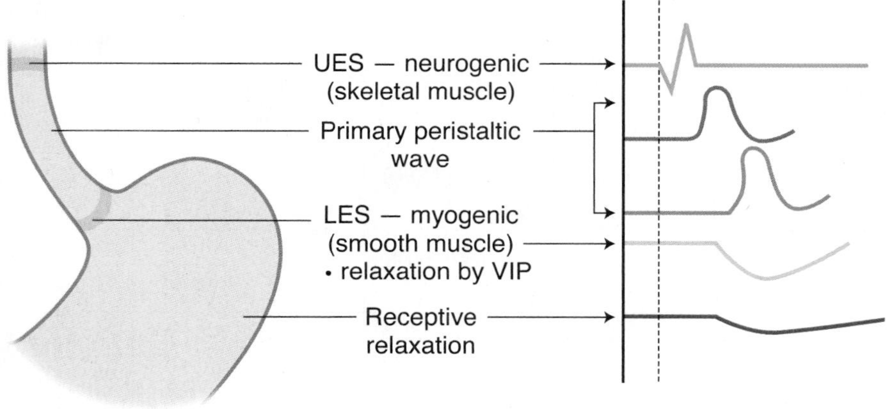

Figure XI-1-2. Swallowing, the Peristaltic Wave

Note

Sympathetic slows parasympathetic speeds.

An increase in sympathetic activity slows processes.

Events during swallowing:

- Relaxation of upper esophageal skeletal muscle sphincter (UES)
- Primary peristaltic wave
- Relaxation of lower esophageal smooth muscle sphincter (LES) via VIP, which relaxes smooth muscle via NO
- Relaxation of proximal stomach (receptive relaxation)

Bridge to Pathology

Barrett esophagus is the term used to describe alterations in the esophageal epithelium that accompany GERD.

If the primary peristaltic wave is not successful, a secondary peristaltic wave is initiated by local distension of the esophagus. The secondary wave is not "conscious."

Disorders of the Esophagus

Achalasia

- Failure of the LES to relax, resulting in swallowed food being retained in the esophagus
- Caused by abnormalities in the enteric nerves
- Peristaltic waves are weak

Gastroesophageal reflux disease (GERD)

- LES doesn't maintain tone
- Acid reflux damages esophageal epithelium

Diffuse esophageal spasm

- Spasms of esophageal muscle
- Presents with characteristics of a heart attack (e.g., chest pain)
- Barium swallow shows repeated, spontaneous waves of contraction

Note

Dysphagia refers to difficulty in swallowing.

Gastric Motility

The primary factors and additional aspects are illustrated in Figure XI-1-3.

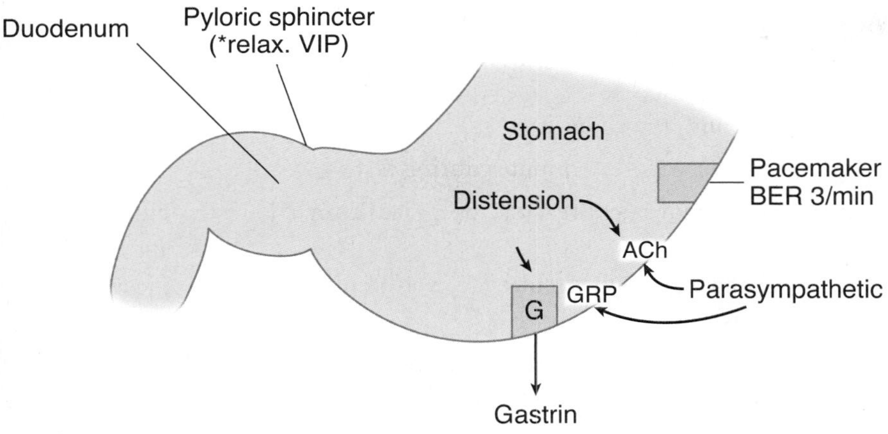

Figure XI-1-3. Endocrine and Neural Control of the Stomach

ACh: Acetylcholine

BER: Basic electrical rhythm

GRP: Gastrin-releasing peptide

VIP: Vasoactive intestinal polypeptide

Stimulation

- Acetylcholine released in response to activation of parasympathetics
- Local distension

Inhibition

- Low pH of stomach contents inhibits the release of gastrin
- Feedback from duodenal release of hormones (CCK, secretin, and GIP)

Stomach emptying

- Liquids > CHO > protein > fat (> = faster than)
- The pyloris of the stomach acts as a sphincter to control the rate of stomach emptying. A wave of contraction closes the sphincter so that only a small volume is moved forward into the duodenum. CCK, GIP, and secretin increase the degree of pyloric constriction and slow stomach emptying.

Small Intestinal Motility

- Rhythmic contractions in adjacent sections create segmentation contractions, which are mixing movements.
- Waves of contractions preceded by a relaxation of the muscle (peristaltic movements) are propulsive.
- The ileocecal sphincter, or valve between the small and large intestine, is normally closed.
- Distension of the ileum creates a muscular wave that relaxes the sphincter.
- Distension of the colon creates a nervous reflex to constrict the sphincter.

Colon Motility

- Segmentation contractions create bulges (haustrations) along the colon.
- Mass movements, which are propulsive, are more prolonged than the peristaltic movements of the small intestine.

Migrating Motor Complex (MMC)

- A propulsive movement initiated during fasting that begins in the stomach and moves undigested material from the stomach and small intestine into the colon.
- Repeats every 90–120 minutes during fasting.
- When one movement reaches the distal ileum, a new one starts in the stomach.
- Correlated with high circulating levels of motilin, a hormone of the small intestine
- This movement prevents the backflow of bacteria from the colon into the ileum and its subsequent overgrowth in the distal ileum.

Defecation

- Defecation is a reflex involving the central nervous system.
- A mass movement in the terminal colon fills the rectum and causes a reflex relaxation of the internal anal sphincter and a reflex contraction of the external anal sphincter.
- Voluntary relaxation of the external sphincter accompanied with propulsive contraction of the distal colon complete defecation.
- Lack of a functional innervation of the external sphincter causes involuntary defecation when the rectum fills.

SECRETIONS

Salivary Secretions

- Parotid gland secretions are entirely serous (lack mucin).
- Submandibular and sublingual gland secretions are mixed mucus and serous.
- They are almost entirely under the control of the parasympathetic system, which promotes secretion.
- The initial fluid formation in the acinus is via an indirect chloride pump (secondary active transport powered by the Na/K ATPase pump), and the electrolyte composition is isotonic and similar to interstitial fluid.

Duct cells modify the initial acinar secretion (Figure XI-1-4).

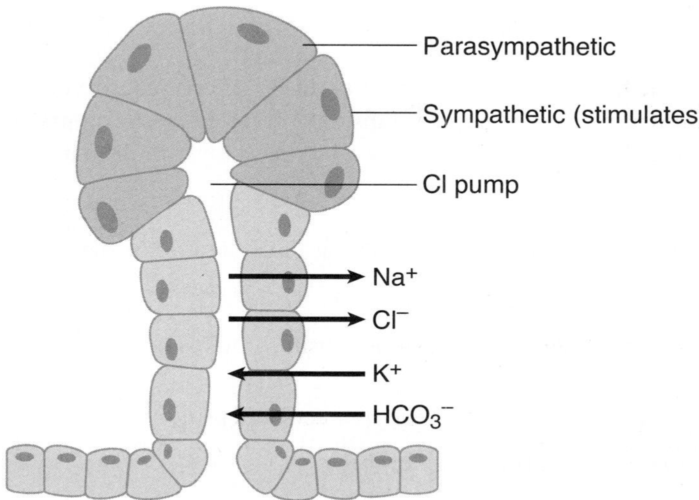

Figure XI-1-4. Salivary Secretion

Composition of salivary secretions

- Low in Na^+, Cl^- because of reabsorption
- High in K^+, HCO3 because of secretion (pH = 8)
- Low tonicity: Salivary fluid is hypotonic because of reabsorption of NaCl and impermeability of ducts to water.
- α-Amylase (ptyalin): secreted in the active form and begins the digestion of carbohydrates
- Mucus, glycoprotein
- Immunoglobulins and lysozymes

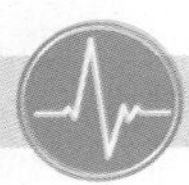

Gastric Secretions

- The epithelial cells that cover the gastric mucosa secrete a highly viscous alkaline fluid (mucin plus bicarbonate) that protects the stomach lining from the caustic action of HCl.
- Fluid needs both mucin and bicarbonate to be protective.
- Nonsteroidal anti-inflammatory drugs such as aspirin decrease the secretion of the mucin and bicarbonate.
- Surface of the mucosa studded with the openings of the gastric glands
- Except for the upper cardiac region and lower pyloric region whose glands secrete mainly a mucoid fluid, gastric glands secrete a fluid whose pH can be initially as low as 1.0.

Secretions of the main cells composing the oxyntic gastric glands

Parietal cells

- HCl
- Intrinsic factor combines with vitamin B_{12} and is reabsorbed in the distal ileum. This is the only substance secreted by the stomach that is required for survival. It is released by the same stimuli that release HCl.

Chief Cells

Pepsinogen is converted to pepsin by H^+, as illustrated in the diagram below.

$$\text{Pepsinogen} \xrightarrow{H^+} \text{pepsin (proteins to peptides)}$$

- Pepsinogen is initially converted to active pepsin by acid.
- Active pepsin continues the process.
- Pepsin is active only in the acid pH medium of the stomach.
- Pepsin begins the digestion of protein but is not essential for life.

Mucous Neck Cells

- Secrete the protective mucus, HCO_3 combination

+ Stimulates secretion
– Inhibits secretion

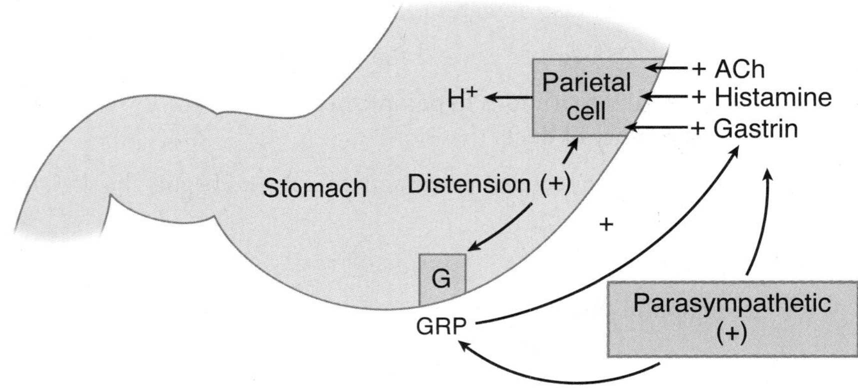

Figure XI-1-5. Control of Gastric Acid Secretion

Control of acid secretion

There are 3 natural substances that stimulate parietal cells:

- Acetylcholine (ACh), acting as a transmitter; release is stimulated by sight/smell of food and reflexly in response to stomach distension (vago-vagal reflex).
- Locally released histamine; stimulated by Ach and gastrin
- The hormone gastrin; stimulated by release of GRP

As stomach pH falls, somatostatin (SST) is released, which inhibits gastrin and reduces acid secretion (feedback regulation of acid secretion).

Cellular mechanisms of acid secretion

- Within the cell, carbonic anhydrase facilitates the conversion of CO_2 into H^+ and HCO_3^-.
- The demand for CO_2 can be so great following a meal that the parietial cells extract CO_2 from the arterial blood. This makes gastric venous blood the most basic in the body.
- Hydrogen ions are secreted by a H/K-ATPase pump similar to that in the distal nephron.
- The pumping of H^+ raises intracellular HCO_3^- and its gradient across the basal membrane and provides the net force for pumping Cl^- into the cell.
- The chloride diffuses through channels across the apical membrane, creating a negative potential in the stomach lumen.
- Because of the extraction of CO_2 and secretion of HCO_3^- , the venous blood leaving the stomach following a meal is alkaline.
- Compared with extracellular fluid, gastric secretions are high in H^+, K^+, Cl^-, but low in Na^+.
- The greater the secretion rate, the higher the H^+ and the lower the Na^+.
- Vomiting stomach contents produces a metabolic alkalosis and a loss of body potassium (hypokalemia mainly due to the alkalosis effect on the kidney).

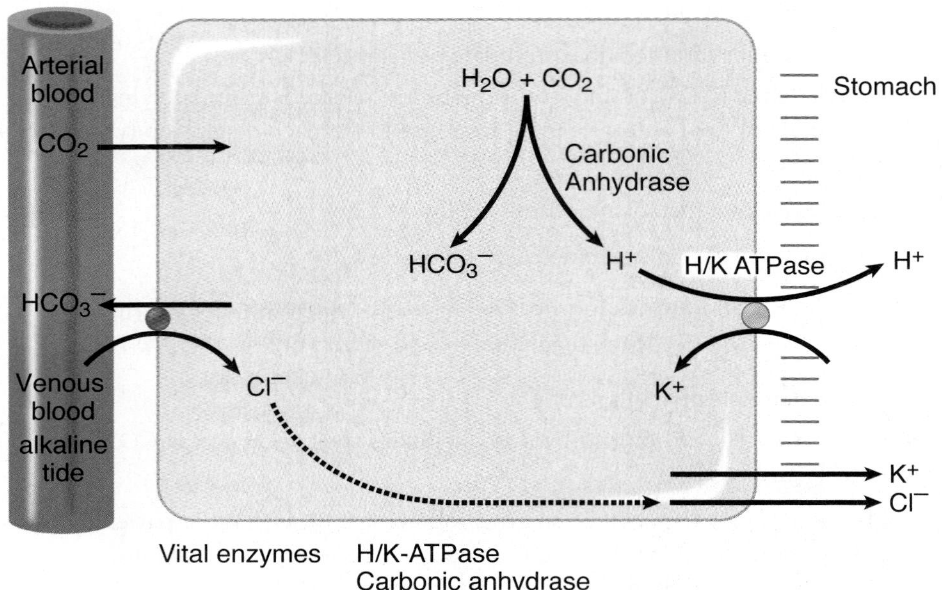

Figure XI-1-6. Regulation of Parietal Cell Secretion

Pancreatic Secretions

- Exocrine tissue is organized into acini and ducts very similar to that of the salivary glands.
- Cholinergic nerves to the pancreas stimulate the secretion of both the enzyme and aqueous component.
- Food in the stomach stimulates stretch receptors and, via vagovagal reflexes, stimulates a small secretory volume.
- Sympathetics inhibit secretion but are a minor influence.
- **Most of the control is via secretin and CCK.**

Enzymatic components

- Trypsin inhibitor, a protein present in pancreatic secretions, prevents activation of the proteases within the pancreas.
- In addition to the following groups of enzymes, pancreatic fluid contains ribonucleases and deoxyribonucleases.
- A diet high in one type of food (protein, CHO, fat) results in the preferential production of enzymes for that particular food.

Pancreatic amylases are secreted as active enzymes:

- Hydrolyze α-1,4-glucoside linkage of complex carbohydrates, forming three smaller compounds:
  - α-Limit dextrins: still a branched polysaccharide
  - Maltotriose, a trisaccharide
  - Maltose, a disaccharide
- Cannot hydrolyze β linkages of cellulose

Pancreatic lipases are mainly secreted as active enzymes. Glycerol ester lipase (pancreatic lipase) needs colipase to be effective. Colipase displaces bile salt from the surface of micelles. This allows pancreatic lipase to attach to the droplet and digest it, leading to formation of two free fatty acids and one monoglyceride (a 2-monoglyceride, i.e., an ester on carbon 2).

Cholesterol esterase (sterol lipase) hydrolyzes cholesterol esters to yield cholesterol and fatty acids. **Pancreatic proteases** are secreted as inactive zymogens. They include trypsinogen, chymotrypsinogen, and procarboxypeptidase.

Activation sequence. The activation sequences are summarized below.

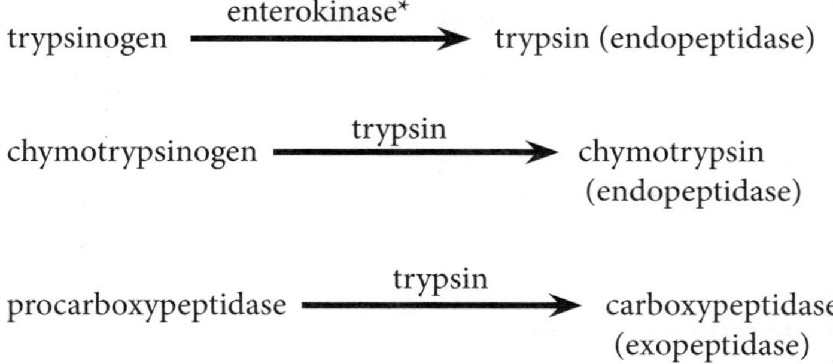

*Enterokinase (also known as enteropeptidase) is an enzyme secreted by the lining of the small intestine. It is not a brush border enzyme. It functions to activate some trypsinogen, and the active trypsin generated activates the remaining proteases.

Fluid and electrolyte components

- Aqueous component is secreted by epithelial cells which line the ducts.
- Fluid is isotonic due to the high permeability of the ducts to water and the concentrations of Na and K are the same as plasma.
- Duct cells secrete chloride into the lumen via the cystic fibrosis transmembrane conductance regulator (CFTR). This chloride is then removed from the lumen in exchange for bicarbonate. Thus, bicarbonate secretion is dependent upon chloride secretion.
- CFTR is activated by cAMP (see below).
- In cystic fibrosis there is a mutation in the gene that encodes this CFTR channel, resulting in less chloride and a reduced fluid component of pancreatic secretions. The smaller volume of highly viscous fluid may also contain few enzymes.

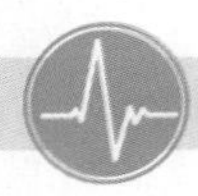

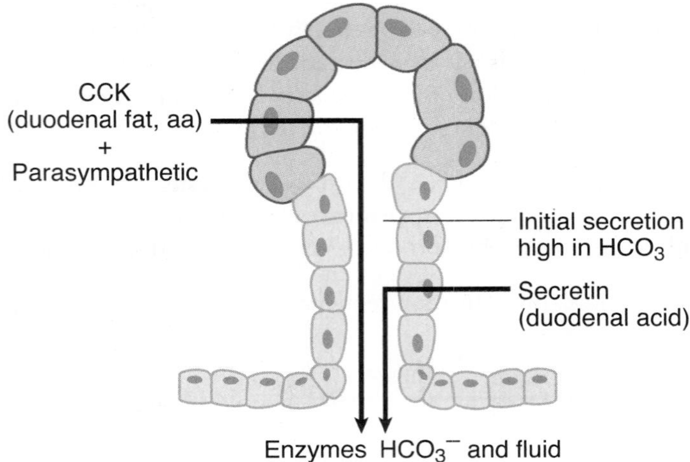

Figure XI-1-7. Control of the Exocrine Pancreas

Control of pancreatic secretions

Most of the regulation is via two hormones: secretin and cholecystokinin

Secretin

- Released from the duodenum in response to acid entering from the stomach.
- Action on the pancreas is the release of fluid high in HCO_3^-. Secretin is a peptide hormone that stimulates chloride entry into the lumen from duct cells. Secretin activates Gs–cAMP, which in turn activates CFTR.
- This released HCO_3^--rich fluid is the main mechanism that neutralizes stomach acid entering the duodenum.

Cholecystokinin (CCK)

- Released from the duodenum in response to partially digested materials (e.g., fat, petides, and amino acids)
- Action on the pancreas is the release of enzymes (amylases, lipases, proteases).

Composition and Formation of Bile

Figure XI-1-8 summarizes the major components of bile.

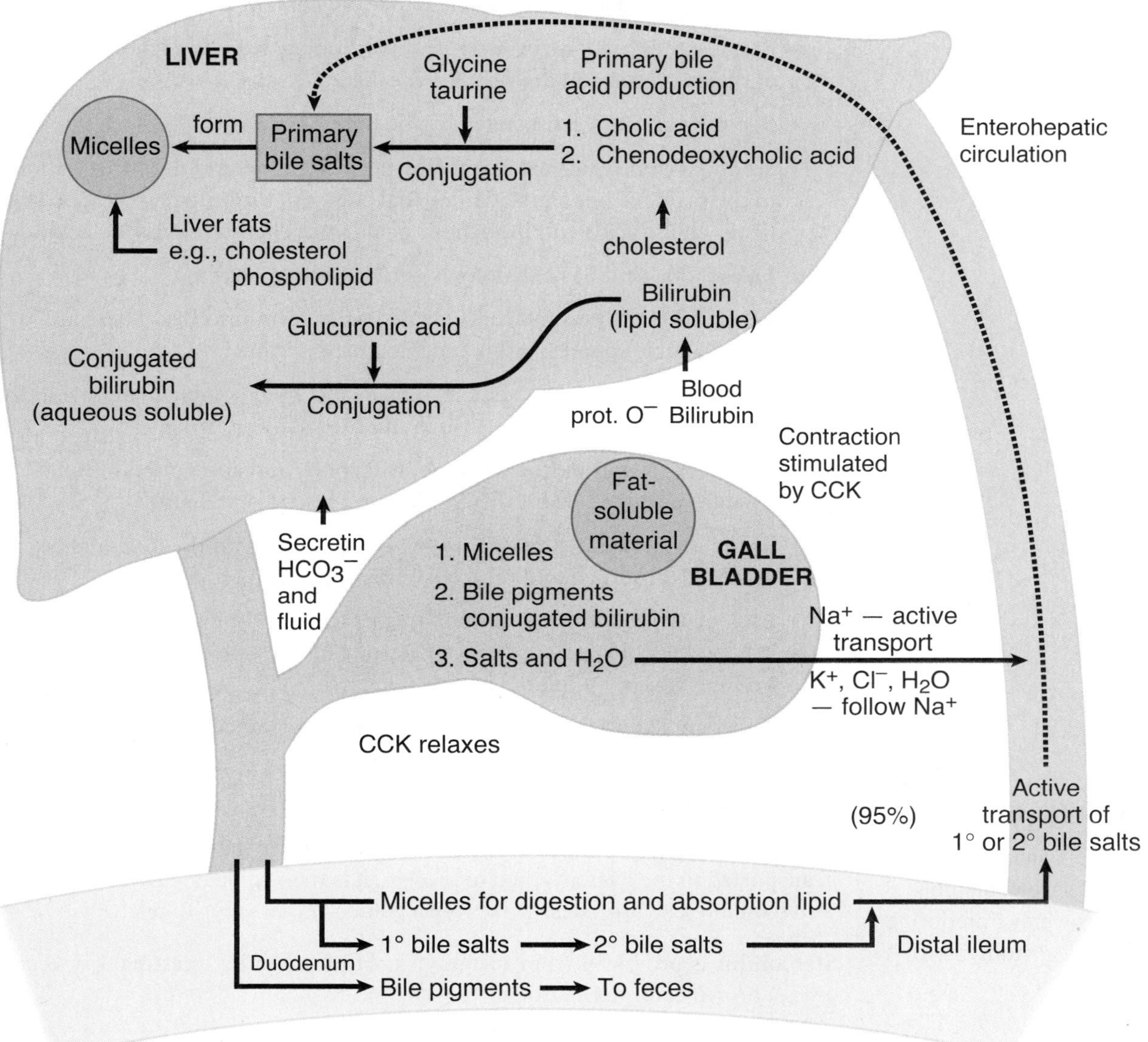

Figure XI-1-8. Production and Metabolism of Bile

Bile salts and micelles

- Primary bile acids known as cholic acid and chenodeoxycholic acid are synthesized by the liver from cholesterol.
- The lipid-soluble bile acids are then conjugated primarily with glycine.
- The conjugated forms are water-soluble but contain a lipid-soluble segment.
- Because they are ionized at neutral pH, conjugated bile acids exist as salts of cations (Na^+) and are, therefore, called bile salts.
- Bile salts are actively secreted by the liver.
- Secondary bile acids are formed by deconjugation and dehydroxylation of the primary bile salts by intestinal bacteria, forming deoxycholic acid (from cholic acid) and lithocholic acid (from chenodeoxycholic acid).
- Lithocholic acid has hepatotoxic activity and is excreted.
- When bile salts become concentrated, they form micelles. These are water-soluble spheres with a lipid-soluble interior.
- As such, they provide a vehicle to transport lipid-soluble materials in the aqueous medium of the bile fluid and the small intestine.
- Micelles are vital in the digestion, transport, and absorption of lipid-soluble substances from the duodenum to the distal ileum.
- In the distal ileum, and only in the distal ileum, can the bile salts be actively reabsorbed and recycled (enterohepatic circulation).
- Lack of active reabsorbing mechanisms (or a distal ileal resection) causes loss in the stool and a general deficiency in bile salts, as the liver has a limited capacity to manufacture them.
- This deficiency can lead to fat malabsorption and cholesterol gallstones.

Bile pigments

A major bile pigment, **bilirubin** is a lipid-soluble metabolite of hemoglobin. Transported to the liver attached to protein, it is then conjugated and excreted as water-soluble glucuronides. These give a golden yellow color to bile.

Stercobilin is produced from metabolism of bilirubin by intestinal bacteria. It gives a brown color to the stool.

Bridge to Pathology

Increased levels of plasma bilirubin produce jaundice. If severe, bilirubin can accumulate in the brain, producing profound neurological disturbances (kernicterus).

Salts and water

The HCO_3^- component is increased by the action of secretin on the liver.

The active pumping of sodium in the gallbladder causes electrolyte and water reabsorption, which concentrates the bile.

Bile pigments and bile salts are not reabsorbed from the gallbladder.

Phospholipids (mainly lecithin)

Insoluble in water but are solubilized by bile salt micelles

Cholesterol

Present in small amounts. It is insoluble in water and must be solubilized by bile salt micelles before it can be secreted in the bile.

Control of bile secretion and gallbladder contraction

- Secretin causes secretion of HCO_3^- and fluid into bile canalicular ducts.
- Secretion of bile salts by hepatocytes is directly proportional to hepatic portal vein concentration of bile salts.
- CCK causes gallbladder contraction and sphincter of Oddi relaxation.

Enterohepatic circulation

- The distal ileum has high-affinity uptake of bile acids/salt (symport with Na^+).
- These bile acids/salts enter the portal vein and travel to the liver, which in turn secretes them into the cystic duct, from which they re-enter the duodenum.
- This recycling occurs many times during the digestion of a meal and plays a significant role in fat digestion.
- The synthesis of bile acids by the liver is directly related to the concentration of bile acids in the portal vein.

Small Intestinal Secretions

- Most prominent feature of the small intestine is the villi.
- Surface epithelial cells display microvilli.
- Water and electrolyte reabsorption greatest at the villus tip.
- Water and electrolyte secretion greatest at the bottom in the crypts of Lieberkuhn.

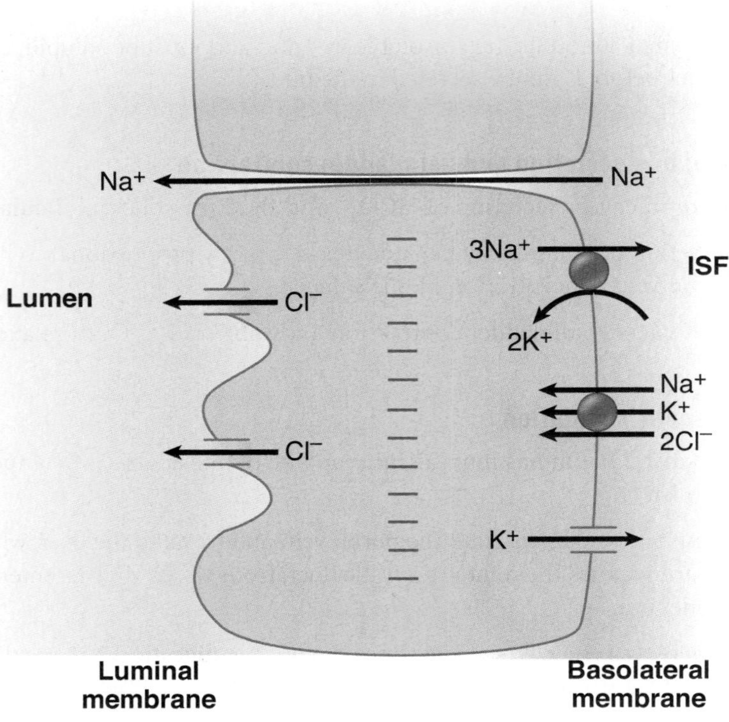

Figure XI-1-9. Secretion of Electrolytes by a Crypt Cell of the Small Intestine

Bridge to Pathology

Cholera toxin binds and activates Gs, resulting in very high levels of intracellular cAMP. This rise in cAMP opens luminal Cl^- channels, causing a massive secretory diarrhea.

Crypt secretion

- A Na^+-K^+-$2Cl^-$ transporter in the basolateral membrane facilitates the ion uptake by secondary active transport.
- Na^+ entry drives the entry of K^+ and Cl^- into the cell.
- The elevated intracellular Cl and negative intracellular potential drives the diffusion of chloride through channels on the apical membrane.
- Luminal Cl then pulls water, Na, and other ions into the lumen, creating the isotonic secretion. This is the general scheme of the chloride pump.
- Neurotransmitter secretagogues include VIP and ACh.
- The Cl^- channels are opened by increases in cytosolic Ca^{2+} and/or cAMP. The cAMP-dependent Ca^{2+} channels are CFTR channels.

DIGESTION

Figure XI-1-10 summarizes the regional entry of the major digestive enzymes proceeding from the mouth, stomach, and through the small intestine.

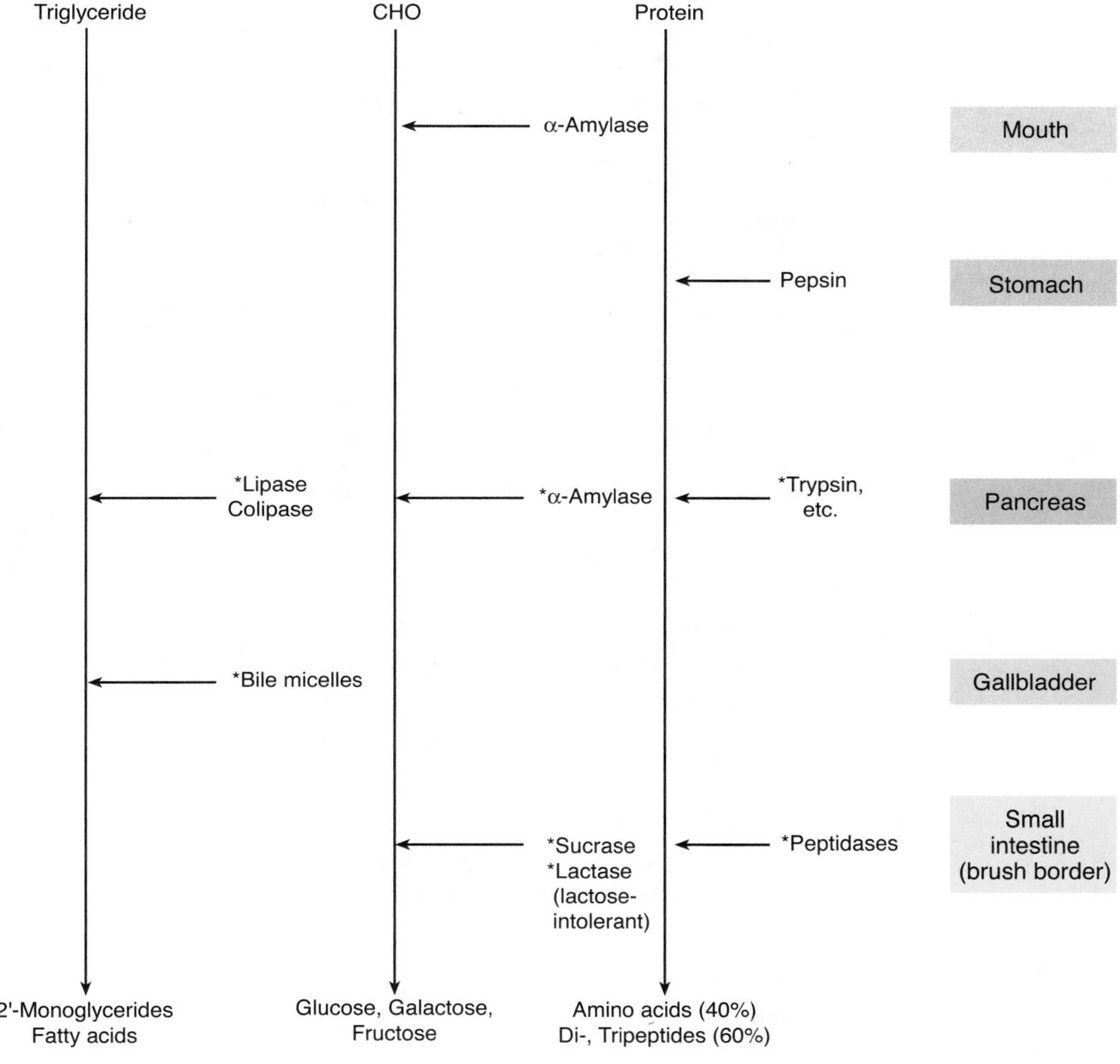

Figure XI-1-10. Summary of Digestive Processes

Digestive Enzymes and End Products

Triglycerides

Stomach: Fatty materials are pulverized to decrease particle size and increase surface area.

Small intestine: Bile micelles emulsify the fat, and pancreatic lipases digest it. Micelles and pancreatic lipase are required for triglyceride digestion. The major end products are 2-monoglycerides and fatty acids.

Carbohydrates

Mouth: Salivary α-amylase begins the digestion, and its activity continues in the stomach until acid penetrates the bolus; however, it is not a required enzyme.

Small intestine: Pancreatic α-amylase, a required enzyme for CHO digestion, continues the process. Hydrolysis of starch by α-amylase goes on in solution in the lumen of the small intestine, mostly in the duodenum. Further processing or splitting of these trisaccharides, disaccharides, and oligosaccharides is necessary but does not take place in solution; rather, it occurs on the brush border. The enzymes—α-dextrinase (or α-glucoamylase), isomaltase, and maltase—are all bound to the brush border (apical membrane of enterocytes). Brush border enzymes have their highest activity in the jejunum (upper). These brush border enzymes are required for digestion mainly because disaccharides—e.g., sucrose, lactose—are not absorbed from the gut.

- The α-dextrinase cleaves terminal α-1,4 bonds, producing free glucose.
- Lactase hydrolyzes lactose into glucose and galactose. Lactase deficiency (lactose intolerance) leads to osmotic diarrhea.
- Sucrase splits sucrose into glucose and fructose.
- Maltase (also a brush border enzyme) breaks down the maltose and maltotriose to form 2 and 3 glucose units, respectively.
- The monosaccharide end products—glucose, galactose, and fructose—are readily absorbed from the small intestine, also mainly in the jejunum.

Proteins

Stomach: Pepsin begins the digestion of protein in the acid medium of the stomach; however, it is not an essential enzyme.

Small intestine: Digestion continues with the pancreatic proteases (trypsin, chymotrypsin, elastase, and carboxypeptidases A and B), which are essential enzymes.

Protein digestion is completed by the small intestinal brush border enzymes, dipeptidases, and an aminopeptidase. The main end products are amino acids (40%) and dipeptides and tripeptides (60%).

Pancreatic enzymes are required for triglyceride, CHO, and protein digestion. Circulating CCK is almost totally responsible for their secretion following a meal.

ABSORPTION

Carbohydrate and Protein

Figure XI-1-11 illustrates the major transport processes carrying sugars and amino acids across the luminal and basal membranes of cells lining the small intestine.

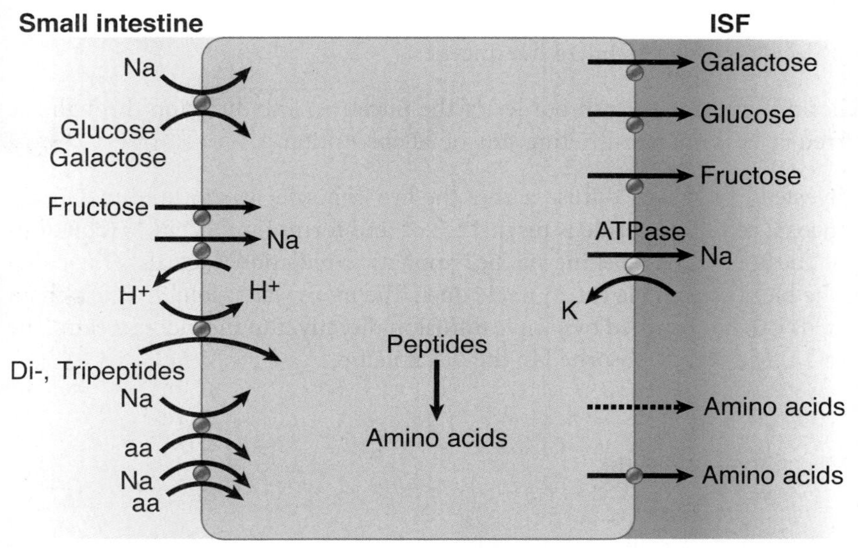

Figure XI-1-11. Absorption of Carbohydrates and Proteins

Bridge to Pathology

Celiac disease is an immune reaction to gluten (protein found in wheat) that damages intestinal cells; the end result is diminished absorptive capacity of the small intestine.

Bridge to Pathology

Many of the amino acid transporters are selective for specific amino acids. Hartnup's disease is a genetic deficiency in the transporter for tryptophan.

Carbohydrate

- **Luminal membrane:** Glucose and galactose are actively absorbed (secondary active transport linked to sodium) via the sodium-glucose linked transporter 1 (SGLT-1). Fructose is absorbed independently by facilitated diffusion.
- **Basal membrane:** The monosaccharides are absorbed passively mainly via facilitated diffusion.

Protein

- **Luminal membrane:** amino acids are transported by secondary active transport linked to sodium. Small peptides uptake powered by a Na-H antiporter.
- **Basal membrane:** simple diffusion of amino acids, although it is now known some protein-mediated transport also occurs.

Lipids

Figure XI-1-12 summarizes the digestion and absorption of lipid substances. The end products of triglyceride digestion, 2-monoglycerides and fatty acids, remain as lipid-soluble substances that are then taken up by the micelles.

Digestive products of fats found in the micelles and absorbed from the intestinal lumen may include:

- Fatty acids (long chain)
- 2-Monoglyceride
- Cholesterol
- Lysolecithin
- Vitamins A, D, E, K
- Bile salts, which stabilize the micelles

Micelles diffuse to the brush border of the intestine. The diffusion through the unstirred layer is the rate-limiting step of fat absorption.

The digested lipids then diffuse across the brush border in the lipid matrix. In the mucosal cell, triglyceride is resynthesized and forms lipid droplets (chylomicrons). These leave the intestine via the lymphatic circulation (lacteals). They then enter the bloodstream via the thoracic duct. The more water-soluble short-chain fatty acids can be absorbed by simple diffusion directly into the bloodstream. The bile salts are actively reabsorbed in the distal ileum.

Bridge to Biochemistry

Chylomicrons contain apolipoprotein B-48. Once in the systemic circulation, chylomicrons are converted to VLDL (very low-density lipoprotein) and they incorporate apoproteins C-II and E from HDL (high-density liproprotein).

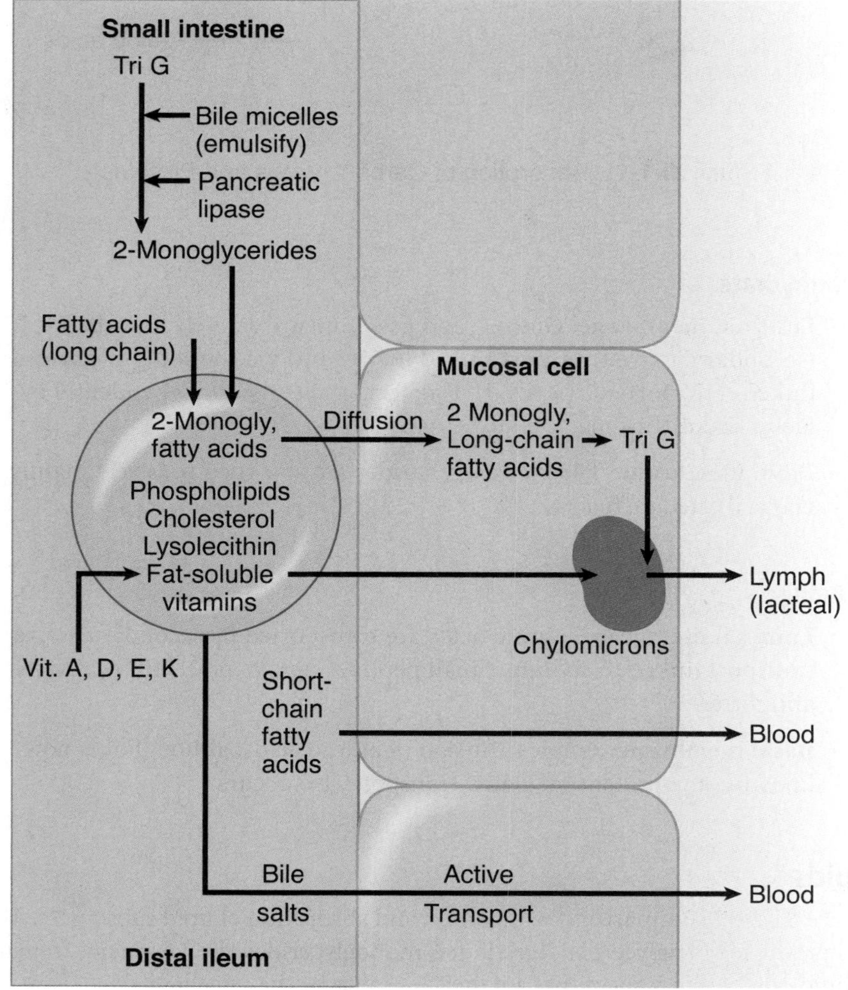

Figure XI-1-12. Absorption of Lipids

Electrolytes

The net transport of electrolytes along the length of the small and large intestine is summarized in Figure XI-1-13.

Duodenum

- Hypertonic fluid enters this region, and following the movement of some water into the lumen, the fluid becomes and remains isotonic (see crypt secretion above).
- The absorption of most divalent ions and water-soluble vitamins begins here and continues through the small intestine.
- Injested iron and calcium tend to form insoluble salts. The acid environment of the stomach redissolves these salts, which facilitates their absorption in the small intestine. Iron and calcium absorption is diminished in individuals with a deficient stomach acid secretion.
- Calcium absorption is enhanced by the presence of calbindin in intestinal cells, and calcitriol (active vitamin D) induces the synthesis of this protein.
- Intestinal cells express the protein ferritin, which facilitates iron absorption.

Jejunum

- Overall, there is a net reabsorption of water and electrolytes.
- The cellular processes involved are almost identical to those described in the renal physiology section for the cells lining the nephron proximal tubule.

Ileum

- Net reabsorption of water, sodium, chloride, and potassium continues, but there begins a net secretion of bicarbonate.
- It is in the distal ileum, and only in the distal ileum, where the reabsorption of bile salts and intrinsic factor with vitamin B_{12} takes place.

Colon

- The colon does not have digestive enzymes or the protein transporters to absorb the products of carbohydrate and protein digestion.
- Also, because bile salts are reabsorbed in the distal ileum, very few lipid-soluble substances are absorbed in the colon.
- There is a net reabsorption of water and sodium chloride, but there are limitations.
- Most of the water and electrolytes must be reabsorbed in the small intestine, or the colon becomes overwhelmed.
- Most of the water and electrolytes are absorbed in the ascending and transverse colon; thereafter, the colon has mainly a storage function.
- The colon is a target for aldosterone, where it increases sodium and water reabsorption and potassium secretion.
- Because there is a net secretion of bicarbonate and potassium, diarrhea usually produces a metabolic acidosis and hypokalemia. It commonly presents as hyperchloremic, nonanion gap metabolic acidosis, as described in the acid-base section.

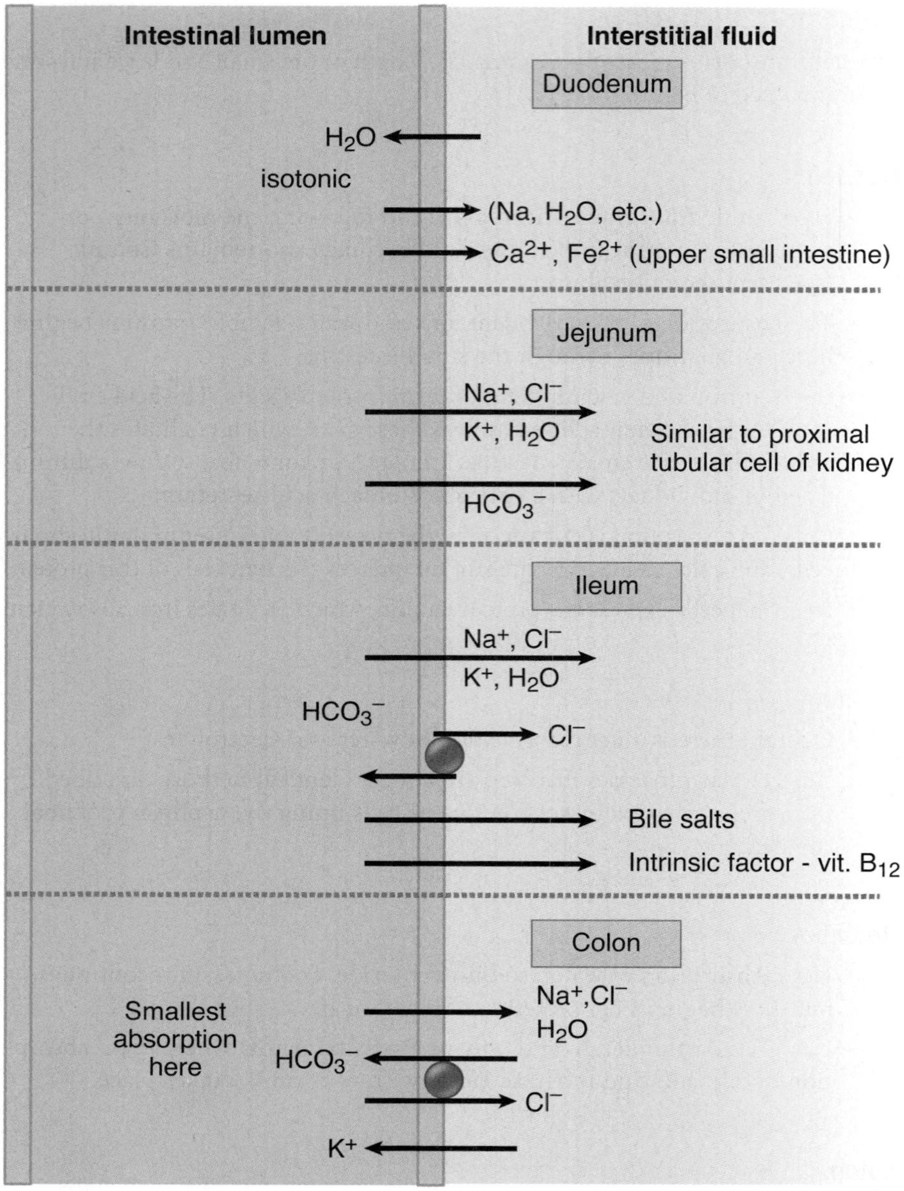

Figure XI-1-13. Transport of Electrolytes

Diarrhea

Except for the infant where it can be hypotonic, diarrhea is a loss of isotonic fluid that is high in bicarbonate and potassium.

Chapter Summary

- Sympathetic activity slows processes in the GI tract, whereas parasympathetic does the opposite.
- Secretin is required for releasing pancreatic bicarbonate, which neutralizes stomach acid entering the duodenum.
- CCK is required to release pancreatic enzymes and for the release of bile into the duodenum.
- Gastric stomach activity and its secretion is inhibited by stomach acid.
- Because of regional pacemaker activity, there is always some basal motor activity in the GI tract.
- Swallowing and defecation are reflexes requiring the central nervous system. Relaxation of the lower esophageal sphincter is due to the release of VIP.
- Following a meal, local distension and parasympathetic activity increase stomach motility. An overload of the duodenum decreases stomach motility.
- There are mixing and propulsive movements in the small intestine and colon.
- Salivary secretions are regulated via parasympathetic input. The reabsorption of sodium chloride produces a fluid that is hypotonic.
- Gastric acid secretion via a hydrogen/potassium-ATPase pump is stimulated by acetylcholine, histamine, and gastrin. A low stomach pH and a duodenal overload inhibit acid secretion.
- Pancreatic enzymes are required for the digestion of carbohydrate, protein, and lipids.
- Pancreatic fluid high in bicarbonate is required to neutralize acid entering the duodenum.
- Bile salts form micelles that are required for the digestion and absorption of lipids. Only in the distal ileum can they be actively reabsorbed. They must be recycled because the liver has a limited ability for their synthesis.
- Bile pigments are water-soluble compounds excreted via the bile and intestine.
- Electrolytes and water, but not bile pigments or bile salts, can be absorbed from the gall bladder lumen.
- Digestion of lipid requires bile micelles and pancreatic lipases. End products absorbed include 2-monoglycerides and fatty acids.
- Digestion of carbohydrate requires pancreatic amylases and the small intestinal brush border enzymes. End products absorbed will be the monosaccharides. Disaccharides cannot be absorbed from the small intestine.
- Digestion of protein requires the pancreatic proteases, which must be initially activated by enterokinase/enteropeptidase and the intestinal brush-border enzymes.
- End products absorbed include amino acids and very small peptides.
- Absorption of carbohydrate, amino acids, and small peptides is mainly by secondary active transport at the luminal membrane in the small intestine.

(*Continued*)

Chapter Summary (*Cont'd*)

- Most of the water and electrolytes are reabsorbed in the small intestine. The distal ileum reabsorbs the bile salts and intrinsic factor–vitamin B_{12} complex.
- The colon does not have digestive enzymes or the transporters to absorb the end products of digestion.
- The colon has a net absorption of water and electrolytes, which is influenced by aldosterone but has a net secretion of bicarbonate and potassium.
- Diarrhea is the loss of isotonic fluid, which is high in bicarbonate and potassium.

Index

I

W

X

Y

Z

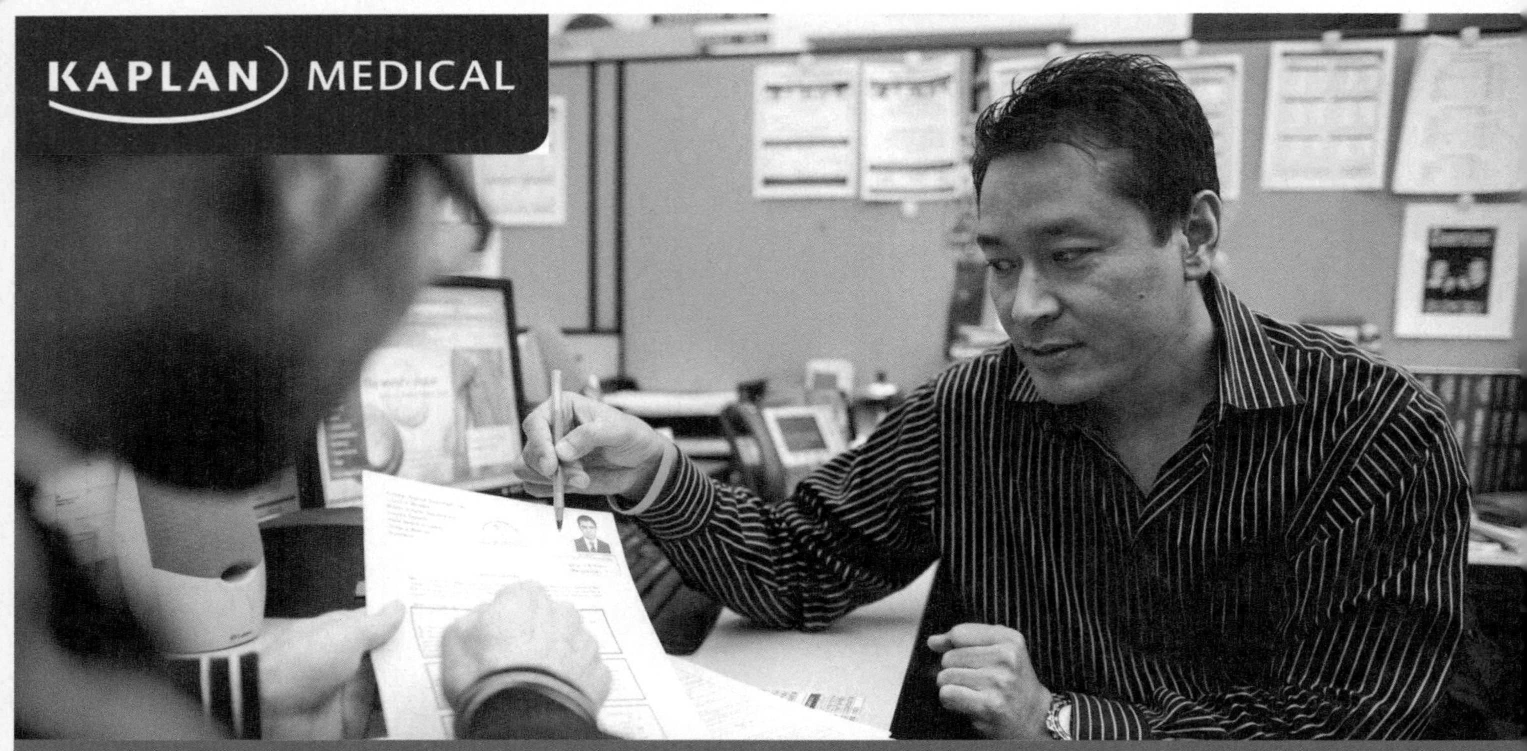
KAPLAN MEDICAL